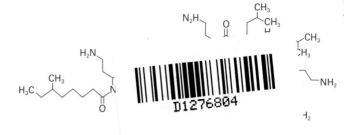

D1276804

2014
Nelson's Pediatric Antimicrobial Therapy

20th Edition

John S. Bradley, MD
Editor in Chief

John D. Nelson, MD
Emeritus

David W. Kimberlin, MD
John A.D. Leake, MD, MPH
Paul E. Palumbo, MD
Pablo J. Sanchez, MD
Jason Sauberan, PharmD
William J. Steinbach, MD
Contributing Editors

American Academy of Pediatrics

DEDICATED TO THE HEALTH OF ALL CHILDREN™

American Academy of Pediatrics Department of Marketing and Publications Staff

Maureen DeRosa, MPA, Director, Department of Marketing and Publications
Mark Grimes, Director, Division of Product Development
Alain Park, Senior Product Development Editor
Carrie Peters, Editorial Assistant
Sandi King, MS, Director, Division of Publishing and Production Services
Shannan Martin, Publishing and Production Services Specialist
Linda Diamond, Manager, Art Direction and Production
Jason Crase, Manager, Editorial Services
Julia Lee, Director, Division of Marketing and Sales
Linda Smessaert, MSIMC, Brand Manager, Clinical and Professional Publications

ISSN: 2164-9278 (print)
ISSN: 2164-9286 (electronic)
ISBN: 978-1-58110-848-4
eISBN: 978-1-58110-853-8
MA0701

The recommendations in this publication do not indicate an exclusive course of treatment or serve as a standard of care. Variations, taking into account individual circumstances, may be appropriate.

Every effort has been made to ensure that the drug selection and dosage set forth in this text are in accordance with the current recommendations and practice at the time of the publication. It is the responsibility of the health care provider to check the package insert of each drug for any change in indications or dosage and for added warnings and precautions.

Brand names are furnished for identifying purposes only. No endorsement of the manufacturers or products listed is implied.

First edition published in 1975.
9-322

1 2 3 4 5 6 7 8 9 10

iii

Editor in Chief
John S. Bradley, MD
Professor of Pediatrics
Chief, Division of Infectious Diseases,
    Department of Pediatrics
University of California San Diego,
    School of Medicine
Director, Division of Infectious Diseases,
    Rady Children's Hospital San Diego
San Diego, CA

Emeritus
John D. Nelson, MD
Professor Emeritus of Pediatrics
The University of Texas
Southwestern Medical Center at Dallas
Southwestern Medical School
Dallas, TX

Contributing Editors
David W. Kimberlin, MD
Professor of Pediatrics
Codirector, Division of Pediatric Infectious Diseases
Sergio Stagno Endowed Chair in Pediatric Infectious Diseases
University of Alabama at Birmingham
Birmingham, AL

John A.D. Leake, MD, MPH
Professor of Pediatrics
Division of Infectious Diseases, Department of Pediatrics
University of California San Diego, School of Medicine
Division of Infectious Diseases, Rady Children's Hospital San Diego
San Diego, CA

Paul E. Palumbo, MD
Professor of Pediatrics and Medicine
Geisel School of Medicine at Dartmouth
Director, International Pediatric HIV Program
Dartmouth-Hitchcock Medical Center
Lebanon, NH

Pablo J. Sanchez, MD
Professor, Department of Pediatrics
Division of Neonatal-Perinatal Medicine and Infectious Diseases
Ohio State University, Nationwide Children's Hospital
Columbus, OH

Jason Sauberan, PharmD
Assistant Clinical Professor
University of California San Diego, Skaggs School of Pharmacy and Pharmaceutical Sciences
Rady Children's Hospital San Diego
San Diego, CA

William J. Steinbach, MD
Associate Professor of Pediatrics
Assistant Professor of Molecular Genetics and Microbiology
Duke University School of Medicine
Durham, NC

Table of Contents

Introduction

Welcome to the 20th Edition of *Nelson's Pediatric Antimicrobial Therapy!* The past 2 years have demonstrated how exceptionally productive and collaborative our relationship with the American Academy of Pediatrics (AAP) has become. While the book now just barely fits into a pocket, we believe that all of the additional information included in the newer chapters enhances the value of the book while maintaining the original "feel" of the book as advice given by a colleague. Of course, many of our friends are very tech savvy and prefer to use the Nelson's book app for Apple and Android devices, among others, but John and I still prefer the book format, so do not expect the book format to disappear anytime soon.

While the book has traditionally been updated every 2 years, rapidly increasing advances in clinical pharmacology and clinical investigation into community-acquired infections as well as infections in immunocompromised hosts lead our editors and the AAP to the conclusion that an annual edition was now needed. We are now committed to providing pediatric health care providers with the most current advice each year, starting with this 2014 edition.

Our collective advice is again backed up by our honest assessment of how strongly we feel about a recommendation and the strength of the evidence to support our recommendation (noted below), and includes new information of relevance in each area of therapeutics since the last publication 2 years ago.

Strength of Recommendation	Description
A	Strongly recommended
B	Recommended as a good choice
C	One option for therapy that is adequate, perhaps among many other adequate therapies

Level of Evidence	Description
I	Based on well-designed, prospective, randomized, and controlled studies in an appropriate population of children
II	Based on data derived from prospectively collected, small comparative trials, or noncomparative prospective trials, or reasonable retrospective data from clinical trials in children, or data from other populations (eg, adults)
III	Based on case reports, case series, consensus statements, or expert opinion for situations in which sound data do not exist

As many of you have probably seen, our AAP editorial staff has created a monthly update "post" with David, Bill, John L, Jason, Paul, Pablo, and John B, in turn, contributing a short and interesting report (www.aap.org/en-us/aap-store/Nelsons/Pages/Whats-New.aspx), so that you don't need to wait a full year to see our suggestions about the most important advances!

The field of neonatal pharmacology and infectious diseases is expanding rapidly. To help with the neonatal section, another Dallas-based, double-trained infectious diseases/neonatologist, JB Cantey, is joining our Nelson's group. In addition, a neonatologist/pharmacologist who is the director of pediatric clinical pharmacology at the Children's National Medical Center, John van den Anker, is reviewing the Antimicrobial Dosages for Neonates table with our editors. We are very grateful to have such expertise for the new edition of the book!

We continue to admire the work of the US Food and Drug Administration (FDA) in reviewing new data on the safety and efficacy of anti-infective compounds, and applaud the collaborations of the National Institute of Child Health and Human Development and FDA to study antimicrobial drug behavior for a number of generic antimicrobial products in all the pediatric age groups, including neonates. However, since all potential infectious disease scenarios cannot possibly be investigated, presented, and reviewed, we are continuing to follow the tradition started with the first edition in 1975, to make recommendations that are "off-label." This is not the same as our making recommendations that are in conflict with the FDA, but, instead, our making recommendations for situations that it has not routinely considered (and the FDA freely states that it has no opinion about the safety and efficacy of data that it has not officially reviewed). Off-label recommendations are often supported by clinical trial data, which we cite.

We are deeply grateful for the hard and innovative work by our AAP partners. Alain Park is now our AAP liaison as senior product development editor (we will miss Martha Cook), and we continue to work very closely and enthusiastically with Jeff Mahoney, Mark Grimes, Linda Smessaert, and Maureen DeRosa.

John S. Bradley, MD, FAAP

John D. Nelson, MD

1. Choosing Among Antibiotics Within a Class: Beta-Lactams, Macrolides, Aminoglycosides, and Fluoroquinolones

New drugs should be compared with others in the same class regarding (1) antimicrobial spectrum; (2) degree of antibiotic exposure (a function of the pharmacokinetics of the nonprotein-bound drug at the site of infection, and the pharmacodynamic properties of the drug); (3) demonstrated efficacy in adequate and well-controlled clinical trials; (4) tolerance, toxicity, and side effects; and (5) cost. If there is no substantial benefit for efficacy or safety, one should opt for using an older, more familiar, and less expensive drug with the most narrow spectrum of activity required to treat the infection.

Beta-Lactams

Oral Cephalosporins (cephalexin, cefadroxil, cefaclor, cefprozil, cefuroxime, cefixime, cefdinir, cefpodoxime, cefditoren [tablet only], and ceftibuten). As a class, the oral cephalosporins have the advantages over oral penicillins of somewhat greater safety and greater palatability of the suspension formulations (penicillins have a bitter taste). The serum half-lives of cefpodoxime, ceftibuten, and cefixime are greater than 2 hours. This pharmacokinetic feature accounts for the fact that they may be given in 1 or 2 doses per day for certain indications, particularly otitis media, where the middle-ear fluid half-life is likely to be much longer than the serum half-life. Cefaclor, cefprozil, cefuroxime, cefdinir, cefixime, cefpodoxime, and ceftibuten have the advantage over cephalexin and cefadroxil (the "first-generation cephalosporins") of enhanced coverage for *Haemophilus influenzae* (including beta-lactamase–producing strains) and some enteric gram-negative bacilli; however, ceftibuten and cefixime in particular have the disadvantage of less activity against *Streptococcus pneumoniae* than the others, particularly against penicillin (beta-lactam) non-susceptible strains. The palatability of generic versions of these products may not have the same pleasant characteristics as the original products.

Parenteral Cephalosporins. First-generation cephalosporins, such as cefazolin, are used mainly for treatment of gram-positive infections (excluding methicillin-resistant *Staphylococcus aureus* [MRSA]) and for surgical prophylaxis; the gram-negative spectrum is limited. Cefazolin is well tolerated on intramuscular or intravenous injection.

A second-generation cephalosporin (cefuroxime) and the cephamycins (cefoxitin and cefotetan) provide increased activity against many gram-negative organisms. Cefoxitin has, in addition, activity against approximately 80% of strains of *Bacteroides fragilis* and can be considered for use in place of metronidazole, clindamycin, or carbapenems when that organism is implicated in non–life-threatening disease.

Third-generation cephalosporins (cefotaxime, ceftriaxone, and ceftazidime) all have enhanced potency against many gram-negative bacilli. They are inactive against enterococci and *Listeria* and only ceftazidime has significant activity against *Pseudomonas*. Cefotaxime and ceftriaxone have been used very successfully to treat meningitis caused by pneumococcus (mostly penicillin-susceptible strains), *Haemophilus influenzae type b* (Hib), meningococcus, and small numbers of young infants with susceptible strains of *Escherichia coli* meningitis. These drugs have the greatest usefulness for treating gram-negative bacillary infections due to their safety, compared with other classes of antibiotics. Because ceftriaxone is excreted to a large extent via the liver, it can be used with little dosage adjustment in patients with renal failure. Further, it has a serum half-life of 4 to 7 hours and can be given once a day for all infections, including meningitis, caused by susceptible organisms.

Cefepime, a fourth-generation cephalosporin approved for use in children, exhibits the antipseudomonal activity of ceftazidime, the gram-positive activity of second-generation cephalosporins, and better activity against gram-negative enteric bacilli such as *Enterobacter* and *Serratia* than is documented with cefotaxime and ceftriaxone.

Ceftaroline is a fifth-generation cephalosporin, the first of the cephalosporins with activity against MRSA. Ceftaroline was approved by the US Food and Drug Administration (FDA) in December 2010 for adults with complicated skin infections (including MRSA) and community-acquired pneumonia (with insufficient numbers of adult patients with MRSA pneumonia to be able to comment on efficacy). Studies are currently underway for children.

Penicillinase-Resistant Penicillins (dicloxacillin [capsules only]; nafcillin and oxacillin [parenteral only]). "Penicillinase" refers specifically to the beta-lactamase produced by *S aureus* in this case, and not those produced by gram-negative bacteria. These antibiotics are active against penicillin-resistant *S aureus*, but not against MRSA. Nafcillin differs pharmacologically from the others in being excreted primarily by the liver rather than by the kidneys, which may explain the relative lack of nephrotoxicity compared with methicillin, which is no longer available in the United States. Nafcillin pharmacokinetics are erratic in persons with liver disease.

Antipseudomonal Beta-Lactams (ticarcillin/clavulanate, piperacillin, piperacillin/tazobactam, aztreonam, ceftazidime, cefepime, meropenem, imipenem, and doripenem). Timentin (ticarcillin/clavulanate) and Zosyn (piperacillin/tazobactam) represent combinations of 2 beta-lactam drugs. One beta-lactam drug in the combination, known as a "beta-lactamase inhibitor" (clavulanic acid or tazobactam in these combinations), binds irreversibly to and neutralizes specific beta-lactamase enzymes produced by the organism, allowing the second beta-lactam drug (ticarcillin or piperacillin) to act as the active antibiotic to bind effectively to the intracellular target site, resulting in death of the organism. Thus the combination only adds to the spectrum of the original antibiotic when the mechanism of resistance is a beta-lactamase enzyme, and only when the beta-lactamase inhibitor is capable of binding to and inhibiting that particular organism's beta-lactamase. Timentin and Zosyn have no significant activity against *Pseudomonas* beyond that of ticarcillin or piperacillin because their beta-lactamase inhibitors do not effectively inhibit all of the relevant beta-lactamases of *Pseudomonas*. However, the combination does extend the spectrum of activity to include many other beta-lactamase–positive bacteria, including some strains of enteric gram-negative bacilli (*E coli, Klebsiella,* and *Enterobacter), S aureus,* and *B fragilis.*

Pseudomonas has an intrinsic capacity to develop resistance following exposure to any beta-lactam, based on inducible chromosomal beta-lactamases, upregulated efflux pumps, and changes in the cell wall. Because development of resistance is not uncommon during single drug therapy with these agents, an aminoglycoside such as tobramycin is often used in combination. Cefepime, meropenem, and imipenem are relatively stable to the beta-lactamases induced while on therapy and can be used as single agent therapy for most *Pseudomonas* infections, but resistance may still develop to these agents based on other mechanisms of resistance. For *Pseudomonas* infections in compromised hosts or in life-threatening infections, these drugs, too, should be used in combination with an aminoglycoside or a second active agent.

Aminopenicillins (amoxicillin and amoxicillin/clavulanate [oral formulations only, in the United States], ampicillin [oral and parenteral], and ampicillin/sulbactam [parenteral only]). Amoxicillin is very well absorbed, good tasting, and associated with very few side effects. Augmentin is a combination of amoxicillin and clavulanate (see previous text regarding beta-lactam/beta-lactamase inhibitor combinations) that is available in several fixed proportions that permit amoxicillin to remain active against many beta-lactamase–producing bacteria, including *H influenzae* and *S aureus* (but not MRSA). Amoxicillin/clavulanate has undergone many changes in formulation since its introduction. The ratio of amoxicillin to clavulanate was originally 4:1, based on susceptibility data of pneumococcus and *Haemophilus* during the 1970s. With the emergence of penicillin-resistant pneumococcus, recommendations for increasing the dosage of amoxicillin, particularly for upper respiratory tract infections, were made. However, if one increases the dosage of clavulanate even slightly, the incidence of diarrhea increases dramatically. If one keeps the dosage of clavulanate constant while increasing the dosage of amoxicillin, one can treat the relatively resistant pneumococci while not increasing the gastrointestinal side effects. The original 4:1 ratio is present in suspensions containing 125-mg and 250-mg amoxicillin/5 mL, and the 125-mg and 250-mg chewable tablets. A higher 7:1 ratio is present both in the suspensions containing 200-mg and 400-mg amoxicillin/5 mL, and in the 200-mg and 400-mg chewable tablets. A still higher ratio of 14:1 is present in the suspension formulation Augmentin ES-600 that contains 600-mg amoxicillin/5 mL; this preparation is designed to deliver 90 mg/kg/day of amoxicillin, divided twice daily, for the treatment of ear (and sinus) infections. The high serum and middle ear fluid concentrations achieved with 45 mg/kg/dose, combined with the long middle ear fluid half-life of amoxicillin, allow for a therapeutic antibiotic exposure to pathogens in the middle ear with a twice-daily regimen. However, the prolonged half-life in the middle ear fluid is not necessarily found in other infection sites (eg, skin, lung tissue, joint tissue), for which dosing of amoxicillin and Augmentin should continue to be 3 times daily for most susceptible pathogens.

For older children who can swallow tablets, the amoxicillin:clavulanate ratios are as follows: 500-mg tab (4:1); 875-mg tab (7:1); 1,000-mg tab (16:1).

Sulbactam, another beta-lactamase inhibitor like clavulanate, is combined with ampicillin in the parenteral formulation, Unasyn. The cautions regarding spectrum of activity for Timentin and Zosyn with respect to the limitations of the beta-lactamase inhibitor in increasing the spectrum of activity (see Antipseudomonal Beta-Lactams) also apply to Unasyn.

Carbapenems. Meropenem, imipenem, doripenem, and ertapenem are carbapenems with a broader spectrum of activity than any other class of beta-lactam currently available. Meropenem, imipenem, and ertapenem are approved by the FDA for use in children. At present, we recommend them for treatment of infections caused by bacteria resistant to standard therapy, or for mixed infections involving aerobes and anaerobes. While imipenem has the potential for greater central nervous system irritability compared with other carbapenems, leading to an increased risk of seizures in children with meningitis, meropenem was not associated with an increased rate of seizures when compared with cefotaxime in children with meningitis. Both imipenem and meropenem are active against virtually all coliform bacilli, including cefotaxime-resistant (extended spectrum beta-lactamase [ESBL]–producing or ampC-producing) strains, against *P aeruginosa* (including most ceftazidime-resistant strains), and against anaerobes, including *B fragilis*. While ertapenem lacks the excellent activity against *P aeruginosa* of the other carbapenems, it has the advantage of a prolonged serum half-life, which allows for once-daily dosing in adults and children aged 13 years and older and twice-daily dosing in younger children. Newly emergent strains of *Klebsiella pneumoniae* contain *K pneumoniae* carbapenemase enzymes (KPCs) that degrade and inactivate all the carbapenems. While the current strains involve adults predominantly in the Northeast United States, they have begun to spread to other areas of the United States, reinforcing the need to keep track of your local antibiotic susceptibility patterns.

Macrolides

Erythromycin is the prototype of macrolide antibiotics. Almost 30 macrolides have been produced, but only 3 are FDA approved for children in the United States: erythromycin, azithromycin (also called an azalide), and clarithromycin, while a fourth, telithromycin (also called a ketolide), is approved for adults and only available in tablet form. As a class, these drugs achieve greater concentrations in tissues than in serum, particularly with azithromycin and clarithromycin. As a result, measuring serum concentrations is usually not clinically useful. Gastrointestinal intolerance to erythromycin is caused by the breakdown products of the macrolide ring structure. This is much less of a problem with azithromycin and clarithromycin. Azithromycin, clarithromycin, and telithromycin extend the activity of erythromycin to include *Haemophilus;* azithromycin and clarithromycin also have substantial activity against certain mycobacteria. Azithromycin is also active in vitro and effective against many enteric gram-negative pathogens including *Salmonella* and *Shigella*.

Aminoglycosides

Although 5 aminoglycoside antibiotics are available in the United States, only 3 are widely used for systemic therapy of aerobic gram-negative infections and for synergy in the treatment of certain gram-positive infections: gentamicin, tobramycin, and amikacin. Streptomycin and kanamycin have more limited utility due to increased toxicity. Resistance in gram-negative bacilli to aminoglycosides is caused by bacterial enzyme adenylation, acetylation, or phosphorylation. The specific activities of each enzyme in each pathogen are highly variable. As a result, antibiotic susceptibility tests must be done for each aminoglycoside drug separately. There are small differences in comparative toxicities of these aminoglycosides to the kidneys and eighth cranial nerve, although it is uncertain whether these small differences are clinically significant. For all children receiving a full treatment course, it is advisable to monitor peak and trough serum concentrations early in the course of therapy as the degree of drug exposure correlates with toxicity and elevated trough concentrations predict impending drug accumulation. With amikacin, desired peak concentrations are 20 to 35 µg/mL, and trough drug concentrations are less than 10 µg/mL; for gentamicin and tobramycin, depending on the frequency of dosing, peak concentrations should be 5 to 10 µg/mL and trough concentrations less than 2 µg/mL. Children with cystic fibrosis require greater dosages to achieve therapeutic serum concentrations. Inhaled tobramycin has been very successful in children with cystic fibrosis as an adjunctive therapy of gram-negative bacillary infections. The role of inhaled aminoglycosides in other gram-negative pneumonias has not yet been defined.

Once-Daily Dosing of Aminoglycosides. Once-daily dosing of 5 to 7.5 mg/kg gentamicin or tobramycin has been studied in adults and in some neonates and children; peak serum concentrations are greater than those achieved with dosing 3 times daily. Aminoglycosides demonstrate concentration-dependent killing of pathogens, suggesting a potential benefit to higher serum concentrations achieved with once-daily dosing. Regimens giving the daily dosage as a single infusion, rather than as traditionally split doses every 8 hours, are effective and safe for both normal adult hosts and immune-compromised hosts with fever and neu-tropenia, and may be less toxic. Experience with once-daily dosing in children is increasing, with similar results as noted for adults. Once-daily dosing should be considered as effective as multiple, smaller doses per day, and may be safer for children.

Fluoroquinolones

More than 30 years ago, toxicity to cartilage in weight-bearing joints in experimental juvenile animals was documented to be dose and duration of therapy dependent. Pediatric studies were, therefore, not initially undertaken with ciprofloxacin or other fluoroquinolones (FQs). However, with increasing antibiotic resistance in pediatric pathogens and an accumu-lating database in pediatrics suggesting that joint toxicity may be uncommon in humans, the FDA allowed prospective studies to proceed in 1998. As of August 2013, no cases of documented FQ-attributable joint toxicity have occurred in children with FQs that are approved for use in the United States. However, no published data are available from pro-spective, blinded studies to accurately assess this risk. Unblinded studies with levofloxacin for respiratory tract infections and unpublished randomized studies comparing ciprofloxa-cin versus other agents for complicated urinary tract infection suggest the possibility of uncommon, reversible, FQ-attributable arthralgia, but these data should be interpreted with caution. Prospective, randomized, double-blind studies of moxifloxacin, in which cartilage injury is being assessed, are currently underway. The use of FQs in situations of antibiotic resistance where no other agent is available is reasonable, weighing the benefits of treatment against the low risk of toxicity of this class of antibiotics. The use of an oral FQ in situa-tions in which the only alternative is parenteral therapy also represents a reasonable use of this class of antibiotic (American Academy of Pediatrics Committee on Infectious Diseases. The use of systemic fluoroquinolones. *Pediatrics.* 2011;128[4]:e1034–e1045).

Ciprofloxacin usually has very good gram-negative activity (with great regional variation in susceptibility) against enteric bacilli (*E coli, Klebsiella, Enterobacter, Salmonella,* and *Shigella)* and against *P aeruginosa.* However, it lacks substantial gram-positive coverage and should not be used to treat streptococcal, staphylococcal, or pneumococcal infec-tions. Newer-generation FQs are more active against these pathogens; levofloxacin has documented efficacy and short-term safety in pediatric clinical trials for respiratory tract infections (acute otitis media and community-acquired pneumonia). No prospective pediatric clinical data exist for moxifloxacin, currently approved for use in adults, although pediatric studies are underway. None of the newer-generation FQs are more active against gram-negative pathogens than ciprofloxacin. Quinolone antibiotics are bitter tasting. Ciprofloxacin and levofloxacin are currently available in a suspension form; ciprofloxacin is FDA approved in pediatrics for complicated urinary tract infections and inhalation anthrax, while levofloxacin is approved for inhalation anthrax only, as the sponsor chose not to apply for approval for respiratory tract infections. For reasons of safety and to prevent the emer-gence of widespread resistance, FQs should not be used for primary therapy of pediatric infections, and should be limited to situations in which safe and effective oral therapy with other classes of antibiotics does not exist.

2. Choosing Among Antifungal Agents: Polyenes, Azoles, and Echinocandins

Polyenes. Amphotericin B (AmB) is a polyene antifungal antibiotic that has been available since 1958 for the treatment of invasive fungal infections. Its name originates from the drug's amphoteric property of reacting as an acid as well as a base. Nystatin is another polyene antifungal, but, due to systemic toxicity, it is only used in topical preparations. It was named after the research laboratory where it was discovered, the New York State Health Department Laboratory. AmB remains the most broad-spectrum antifungal available for clinical use. This lipophilic drug binds to ergosterol, the major sterol in the fungal cell membrane, and creates transmembrane pores that compromise the integrity of the cell membrane and create a rapid fungicidal effect through osmotic lysis. Toxicity is likely due to the cross-reactivity with the human cholesterol bi-lipid membrane, which resembles ergosterol. The toxicity of the conventional formulation, AmB deoxycholate (AmB-D), is substantial from the standpoints of both systemic reactions (fever, rigors) and acute and chronic renal toxicity. Premedication with acetaminophen, diphenhydramine, and meperidine is often required to prevent systemic reactions during infusion. Renal dysfunction manifests primarily as decreased glomerular filtration with a rising serum creatinine concentration, but substantial tubular nephropathy is associated with potassium and magnesium wasting, requiring supplemental potassium for many neonates and children, regardless of clinical symptoms associated with infusion. Fluid loading with saline pre– and post–AmB-D infusion seems to mitigate renal toxicity.

Three lipid preparations approved in the mid-1990s decrease toxicity with no apparent decrease in clinical efficacy. Decisions on which lipid AmB preparation to use should, therefore, largely focus on side effects and costs. Two clinically useful lipid formulations exist: one in which ribbonlike lipid complexes of AmB are created (amphotericin B lipid complex; ABLC), Abelcet; and one in which AmB is incorporated into true liposomes (liposomal amphotericin B; L-AmB), AmBisome. The standard dosage used of these preparations is 5 mg/kg/day, in contrast to the 1 mg/kg/day of AmB-D. In most studies, the side effects of L-AmB were somewhat less than those of ABLC, but both have significantly fewer side effects than AmB-D. The advantage of the lipid preparations is the ability to safely deliver a greater overall dose of the parent AmB drug. The cost of conventional AmB-D is substantially less than either lipid formulation. A colloidal dispersion of AmB in cholesteryl sulfate, Amphotec, is also available, with decreased nephrotoxicity, but infusion-related side effects are closer to AmB-D than to the lipid formulations. The decreased nephrotoxicity of the 3 lipid preparations is thought to be due to the preferential binding of its AmB to high-density lipoproteins, compared to AmB-D binding to low-density lipoproteins. Despite in vitro concentration-dependent killing, a clinical trial comparing L-AmB at doses of 3 mg/kg/day versus 10 mg/kg/day found no efficacy benefit for the higher dose and only greater toxicity.[1] Therefore, it is generally not recommended to use any AmB preparations at higher dosages (>5 mg/kg/day), as it will likely only incur greater toxicity with no real therapeutic advantage. AmB has a long terminal half-life and, coupled with the concentration-dependent killing, the agent is best used as single daily doses. If the overall AmB exposure needs to be decreased due to toxicity, it is best to increase the dosing interval (eg, 3 times weekly) but retain the mg/kg dose for optimal pharmacokinetics.

AmB-D has been used for nonsystemic purposes, such as in bladder washes, intraventricular instillation, intrapleural instillation, and other modalities, but there are no firm data supporting those clinical indications, and it is likely that the local toxicities outweigh the theoretical benefits. Due to the lipid chemistry, the L-AmB does not interact well with renal tubules, so there is a theoretical concern with using a lipid formulation, as opposed to AmB-D, when treating isolated urinary fungal disease. Importantly, there are several pathogens that are either inherently or functionally resistant to AmB, including *Candida lusitaniae, Trichosporon* spp, *Aspergillus terreus, Fusarium* spp, and *Pseudallescheria boydii (Scedosporium apiospermum)* or *Scedosporium prolificans*.

Azoles. This class of systemic agents was first approved in 1981 and is divided into imidazoles (ketoconazole), triazoles (fluconazole, itraconazole), and second-generation triazoles (voriconazole, posaconazole, and isavuconazole) based on the number of nitrogens in the azole ring. All of the azoles work by inhibition of ergosterol synthesis (fungal cytochrome P450 [CYP] sterol 14-demethylation), required for fungal cell membrane integrity. While the polyenes are rapidly fungicidal, the azoles are fungistatic against yeasts and fungicidal against molds. However, it is important to note that ketoconazole and fluconazole have no mold activity. The only systemic imidazole is ketoconazole, which is primarily active against *Candida* spp, and is available in an oral formulation.

Fluconazole is active against a broader range of fungi than ketoconazole, and includes clinically relevant activity against *Cryptococcus, Coccidioides,* and *Histoplasma*. Like most other azoles, fluconazole requires a loading dose—which has been nicely studied in neonates[2] and is likely also required, but not definitively proven yet, in children. Fluconazole achieves relatively high concentrations in urine and cerebrospinal fluid compared with AmB due to its low lipophilicity, with urinary concentrations often so high that treatment against even "resistant" pathogens that are isolated only in the urine is possible. Fluconazole remains one of the most active, and so far the safest, systemic antifungal agent for the treatment of most *Candida* infections. *Candida albicans* remains generally sensitive to fluconazole, although some resistance is present in many non-*albicans Candida* spp as well as in *C albicans* in children repeatedly exposed to fluconazole. *Candida krusei* is considered inherently resistant to fluconazole, and *Candida glabrata* demonstrates dose-dependent resistance to fluconazole. Available in both parenteral and oral (with >90% bioavailability) formulations, clinical data and pharmacokinetics have been generated to include premature neonates. Toxicity is unusual and primarily hepatic.

Itraconazole is active against an even broader range of fungi and, unlike fluconazole, includes molds such as *Aspergillus*. It is currently available as a capsule or oral solution (the intravenous form was discontinued); the oral solution provides higher, more consistent serum concentrations than capsules and should be used preferentially. Absorption using itraconazole oral solution is improved on an empty stomach, and monitoring itraconazole serum concentrations, like most azole antifungals, is a key principal in management. Itraconazole is indicated in adults for therapy of mild/moderate disease with blastomycosis, histoplasmosis, and others. Although it possesses antifungal activity, itraconazole is not indicated as primary therapy against invasive aspergillosis, as voriconazole is now a far better option. Limited pharmacokinetic data are available in children; itraconazole has not been approved by the US Food and Drug Administration (FDA) for pediatric indications. Toxicity in adults is primarily hepatic.

Voriconazole was approved in 2002 and is not yet FDA approved for children younger than 12 years, although limited pharmacokinetic data for children aged 2 to 12 years are included in the package label. Voriconazole is a fluconazole derivative, so think of it as having the greater tissue and cerebrospinal fluid penetration of fluconazole, but the added antifungal spectrum to include molds. While the bioavailability of voriconazole in adults is approximately 96%, it is only approximately 50% in children—requiring clinicians to carefully monitor voriconazole trough concentrations, especially in patients taking the oral formulation. Voriconazole serum concentrations are tricky to interpret, confounded by great interpatient variability, but monitoring concentrations is essential to using this drug, like all azole antifungals, and especially important in circumstances of suspected treatment failure or possible toxicity. Most experts suggest voriconazole trough concentrations of 1 to 2 μg/mL or greater, which would generally exceed the pathogen's minimum inhibitory concentration. One important point is the acquisition of an accurate trough concentration, one obtained just before the next dose is due and not obtained through a catheter infusing the drug. These simple trough requirements will make interpretation possible. The fundamental voriconazole pharmacokinetics are different in adults versus children; in adults, voriconazole is metabolized in a nonlinear fashion, whereas, in children, the drug is metabolized in a linear fashion. Children require higher dosages of the drug and also have a larger therapeutic window for dosing. Given the poor clinical and microbiological response of *Aspergillus* infections to AmB, voriconazole is now the treatment of choice for invasive aspergillosis and many other mold infections. Importantly, infections with *Zygomycetes* (eg, mucormycosis) are resistant to voriconazole. Voriconazole retains activity against most *Candida* spp, including some that are fluconazole resistant, but it is unlikely to replace fluconazole for treatment of fluconazole-susceptible *Candida* infections. However, there are increasing reports of *C glabrata* resistance to voriconazole. Voriconazole produces some unique transient visual field abnormalities in about 10% of adults and children. Hepatotoxicity is uncommon, occurring only in 2% to 5% of patients. Voriconazole is CYP metabolized (CYP2C19), and allelic polymorphisms in the population have shown that some Asian patients can achieve higher toxic serum concentrations than other patients. Voriconazole also interacts with many similarly P450 metabolized drugs to produce some profound changes in serum concentrations of many concurrently administered drugs.

Posaconazole, an itraconazole derivative, was approved in 2006 and is also not currently FDA approved for children younger than 13 years. An extended-release tablet formulation was recently approved (November 2013) to complement the oral suspension, and an intravenous formulation will be available in the future. Effective absorption of the oral suspension requires taking the medication with food, ideally a high-fat meal; the tablet formulation has better absorption, but absoprtion will still be increased with food. If the patient is unable to take food with the medication, the tablet is recommended. The pediatric dosing for posaconazole has not been completely determined and requires consultation with a pediatric antifungal expert. The in vitro activity of posaconazole against *Candida* spp is better than that of fluconazole and similar to voriconazole. Overall activity against *Aspergillus* is also equivalent to voriconazole, but notably it is the first triazole with substantial activity against some zygomycetes, including *Rhizopus* spp and *Mucor* spp, as well as activity against *Coccidioides, Histoplasma,* and *Blastomyces* and the pathogens of phaeohyphomycosis. Posaconazole has had some anecdotal success against invasive aspergillosis, especially in patients with chronic granulomatous disease, where voriconazole does not seem to be as effective as posaconazole in this specific patient population for an unknown reason. Posaconazole is eliminated by hepatic glucuronidation but does demonstrate inhibition of the CYP 3A4 enzyme system, leading to many drug interactions with other P450 metabolized drugs. It is currently approved for prophylaxis of *Candida* and *Aspergillus* infections in high-risk adults, and for treatment of *Candida* esophagitis in adults.

Isavuconazole is a new triazole that is not yet FDA approved for clinical use at the time of this writing, yet is anticipated in 2014 with both oral and intravenous formulations. Isavuconazole has a similar antifungal spectrum as voriconazole and some activity against the zygomycetes (yet not as potent against zygomycetes as posaconazole). No pediatric dosing data exist for isavuoncaozle yet.

Echinocandins. This entirely new class of systemic antifungal agents was first approved in 2001. The echinocandins inhibit cell wall formation (in contrast to acting on the cell membrane by the polyenes and azoles) by noncompetitively inhibiting beta-1,3-glucan synthase, an enzyme present in fungi but absent in mammalian cells.[3] These agents are generally very safe, as there is no beta-1,3-glucan in humans. The echinocandins are not metabolized through the CYP system, so fewer drug interactions are problematic, compared with the azoles. There is no need to dose-adjust in renal failure, but one needs a lower dosage in the setting of very severe hepatic dysfunction. While the 3 clinically available echinocandins each have unique and important dosing and pharmacokinetic parameters, including limited penetration into the cerebrospinal fluid, efficacy is generally equivalent. Opposite the azole class, the echinocandins are fungicidal against yeasts but fungistatic against molds. The fungicidal activity against yeasts has elevated the echinocandins to the preferred therapy against *Candida* in a neutropenic or critically ill patient. Improved efficacy with combination therapy with the echinocandins and the triazoles against *Aspergillus* infections is unclear, with disparate results in multiple smaller studies, and a definitive clinical trial demonstrating no clear benefit over voriconazole monotherapy.

Caspofungin received FDA approval for children aged 3 months to 17 years in 2008 for empiric therapy of presumed fungal infections in febrile, neutropenic children; treatment of candidemia as well as *Candida* esophagitis, peritonitis, and empyema; and for salvage therapy of invasive aspergillosis. Caspofungin dosing in children is calculated according to body surface area, with a loading dose on the first day of 70 mg/m^2, followed by daily maintenance dosing of 50 mg/m^2.

Micafungin was approved in adults in 2005 for treatment of candidemia, *Candida* esophagitis and peritonitis, and prophylaxis of *Candida* infections in stem cell transplant recipients, and in 2013 for pediatric patients aged 4 months and older. Efficacy studies in pediatric age groups are currently underway, but some pediatric pharmacokinetic data have been published.[4–6] Micafungin dosing in children is age dependent, as clearance increases dramatically in the younger age groups (especially neonates), necessitating higher doses for younger children. Doses in children are generally 2 to 4 mg/kg/day, with premature neonates dosed at 10 mg/kg/day.

Anidulafungin was approved for adults for candidemia and *Candida* esophagitis in 2006. Like the other echinocandins, anidulafungin is not P450 metabolized and has not demonstrated significant drug interactions. Limited clinical efficacy data are available in children, with only some pediatric pharmacokinetic data suggesting weight-based dosing.[7]

3. How Antibiotic Dosages Are Determined Using Susceptibility Data, Pharmacodynamics, and Treatment Outcomes

Factors Involved in Dosing Recommendations. Our view of how to use antimicrobials is continually changing. As the published literature and our experience with each drug increase, our recommendations evolve as we compare the efficacy, safety, and cost of each drug in the context of current and previous data. Every new antibiotic must demonstrate some degree of efficacy and safety before we attempt to treat children. Occasionally, unanticipated toxicities and unanticipated clinical failures modify our initial recommendations.

Important considerations in any new recommendations we make include (1) the susceptibilities of pathogens to antibiotics, which are constantly changing, are different from region to region, and are hospital- and unit-specific; (2) the antibiotic concentrations achieved at the site of infection over a 24-hour dosing interval; (3) the mechanism of how antibiotics kill bacteria; (4) how often the dose we select produces a clinical and microbiological cure; (5) how often we encounter toxicity; and (6) how likely the antibiotic exposure leads to antibiotic resistance in the treated child and in the population in general.

Susceptibility. Susceptibility data for each bacterial pathogen against a wide range of antibiotics are available from the microbiology laboratory of virtually every hospital. This antibiogram can help guide you in antibiotic selection for empiric therapy. Many hospitals can separate the inpatient culture results from outpatient results, and many can give you the data by ward of the hospital (eg, pediatric ward vs neonatal intensive care unit vs adult intensive care unit). Susceptibility data are also available by region and by country from reference laboratories or public health laboratories. The recommendations made in *Nelson's Pediatric Antimicrobial Therapy* reflect overall susceptibility patterns present in the United States. Wide variations may exist for certain pathogens in different regions of the United States and the world.

Drug Concentrations at the Site of Infection. With every antibiotic, we can measure the concentration of antibiotic present in the serum. We can also directly measure the concentrations in specific tissue sites, such as spinal fluid or middle ear fluid. Since free, nonprotein-bound antibiotic is required to kill pathogens, it is also important to calculate the amount of free drug available at the site of infection. While traditional methods of measuring antibiotics focused on the peak concentrations in serum and how rapidly the drugs were excreted, complex models of drug distribution and elimination now exist, not only for the serum, but for other tissue compartments as well. Antibiotic exposure to pathogens at the site of infection can be described in many ways: (1) the percentage of time in a 24-hour dosing interval that the antibiotic concentrations are above the minimum inhibitory concentration (MIC, the antibiotic concentration required for inhibition of growth of an organism) at the site of infection; (2) the mathematically calculated area below the serum concentration-versus-time curve (area under the curve, AUC); and (3) the maximal concentration of drug achieved at the tissue site (Cmax). For each of these 3 values, a ratio of that value to the MIC of the pathogen in question can be calculated and provides more useful information on specific drug activity against a specific pathogen than simply looking at the MIC. It allows us to compare the exposure of different antibiotics (that achieve quite different concentrations in tissues) to a pathogen (where the MIC for each drug may be different), and to compare the activity of the same antibiotic to many different pathogens.

Pharmacodynamics. Pharmacodynamic data provide the clinician with information on how the bacterial pathogens are killed (see Suggested Reading). Beta-lactam antibiotics tend to eradicate bacteria following prolonged exposure of the antibiotic to the pathogen at the site of infection, usually expressed as the percent of time over a dosing interval that the antibiotic is present at the site of infection in concentrations greater than the MIC (%T>MIC). For example, amoxicillin needs to be present at the site of pneumococcal infection at a concentration above the MIC for only 40% of a 24-hour dosing interval. Remarkably, neither higher concentrations of amoxicillin nor a more prolonged exposure will substantially increase the cure rate. On the other hand, gentamicin's activity against *Escherichia coli* is based primarily on the absolute concentration of free antibiotic at the site of infection. The more antibiotic you can deliver to the site of infection, the more rapidly you can sterilize the tissue; we are only limited by the toxicities of gentamicin. For fluoro-quinolones like ciprofloxacin, antibiotic exposure is best predicted by the AUC.

Assessment of Clinical and Microbiological Outcomes. In clinical trials of anti-infective agents, most children will hopefully be cured, but a few will fail therapy. For those few, we may note inadequate drug exposure (eg, more rapid drug elimination in a particular child) or infection caused by a pathogen with a particularly high MIC. By analyzing the successes and the failures based on the appropriate exposure parameters outlined previously (%T>MIC, AUC, or Cmax), linked to the MIC, we can often observe a particular value of exposure, above which we observe a very high rate of cure and below which the cure rate drops quickly. Knowing this target value (the "antibiotic exposure break point") allows us to calculate the dosage that will create treatment success in most children. It is this dosage that we subsequently offer to you (if we have it) as one likely to cure your patient.

Suggested Reading

Bradley JS, Garonzik SM, Forrest A, Bhavnani SM. Pharmacokinetics, pharmacodynamics, and Monte Carlo simulation: selecting the best antimicrobial dose to treat an infection. *Pediatr Infect Dis J.* 2010;29(11):1043–1046. PMID: 20975453

4. Community-Associated Methicillin-Resistant *Staphylococcus aureus*

Community-associated methicillin-resistant *Staphylococcus aureus* (CA-MRSA) is a community pathogen for children (that can also spread from child to child in hospitals) that first appeared in the United States in the mid-1990s and currently represents 30% to 80% of all community isolates in various regions of the United States (check your hospital microbiology laboratory for your local rate); it is increasingly present in many areas of the world. This CA-MRSA, like the hospital-associated MRSA strain that has been prevalent for the past 40 years, is resistant to methicillin and to all other beta-lactam antibiotics, except for the newly US Food and Drug Administration (FDA)-approved fifth-generation cephalosporin antibiotic, ceftaroline, for which there are only limited published pediatric data on pharmacokinetics, safety, and efficacy (as of August 2013). In contrast to the old strains, CA-MRSA usually does not have multiple antibiotic resistance genes. However, there are an undetermined number of pathogenicity factors that make CA-MRSA more aggressive than its predecessor in the community, methicillin-susceptible *S aureus* (MSSA). Although published descriptions of clinical disease and treatment of the old *S aureus* found in textbooks, the medical literature, and older editions of *Nelson's Pediatric Antimicrobial Therapy* remain accurate for MSSA, CA-MRSA seems to cause greater tissue necrosis, an increased host inflammatory response, an increased rate of complications, and an increased rate of recurrent infections compared with MSSA. Response to therapy with non–beta-lactam antibiotics (eg, vancomycin, clindamycin) seems to be delayed, and it is unknown whether the longer courses of alternative agents that seem to be needed for clinical cure are due to a hardier, better-adapted, more resistant pathogen, or whether alternative agents are not as effective against MRSA as beta-lactam agents are against MSSA.

Therapy for CA-MRSA

Vancomycin (intravenous [IV]) has been the mainstay of parenteral therapy of MRSA infections for the past 4 decades and continues to have activity against more than 98% of strains isolated from children. A few cases of intermediate resistance and "heteroresistance" (transient moderately increased resistance based on thickened staphylococcal cell walls) have been reported, most commonly in adults who are receiving long-term therapy or who have received multiple exposures to vancomycin. Unfortunately, the response to therapy using standard vancomycin dosing of 40 mg/kg/day in the treatment of the new CA-MRSA strains has not been as predictably successful as in the past with MSSA. Increasingly, data in adults suggest that serum trough concentrations of vancomycin in treating serious CA-MRSA infections should be kept in the range of 15 to 20 µg/mL, which frequently causes toxicity in adults. For children, serum trough concentrations of 15 to 20 µg/mL can usually be achieved using the old pediatric "meningitis dosage" of vancomycin of 60 mg/kg/day. Although no prospectively collected data are available, it appears that this dosage in children is reasonably effective and not associated with the degree of nephrotoxicity observed in adults. For vancomycin, the area under the curve/minimum inhibitory concentration (MIC) ratios that best predict a successful outcome are those of about 400, which is achievable for CA-MRSA strains with in vitro MIC values of 1 or less, but difficult to achieve for strains with 2 µg/mL or greater.[2] Strains with MIC values of 4 µg/mL or greater should generally be considered resistant to vancomycin. At the higher "meningitis" treatment dosage, one needs to follow renal function for the development of toxicity.

Clindamycin (oral [PO] or IV) is active against approximately 70% to 90% of strains, with great geographic variability (again, check with your hospital laboratory). The dosage for moderate to severe infections is 30 to 40 mg/kg/day, in 3 divided doses, using the same mg/kg dose PO or IV. Clindamycin is not as bactericidal as vancomycin but achieves higher concentrations in abscesses. Some CA-MRSA strains are susceptible to clindamycin on initial testing but have inducible clindamycin resistance that is usually assessed by the "D-test." Within each population of these CA-MRSA organisms, a rare organism will have a mutation that allows for constant (rather than induced) resistance. Although still somewhat controversial, clindamycin should be effective therapy for infections that have a relatively low organism load (cellulitis, small abscesses) and are unlikely to contain these mutants. Infections with a high organism load (empyema) may have a greater risk of failure against strains positive on a D-test (as the likelihood of having a few truly resistant organisms is greater, given the greater numbers of organisms), and clindamycin should not be used as the preferred agent.

Clindamycin is used to treat most CA-MRSA infections that are not life-threatening, and, if the child responds, therapy can be switched from IV to PO (although the oral solution is not very well tolerated). *Clostridium difficile* enterocolitis is a concern as a clindamycin-associated complication; however, despite a great increase in the use of clindamycin in children during the past decade, there are no recent published reports on any clinically significant increase in the rate of this complication in children.

Trimethoprim/sulfamethoxazole (TMP/SMX) (PO, IV), Bactrim/Septra, is active against CA-MRSA in vitro. New, prospective comparative data on treatment of skin or skin structure infections (IDWeek, October 2013) in adults and children document efficacy equivalent to clindamycin. Given our current lack of prospective, comparative information in MRSA bacteremia, pneumonia, and osteomyelitis, TMP/SMX should not be used routinely to treat these more serious infections.

Linezolid, Zyvox (PO, IV), active against virtually 100% of CA-MRSA strains, is another reasonable alternative but is considered bacteriostatic, and has relatively frequent hematologic toxicity in adults (neutropenia, thrombocytopenia) and some infrequent neurologic toxicity (peripheral neuropathy, optic neuritis), particularly when used for courses of 2 weeks or longer (a complete blood cell count should be checked every week or 2 in children receiving prolonged linezolid therapy). It is still under patent, so the cost is substantially more than clindamycin or vancomycin.

Daptomycin (IV), FDA approved for adults for skin infections and bacteremia/endocarditis, is a new class of antibiotic, a lipopeptide, and is highly bactericidal against bacterial cell membrane depolarization. Daptomycin should be considered for treatment of these infections in failures with other better studied antibiotics. However, daptomycin demonstrated relatively poor outcomes in the treatment of adults with community-acquired pneumonia due to binding of the drug to surfactant in the lung. Pediatric studies for skin infections, bacteremia, and osteomyelitis are underway.

Tigecycline and fluoroquinolones, both of which may show in vitro activity, are not generally recommended for children if other agents are available and are tolerated, due to potential toxicity issues for children with tetracyclines and fluoroquinolones.

Ceftaroline, a fifth-generation cephalosporin antibiotic for adults for skin and skin structure infections (including CA-MRSA) and community-acquired pneumonia, is the first FDA-approved beta-lactam antibiotic to have been chemically modified to be able to bind to the altered MRSA protein (PBP2a) that confers resistance to all other beta-lactams. The gram-negative coverage is similar to cefotaxime, with no activity against *Pseudomonas.* As of August 2013, pediatric pharmacokinetic data have been collected for all age groups, and studies for skin and skin structure infections and community-acquired pneumonia are underway. The efficacy and toxicity profile in adults is what one would expect from most cephalosporins.

Combination therapy for serious infections, with vancomycin and rifampin (for deep abscesses) or vancomycin and gentamicin (for bacteremia), is often used, but no data exist on improved efficacy over single antibiotic therapy. Some experts use vancomycin and clindamycin in combination, particularly for children with a toxic-shock clinical presentation (with clindamycin, a ribosomal agent, theoretically decreasing toxin production more quickly than vancomycin), but no data are currently available to compare one antibiotic against another for CA-MRSA, let alone one combination against another.

Recommendations for treatment of staphylococcal infections are given for 2 situations in Chapter 6: standard (eg, MSSA) and CA-MRSA. Cultures should be obtained whenever possible. If cultures demonstrate MSSA, then CA-MRSA antibiotics can be discontinued, continuing with the preferred beta-lactam agents like cephalexin. Rapid tests are becoming widely available to allow for identification of CA-MRSA within a few hours of obtaining a sample, rather than taking 1 to 3 days for the culture report.

Life-threatening and Serious Infections. If any CA-MRSA is present in your community, empiric therapy for presumed staphylococcal infections that are either life-threatening or infections for which any risk of failure is unacceptable (eg, meningitis) should follow the recommendations for CA-MRSA and include high-dose vancomycin, clindamycin, or linezolid, as well as nafcillin or oxacillin (beta-lactam antibiotics are considered better than vancomycin or clindamycin for MSSA).

Moderate Infections. If you live in a location with greater than 10% methicillin resistance, consider using the CA-MRSA recommendations for hospitalized children with presumed staphylococcal infections of any severity, and start empiric therapy with clindamycin (usually active against >90% of CA-MRSA), vancomycin, or linezolid IV. Standard empiric therapy can still be used for less severe infections in these regions, realizing that a certain low percentage of children who are actually infected by CA-MRSA may fail standard therapy for MSSA.

In skin and skin structure abscesses, drainage of the abscess seems to be completely curative in some children, and antibiotics may not be necessary following incision and drainage.

Mild Infections. For nonserious, presumed staphylococcal infections in regions with significant CA-MRSA, empiric topical therapy with either mupirocin (Bactroban) or retapamulin (Altabax) ointment, or oral therapy with trimethoprim/sulfamethoxazole or clindamycin are preferred. For older children, doxycycline and minocycline are also options based on data in adults. Again, using standard empiric therapy with erythromycins, oral cephalosporins, or amoxicillin/clavulanate may be acceptable in areas with a low prevalence of CA-MRSA and a high likelihood of MSSA as the local staphylococcal pathogen, for which these antimicrobials are usually effective.

Recurrent Infections. For children with problematic, recurrent infections, no well-studied prospectively collected data provide a solution. Bleach baths (one-half cup of bleach in one-quarter–filled bathtub[3]) seem to be able to transiently decrease the numbers of colonizing organisms. Bathing with chlorhexidine (Hibiclens, a preoperative antibacterial skin disinfectant) daily or a few times each week should provide topical anti-MRSA activity for several hours following a bath. Nasal mupirocin ointment (Bactroban) designed to eradicate colonization may also be used. All of these measures have advantages and disadvantages and need to be used together with environment measures (eg, washing towels frequently, using hand sanitizers, not sharing items of clothing). Helpful advice can be found on the Centers for Disease Control and Prevention Web site at www.cdc.gov/mrsa.

The Future. A number of new antibiotics are in clinical trials for adults, including a number of oxazolidinones, glycopeptides, and lipopeptides that have advantages over currently approved drugs in activity, safety, or dosing regimens. It will be important to see how these drugs perform in adults before recommending them for children. Vaccines against staphylococcal infections have not been successful to date. Immune globulin and antibody products with activity against CA-MRSA are also under investigation.

5. Antimicrobial Therapy for Newborns

NOTES

- Prospectively collected data in newborns continue to become available, thanks in large part to federal legislation (including the Food and Drug Administration Safety and Innovation Act of 2012 that mandates neonatal studies). In situations of inadequate data, suggested doses are based on efficacy, safety, and pharmacologic data from older children or adults. These may not account for the effect of developmental changes (effect of ontogeny) on drug metabolism that occur during early infancy and among premature and full-term infants.[1] These values may vary widely, particularly for the unstable premature infant. Oral convalescent therapy for neonatal infections has not been well studied but may be used cautiously in non–life-threatening infections, in adherent families with ready access to medical care.[2]

- The recommended antibiotic dosages and intervals of administration are given in the tables at the end of this chapter.

- **Adverse drug reaction:** Neonates should not receive intravenous (IV) ceftriaxone while receiving IV calcium-containing products including parenteral nutrition by the same or different infusion lines, as fatal reactions with ceftriaxone-calcium precipitates in lungs and kidneys in neonates have occurred. There are no data on interactions between IV ceftriaxone and oral calcium-containing products or between intramuscular ceftriaxone and IV or oral calcium-containing products. Current information is available on the US Food and Drug Administration Web site.[3] Cefotaxime is preferred over ceftriaxone for neonates with hyperbilirubinemia.[4]

- **Abbreviations:** ABLC, lipid complex amphotericin; AmB, amphotericin B; amox/clav, amoxicillin/clavulanate; AOM, acute otitis media; bid, twice daily; BSA, body surface area; CA, chronologic age; CBC, complete blood cell count; CLD, chronic lung disease; CMV, cytomegalovirus; CNS, central nervous system; CSF, cerebrospinal fluid; div, divided; ESBL, extended spectrum beta-lactamase; FDA, US Food and Drug Administration; GA, gestational age; GBS, group B streptococcus; GI, gastrointestinal; G-CSF, granulocyte colony stimulating factor; HSV, herpes simplex virus; ID, infectious diseases; IM, intramuscular; IV, intravenous; IVIG, intravenous immune globulin; L-AmB, liposomal AmB; MRSA, methicillin-resistant *Staphylococcus aureus;* MSSA, methicillin-susceptible *S aureus;* NEC, necrotizing enterocolitis; NICU, neonatal intensive care unit; NVP, nev rapine; oxacillin/ nafcillin, oxacillin or nafcillin; PCR, polymerase chain reaction; pip/tazo, piperacillin/ tazobactam; PO, orally; RPR, rapid plasma reagin; RSV, respiratory syncytial virus; ticar/ clav, ticarcillin/clavulanate; tid, 3 times daily; TIG, tetanus immune globulin; TMP/SMX, trimethoprim/sulfamethoxazole; UTI, urinary tract infection; VCUG, voiding cystoure-throgram; VDRL, Venereal Disease Research Laboratories; ZDV, zidovudine.

A. RECOMMENDED THERAPY FOR SELECTED NEWBORN CONDITIONS

Condition	Therapy (evidence grade) See Table 5B–D for Neonatal Dosages	Comments
Conjunctivitis		
– Chlamydial[5–8]	Azithromycin PO for 5 days (AII) or erythromycin ethylsuccinate PO for 10–14 days (AII)	Macrolides PO preferred to prevent development of pneumonia; association of erythromycin and pyloric stenosis in young infants.[9] Alternatives: Oral sulfonamides may be used after the immediate neonatal period for infants who do not tolerate erythromycin.
– Gonococcal[10–14]	Ceftriaxone 25–50 mg/kg (max 125 mg) IV, IM once (AI) (longer treatment may be used for severe cases)	Saline irrigation of eyes. Alternative: cefotaxime may be used in infants with hyperbilirubinemia. Evaluate for chlamydial infection. All infants born to mothers with untreated gonococcal infection (regardless of symptoms) require therapy. Cefixime and ciprofloxacin no longer recommended for empiric maternal therapy.
– *Staphylococcus aureus*[15–17]	Topical therapy sufficient for mild *S aureus* cases (AII), but oral or IV therapy may be considered for moderate to severe conjunctivitis. MSSA: oxacillin/nafcillin IV or cefazolin (for non-CNS infections) IM, IV for 7 days. MRSA: vancomycin IV or clindamycin IV, PO.	Neomycin or erythromycin (BIII) ophthalmic drops or ointment. No prospective data for MRSA conjunctivitis (BIII). Cephalexin PO for mild-to-moderate disease caused by MSSA. Increased *S aureus* resistance with ciprofloxacin/levofloxacin ophthalmic formulations (AII).
– *Pseudomonas aeruginosa*[18–20]	Ceftazidime IM, IV AND tobramycin IM, IV for 7–10 days (alternatives: meropenem, cefepime, pip/tazo) (BII)	Aminoglycoside or polymyxin B-containing ophthalmic drops or ointment as adjunctive therapy
– Other gram-negative	Aminoglycoside or polymyxin B-containing ophthalmic drops or ointment if mild (AII) Systemic therapy if moderate to severe, or unresponsive to topical therapy (AIII)	Duration of therapy dependent on clinical course and may be as short as 5 days if clinically resolved.

Cytomegalovirus	
– Congenital[21–24]	Oral valganciclovir at 16 mg/kg/dose PO bid for 6 mo[24] (AI); intravenous ganciclovir 6 mg/kg/dose IV q12h can be used for some or all of the first 6 wk of therapy if oral therapy contraindicated (eg, necrotizing enterocolitis, extreme prematurity) (AII).	Benefit for hearing loss and neurodevelopmental outcomes (AI). Treatment recommended for neonates with symptomatic congenital CMV disease, with or without CNS involvement. Neutropenia in 20% (oral valganciclovir) to 68% (IV ganciclovir) of infants on long-term therapy (responds to G-CSF or discontinuation of therapy). Treatment for congenital CMV should start within the first month of life. CMV-IVIG not recommended.
– Perinatally or postnatally acquired[23]	Ganciclovir 12 mg/kg/day IV div q12h for 14–21 days (AIII)	Only recommended for acute severe disease with pneumonia, hepatitis, encephalitis, or persistent thrombocytopenia. Observe for possible relapse after completion of therapy (AIII).
Fungal infections (See Chapter 8.)		
– Candidiasis[25–33]	L-AmB/ABLC (3–5 mg/kg/day) or AmB-D (1 mg/kg/day). If urinary tract involvement is excluded, then can use L-AmB/ABLC due to theoretical concerns of lipid formulations not penetrating kidneys adequately for treatment. For susceptible strains, fluconazole is usually effective. For treatment of neonates load with 25 mg/day for day one, then continue with 12 mg/kg/day (BI).[34] For treatment of neonates and young infants (<120 days) on ECMO, fluconazole load with 35 mg/kg on day one, followed by 12 mg/kg/day (BII). For prophylaxis, fluconazole 6 mg/kg/day twice a week in high-risk neonates (birth weight <1,000 g) in centers where incidence of disease is high (generally thought to be >10%). For prophylaxis in neonates and young infants (<120 days) on ECMO, fluconazole 25 mg/kg once weekly (BII).	Prompt removal of all catheters essential (AII). Evaluate for other sites: CSF analysis, cardiac echo, abdominal ultrasound to include bladder; retinal eye examination. Persistent disease requires evaluation of catheter removal or search for disseminated sites. Antifungal susceptibility is suggested with persistent disease. (*Candida krusei* inherently resistant to fluconazole. *Candida parapsilosis* may be less susceptible to echinocandins). No proven benefit for combination antifungal therapy in candidiasis. Change from amphotericin B or fluconazole to micafungin/capsofungin if cultures persistently positive (BII). Role of flucytosine (5-FC) orally in neonates with *Candida* meningitis is not well defined and not routinely recommended due to toxicity concerns. Length of therapy dependent on disease (BIII), usually 3 wk. Limited data in humans exist on echinocandin CSF/brain penetration. Animal studies suggest adequate penetration, but clinical utility in the CSF/brain is unclear. Higher echinocandin doses needed in the smallest infants. Antifungal bladder washes not indicated.

A. RECOMMENDED THERAPY FOR SELECTED NEWBORN CONDITIONS (cont)

Condition	Therapy (evidence grade) See Table 5B for Neonatal Dosages	Comments
– Aspergillosis (usually cutaneous infection with systemic dissemination)[35–37]	Voriconazole (18 mg/kg/day divided q12h load, then continue with 16 mg/kg/day; very important to follow serum concentrations). Duration depends on severity of disease and success of local debridement (BIII).	Aggressive antifungal therapy, early debridement of skin lesions (AIII)
Gastrointestinal infections		
– NEC or peritonitis secondary to bowel rupture[38–43]	Ampicillin IV AND gentamicin IM, IV for ≥10 days (AII). Alternatives: pip/tazo AND gentamicin (AII); ceftazidime/cefotaxime AND gentamicin ± metronidazole (BIII); OR meropenem (BI). ADD fluconazole if known to have gastrointestinal colonization with candida (BIII).	Surgical drainage (AII). Definitive antibiotic therapy based on culture results (aerobic, anaerobic, and fungal); meropenem or cefepime if ceftazidime-resistant gram-negative bacilli isolated. Vancomycin rather than ampicillin if MRSA prevalent. *Bacteroides* not common until several weeks of age (AIII). Duration of therapy dependent on clinical response and risk of persisting intra-abdominal abscess (AII). Probiotics may prevent NEC in infants born <1,500 g but agent, dose, and safety not fully known.
– *Salmonella*[44]	Ampicillin IM, IV (if susceptible) OR cefotaxime IM for 7–10 days (AII)	Observe for focal complications (eg, meningitis, arthritis) (AIII)
Herpes simplex infection		
– CNS and disseminated disease[45–47]	Acyclovir IV for 21 days (AII) (if eye disease present, ADD topical 1% trifluridine, 0.1% iododeoxyuridine, or 0.15% ganciclovir ophthalmic gel) (AII)	For CNS disease, perform CSF HSV PCR near end of 21 days of therapy and continue acyclovir until PCR negative. Serum AST/ALT may help identify early disseminated infection. Foscarnet for acyclovir-resistant disease. Acyclovir PO (300 mg/m²/dose tid) suppression for 6 mo recommended following parenteral therapy (AI).[48] Monitor for neutropenia during suppressive therapy.

– Skin, eye, or mouth disease[45-47]	Acyclovir IV for 14 days (AII) (if eye disease present, ADD topical 1% trifluridine, 0.1% iododeoxyuridine, or 0.15% ganciclovir ophthalmic gel) (AII). Obtain CSF PCR for HSV to assess for CNS infection.	Acyclovir PO (300 mg/m²/dose tid) suppression for 6 mo recommended following parenteral therapy (AI).[48] Monitor for neutropenia during suppressive therapy. For recurrent cutaneous disease, oral acyclovir until lesions crusted (assuming CNS disease at the time of cutaneous recurrence).
Human immunodeficiency virus infection[49,50]	Peripartum presumptive preventive therapy for HIV-exposed newborns: ZDV for the first 6 wk of age (AI). GA ≥35 wk: ZDV 8 mg/kg/day PO div bid OR 6 mg/kg/day IV div q6h for 6 wk. GA <35 wk but >30 wk: ZDV 4 mg/kg/day PO (OR 3 mg/kg/day IV) div q12h. Increase at 2 wk of age to 6 mg/kg/day PO (OR 4.6 mg/kg/day IV) div q12h. GA ≤30 wk: ZDV 3 mg/kg/day IV (OR 4 mg/kg/day PO) div q12h. Increase at 4 wk of age to 6 mg/kg/day PO (OR 4.6 mg/kg/day IV) div q12h. For newborns whose mothers received NO antenatal intervention, add 3 doses of NVP in the first week of life (1st dose at 0–48 h; 2nd dose 48 h later; 3rd dose 96 h after 2nd dose) to the 6 wk of ZDV treatment. NVP dose: Birth weight 1.5–2 kg: 8 mg/dose PO; Birth weight >2 kg: 12 mg/dose PO. (AI).[51] The preventive ZDV doses listed above for neonates are also treatment doses for infants with diagnosed HIV infection. Note that antiretroviral treatment doses for neonates are established only for ZDV and 3TC. Treatment of HIV-infected neonates should be considered only with expert consultation.	For detailed information: http://aidsinfo.nih.gov/Guidelines (accessed November 8, 2013). National Perinatal HIV Hotline (888/448-8765) provides free clinical consultation. Start therapy at 6–8 h of age if possible (AII). Monitor CBC at birth and 4 wk (AII). Some experts consider the use of ZDV in combination with other antiretroviral drugs in certain situations (eg, mothers with minimal intervention before delivery, has high viral load, or with known resistant virus). Since optimal prophylactic regimens have not been formally established, consultation with a pediatric HIV specialist is recommended (BIII). Perform HIV-1 DNA PCR or RNA assays at 14–21 days, 1–2 mo, and 4–6 mo (AI). Initiate prophylaxis for pneumocystis pneumonia at 6 wk of age if HIV infection not yet excluded (AII).
Influenza A and B viruses[52,53]	Preterm, <38 weeks postmenstrual age: 1.0 mg/kg/dose PO BID Preterm, 38 through 40 weeks postmenstrual age: 1.5 mg/kg/dose PO BID Preterm, >40 weeks postmenstrual age: 3.0 mg/kg/dose PO BID[53] Term, birth through 8 months: 3.0 mg/kg/dose PO BID 9 through 11 months: 3.5 mg/kg/dose PO BID 12 through 23 months: 3.5 mg/kg/dose PO BID[54]	Prophylaxis is not recommended unless situation judged critical because of limited data on safety/efficacy in this age group.

A. RECOMMENDED THERAPY FOR SELECTED NEWBORN CONDITIONS (cont)

Condition	Therapy (evidence grade) See Table 5B for Neonatal Dosages	Comments
Omphalitis and funisitis		
– Empiric therapy for omphalitis and necrotizing funisitis direct therapy against coliform bacilli, S aureus (consider MRSA), and anaerobes[55–57]	Cefotaxime OR gentamicin, AND clindamycin for ≥10 days (AII)	Need to culture to direct therapy. Alternatives for coliform coverage if resistance likely: cefepime, meropenem. For suspect MRSA: add vancomycin. Alternatives for combined MSSA and anaerobic coverage: pip/tazo or ticar/clav. Appropriate wound management for infected cord and necrotic tissue (AIII).
– Group A or B streptococci[58]	Penicillin G IV for ≥7–14 days (shorter course for superficial funisitis without invasive infection) (AII)	Group A streptococcus usually causes "wet cord" without pus and with minimal erythema; single dose of benzathine penicillin IM adequate. Consultation with pediatric ID specialist is recommended for necrotizing fasciitis (AII).
– S aureus[57]	MSSA: oxacillin/nafcillin IV, IM for ≥5–7 days (shorter course for superficial funisitis without invasive infection) (AIII) MRSA: vancomycin (AIII)	Assess for bacteremia and other focus of infection. Alternatives for MRSA: linezolid, clindamycin (if susceptible).
– Clostridium spp[59]	Clindamycin OR penicillin G IV for ≥10 days, with additional agents based on culture results (AII)	Crepitance and rapidly spreading cellulitis around umbilicus Mixed infection with other gram-positive and gram-negative bacteria common
Osteomyelitis, suppurative arthritis[60–62] Obtain cultures (aerobic; fungal if NICU) of bone or joint fluid before antibiotic therapy. Duration of therapy dependent on causative organism and normalization of erythrocyte sedimentation rate and C-reactive protein; minimum for osteomyelitis 3 wk and arthritis therapy 2–3 wk if no organism identified (AIII). Surgical drainage of pus (AIII); physical therapy may be needed (BIII).		
– Empiric therapy	Nafcillin/oxacillin IV (or vancomycin if MRSA is a concern) AND cefotaxime or gentamicin IV, IM (AIII)	

Condition / Organism	Therapy	Comments
– Coliform bacteria (eg, *Escherichia coli*, *Klebsiella* spp, *Enterobacter* spp)	For *E coli* and *Klebsiella*: cefotaxime OR gentamicin OR ampicillin (if susceptible) (AIII). For *Enterobacter*, *Serratia*, or *Citrobacter*: ADD gentamicin IV, IM to cefotaxime or ceftriaxone, OR use cefepime or meropenem alone (AIII).	Meropenem for ESBL-producing *E coli* and *Klebsiella* (AIII). Pip/tazo or cefepime are alternatives for susceptible bacilli (BIII).
– Gonococcal arthritis and tenosynovitis[11-14]	Ceftriaxone IV, IM OR cefotaxime IV x 7–10 days (AII)	Cefotaxime is preferred for infants with hyperbilirubinemia.
– *S aureus*	MSSA: oxacillin/nafcillin IV (AII) MRSA: vancomycin IV (AIII)	Alternative for MSSA: cefazolin (AIII) Alternatives for MRSA: linezolid, clindamycin (if susceptible) (BIII), daptomycin (CIII) Addition of rifampin if persistently positive cultures
– Group B streptococcus	Ampicillin or penicillin G IV (AII)	
– *Haemophilus influenzae*	Ampicillin IV OR cefotaxime IV, IM If ampicillin-resistant	Start with IV therapy, and switch to oral therapy when clinically stable. Amox/clav PO OR amoxicillin PO if susceptible (AII).
Otitis media[63]	No controlled treatment trials in newborns; if no response, obtain middle ear fluid for culture.	In addition to *Pneumococcus* and *Haemophilus*, coliforms and *S aureus* may also cause AOM in neonates (AIII).
– Empiric therapy[64]	Oxacillin/nafcillin AND cefotaxime or gentamicin	Start with IV therapy, and switch to oral therapy when clinically stable. Amox/clav (AIII).
– *E coli* (therapy of other coliforms based on susceptibility testing)	Cefotaxime OR gentamicin	Start with IV therapy, and switch to oral therapy when clinically stable. For ESBL-producing strains, use meropenem (AII). Amox/clav if susceptible (AIII).
– *S aureus*	MSSA: oxacillin/nafcillin IV (MSSA) MRSA: vancomycin or clindamycin IV (If susceptible)	Start with IV therapy, and switch to oral therapy when clinically stable. MSSA: cephalexin PO for 10 days or cloxacillin PO (AIII). MRSA: linezolid PO or clindamycin PO (BIII).

A. RECOMMENDED THERAPY FOR SELECTED NEWBORN CONDITIONS (cont)

Condition	Therapy (evidence grade) See Table 5B for Neonatal Dosages	Comments
Otitis media[63] (cont)		
– Group A or B streptococcus	Penicillin G or ampicillin IV, IM	Start with IV therapy, and switch to oral therapy when clinically stable. Amoxicillin 30–40 mg/kg/day PO div q8h for 10 days.
Parotitis, suppurative[65]	Oxacillin/nafcillin IV AND gentamicin IV, IM for 10 days; consider vancomycin if MRSA suspected (AIII).	Usually staphylococcal but occasionally coliform. Antimicrobial regimen without incision/drainage is adequate in >75% of cases.
Pulmonary infections		
– Empiric therapy of the neonate with early onset of pulmonary infiltrates (within the first 48–72 h of life)	Ampicillin IV/IM AND gentamicin or cefotaxime IV/IM for 10 days; many neonatologists treat low-risk infants for 7 days or less (see Comments).	For newborns with no additional risk factors for bacterial infection (eg, maternal amnionitis) who (1) have negative blood cultures, (2) have no need for >8 h of oxygen, and (3) are asymptomatic at 48 h into therapy, 4 days may be sufficient therapy, based on limited data.[66]
– Aspiration pneumonia[67]	Ampicillin IV, IM AND gentamicin IV, IM for 7–10 days (AIII)	Early onset neonatal pneumonia may represent aspiration of amniotic fluid, particularly if fluid is not sterile. Mild aspiration episodes may not require antibiotic therapy.
– Chlamydia trachomatis[68]	Azithromycin PO, IV q24h for 5 days OR erythromycin ethylsuccinate PO for 14 days (AII)	Association of erythromycin and pyloric stenosis in young infants
– Mycoplasma hominis[69,70]	Clindamycin PO, IV for 10 days (organisms are resistant to macrolides)	Pathogenic role in pneumonia not well defined and clinical efficacy unknown; no association with bronchopulmonary dysplasia (BIII).
– Pertussis[71]	Azithromycin 10 mg/kg PO, IV q24h for 5 days OR erythromycin ethylsuccinate PO for 14 days (AII)	Association of erythromycin and pyloric stenosis in young infants; may also occur with azithromycin Alternatives for >1 mo of age, clarithromycin for 7 days, and for >2 mo of age, TMP/SMX for 14 days

– P aeruginosa[72]	Ceftazidime IV, IM AND tobramycin IV, IM for ≥10–14 days (AIII)	Alternatives: cefepime or meropenem, OR pip/tazo AND tobramycin
– Respiratory syncytial virus[73,74]	Prevention of infection with palivizumab (Synagis) at 15 mg/kg IM, monthly during the RSV season in high-risk infants (AI): 1. Infants <24 mo of age with chronic lung disease and requiring medical therapy (max 5 doses) 2. Infants <24 mo of age with hemodynamically significant congenital heart disease (max 5 doses) 3. Premature infants: (a) GA ≤28 wk, and CA <12 mo at the start of the season; (b) GA 29 to <32 wk, and CA <6 mo at the start of the season; (c) GA from 32 to <35 wk, and CA <3 mo before or during RSV season AND 1 of 2 risk factors (child care attendance, sibling <5 y of age) (max 3 doses) 4. Infants <35 wk GA and <12 mo of age with congenital abnormalities of airway or neuromuscular disorder	Aerosol ribavirin provides little, if any, benefit and should only be used for life-threatening infection with RSV. Difficulties in administration, complications with airway reactivity, and concern for potential toxicities to health care workers preclude routine use. Palivizumab does not provide benefit in the treatment of an active RSV infection. Palivizumab may benefit immunocompromised children and those with cystic fibrosis but is not routinely recommended as benefits not well defined.
– S aureus[17,75–77]	MSSA: oxacillin/nafcillin IV for 21 days minimum (AIII) MRSA: vancomycin IV OR clindamycin IV if susceptible (AIII) for 21 days minimum	Alternative for MSSA: cefazolin IV Addition of rifampin or linezolid if persistently positive cultures (AIII) Thoracostomy drainage of empyema
– Group B streptococcus[78,79]	Penicillin G IV OR ampicillin IV, IM for 10 days (AIII)	For serious infections, ADD gentamicin for synergy until clinically improved. No prospective, randomized data on the efficacy of a 7-day treatment course.
– Ureaplasma spp (urealyticum or parvum)[80]	Azithromycin PO/IV for 5 days or clarithromycin PO for 10 days (BIII)	Pathogenic role of Ureaplasma not well defined and no prophylaxis recommended for CLD Many Ureaplasma spp resistant to erythromycin Association of erythromycin and pyloric stenosis in young infants

5

A. RECOMMENDED THERAPY FOR SELECTED NEWBORN CONDITIONS (cont)

Condition	Therapy (evidence grade) See Table 5B for Neonatal Dosages	Comments
Sepsis and meningitis[78,81,82]	NOTE: Duration of therapy: 10 days for sepsis without a focus (AIII); minimum of 21 days for gram-negative meningitis (or at least 14 days after CSF is sterile) and 14–21 days for GBS meningitis and other gram-positive bacteria (AIII)	There are no prospective, controlled studies on 5- or 7-day courses for mild or presumed sepsis.
– Initial therapy, organism unknown	Ampicillin IV AND cefotaxime IV (AII), OR ampicillin IV AND gentamicin IV, IM (AII)	Cefotaxime preferred if meningitis suspected or cannot be excluded (AIII). Initial empiric therapy of nosocomial infection should be based on each hospital's pathogens and susceptibilities.
– Bacteroides fragilis	Metronidazole or meropenem IV, IM (AIII)	Alternative: clindamycin, but increasing resistance reported
– Enterococcus spp	Ampicillin IV, IM AND gentamicin IV, IM (AIII); for ampicillin-resistant organisms: vancomycin AND gentamicin (AIII)	Gentamicin needed with either ampicillin or vancomycin for bactericidal activity; continue until clinical and microbiological response documented (AIII) For vancomycin-resistant enterococci that are also ampicillin resistant: linezolid (AIII)
– E coli[81,82]	Cefotaxime IV, IM or gentamicin IV, IM (AII) if no CNS infection	Meropenem or cefepime for gentamicin/cefotaxime-resistant coliforms (eg, Enterobacter, Serratia) (AIII) Meropenem for ESBL-producing coliforms (AIII)
– Gonococcal[11–14]	Ceftriaxone IV, IM OR cefotaxime IV, IM (AII)	Duration of therapy not well defined, consider 5 days Cefotaxime is preferred for infants with hyperbilirubinemia.
– Listeria monocytogenes[83]	Ampicillin IV AND gentamicin IV, IM (AIII)	Gentamicin is synergistic in vitro with ampicillin. Continue until clinical and microbiological response documented (AIII).
– P aeruginosa	Ceftazidime IV, IM AND tobramycin IV, IM (AIII)	Meropenem, cefepime, and tobramycin are suitable alternatives (AIII). Pip/tazo should not be used for CNS infection.
– S aureus[17,75–77,84,85]	MSSA: oxacillin/nafcillin IV, IM, or cefazolin IV, IM (AII) MRSA: vancomycin IV (AIII)	Alternatives for MRSA: clindamycin, linezolid

– Staphylococcus epidermidis (or any coagulase-negative staphylococci)	Vancomycin IV (AIII)	If organism susceptible and infection not severe, oxacillin/nafcillin or cefazolin are alternatives for methicillin-susceptible strains. Cefazolin does not enter CNS. Add rifampin if cultures persistently positive. Alternative: linezolid.
– Group A streptococcus	Penicillin G or ampicillin IV (AII)	
– Group B streptococcus[78]	Ampicillin or penicillin G IV AND gentamicin IV, IM (AI)	Continue gentamicin until clinical and microbiological response documented (AIII). Duration of therapy: 10 days for bacteremia/sepsis (AII); minimum of 14 days for meningitis (AII).
Skin and soft tissues		
– Breast abscess[86]	Vancomycin IV (for MRSA) or oxacillin/nafcillin IV, IM (MSSA) AND cefotaxime OR gentamicin if gram-negative rods seen on Gram stain (AIII)	Gram stain of expressed pus guides empiric therapy; vancomycin if MRSA prevalent in community; alternative to vancomycin: clindamycin, linezolid, may need surgical drainage to minimize damage to breast tissue Treatment duration individualized, until clinical findings have completely resolved (AIII)
– Erysipelas (and other group A streptococcal infections)	Penicillin G IV for 5–7 days, followed by oral therapy (if bacteremia not present) to complete a 10-day course (AIII)	Alternative: ampicillin. GBS may produce similar cellulitis or nodular lesions.
– Impetigo neonatorum	MSSA: oxacillin/nafcillin IV, IM OR cephalexin (AIII) MRSA: vancomycin IV; for 5 days (AIII)	Systemic antibiotic therapy usually not required for superficial impetigo; local chlorhexidine cleansing may help with or without topical mupirocin (MRSA) or bacitracin (MSSA). Alternatives for MRSA: clindamycin IV, PO, or linezolid IV, PO.
– S aureus[17,75,77,87]	MSSA: oxacillin/nafcillin IV, IM (AII) MRSA: vancomycin IV (AIII)	Surgical drainage may be required. MRSA may cause necrotizing fasciitis. Alternatives for MRSA: clindamycin IV or linezolid IV. Convalescent oral therapy if infection responds quickly to IV therapy.
– Group B streptococcus[78]	Penicillin G IV OR ampicillin IV, IM	Usually no pus formed Treatment course dependent on extent of infection, 7–14 days

5

Antimicrobial Therapy for Newborns

A. RECOMMENDED THERAPY FOR SELECTED NEWBORN CONDITIONS (cont)

Condition	Therapy (evidence grade) See Table 5B for Neonatal Dosages	Comments
Syphilis, congenital (<1 mo of age)[88]	During periods when the availability of penicillin is compromised, see www.cdc.gov/std/Treatment/misc/penicillinG.htm.	Evaluation and treatment do not depend on mother's HIV status. Obtain follow-up serology every 2–3 mo until nontreponemal test nonreactive or decreased 4-fold. If CSF positive, repeat spinal tap with CSF VDRL at 6 mo, and if abnormal, re-treat.
– Proven or highly probable disease: (1) abnormal physical examination; (2) serum quantitative nontreponemal serologic titer that is 4-fold higher than the mother's titer; or (3) a positive darkfield or fluorescent antibody test of body fluid(s)	Aqueous penicillin G 50,000 U/kg/dose q12h (day of life 1–7), q8h (>7 days) IV OR procaine penicillin G 50,000 U/kg IM q24h; for 10 days (AII)	Evaluation to determine type and duration of therapy: CSF analysis (VDRL, cell count, protein), CBC and platelet count. Other tests as clinically indicated, including long-bone radiographs, chest radiograph, liver function tests, cranial ultrasound, ophthalmologic examination, and hearing test (auditory brainstem response). If >1 day of therapy is missed, the entire course is restarted.
– Normal physical examination, serum quantitative nontreponemal serologic titer ≤maternal titer and maternal treatment was (1) none, inadequate, or undocumented; (2) erythromycin, azithromycin, or other non-penicillin regimen; or (3) <4 wk before delivery	Evaluation abnormal or not done completely: aqueous penicillin G 50,000 U/kg/dose q12h (day of life 1–7), q8h (>7 days) IV OR procaine penicillin G 50,000 U/kg IM q24h for 10 days (AII) Evaluation normal: aqueous penicillin G 50,000 U/kg/dose q12h (day of life 1–7), q8h (>7 days) IV OR procaine penicillin G 50,000 U/kg IM q24h for 10 days; OR benzathine penicillin G 50,000 units/kg/dose IM in a single dose (AIII)	Evaluation: CSF analysis, CBC with platelets, long-bone radiographs. If >1 day of therapy is missed, the entire course is restarted. Reliable follow-up important if only a single dose of benzathine penicillin given.

– Normal physical examination, serum quantitative non-treponemal serologic titer ≤maternal titer: mother treated adequately during pregnancy and >4 wk before delivery; no evidence of reinfection or relapse in mother	Benzathine penicillin G 50,000 units/kg/dose IM in a single dose (AIII)	No evaluation required. Some experts would not treat but provide close serologic follow-up.
– Normal physical examination, serum quantitative non-treponemal serologic titer ≤maternal titer, and the mother's treatment was adequate before pregnancy	No treatment	No evaluation required. Some experts would treat with benzathine penicillin G 50,000 units/kg as a single IM injection, particularly if follow-up is uncertain.
Syphilis, congenital (>1 mo of age)[88]	Aqueous crystalline penicillin G 200,000–300,000 units/kg/day IV div q4–6h for 10 days (All)	Evaluation to determine type and duration of therapy: CSF analysis (VDRL, cell count, protein), CBC and platelet count. Other tests as clinically indicated, including long-bone radiographs, chest radiographs, liver function tests, neuroimaging, ophthalmologic examination, and hearing evaluation. If no clinical manifestations of disease, the CSF examination is normal, and the CSF VDRL test result is nonreactive, some specialists would treat with up to 3 weekly doses of benzathine penicillin G, 50,000 U/kg IM. Some experts would provide a single dose of benzathine penicillin G, 50,000 U/kg IM after the 10 days of parenteral treatment, but the value of this additional therapy is not well documented.
Tetanus neonatorum[89]	Metronidazole IV/PO (alternative: penicillin G [IV] for 10–14 days (AIII) Human TIG 3,000–6,000 U IM for 1 dose (AIII)	Wound cleaning and debridement vital; IVIG (200–400 mg/kg) is an alternative if TIG not available; equine tetanus antitoxin not available in the United States but is alternative to TIG.

A. RECOMMENDED THERAPY FOR SELECTED NEWBORN CONDITIONS (cont)

Condition	Therapy (evidence grade) See Table 5B for Neonatal Dosages	Comments
Toxoplasmosis, congenital[90,91]	Sulfadiazine 100 mg/kg/day PO div q12H AND pyrimethamine 2 mg/kg PO daily for 2 days (loading dose), then 1 mg/kg PO q24H for 2–6 mo, then 3 times weekly (M-W-F) up to 1 y (AII) Folinic acid (leukovorin) 10 mg 3 times weekly (AII)	Corticosteroids (1 mg/kg/day div q12h) if active chorioretinitis or CSF protein >1 g/dL (AIII). Start sulfa after neonatal jaundice has resolved. Therapy is only effective against active trophozoites, not cysts.
Urinary tract infection[92]	Initial empiric therapy with ampicillin AND gentamicin; OR ampicillin AND cefotaxime pending culture and susceptibility test results for 7–10 days	Investigate for kidney disease and for abnormalities of urinary tract: VCUG indicated if renal ultrasound abnormal or after 1st UTI. Oral therapy acceptable once infant asymptomatic and culture sterile. No prophylaxis for grades 1–3 reflux.
– Coliform bacteria (eg, E coli, Klebsiella, Enterobacter, Serratia)	Cefotaxime IV, IM OR, in the absence of renal or perinephric abscess, gentamicin IV, IM for 7–10 days (AII)	Ampicillin used for susceptible organisms
– Enterococcus	Ampicillin IV, IM for 7 days for cystitis, may need 10–14 days for pyelonephritis; add gentamicin until cultures are sterile (AIII); for ampicillin resistance, use vancomycin, add gentamicin until cultures are sterile.	Aminoglycoside needed with ampicillin or vancomycin for bactericidal activity (assuming organisms susceptible to an aminoglycoside)
– P aeruginosa	Ceftazidime IV, IM OR, in the absence of renal or perinephric abscess, tobramycin IV, IM for 7–10 days (AIII)	Meropenem or cefepime are alternatives.
– Candida spp[30–32]	AmB-D IV OR fluconazole (if susceptible) (AII)	Because neonatal Candida disease is often systemic with isolated Candida UTI less likely to occur, and given that AmB lipid formulations are similarly effective and less toxic than AmB-D, they are preferred. However, the AmB lipid formulations theoretically have less penetration into the renal system compared with AmB-D. Evaluate for other sites in high-risk neonates: CSF analysis; cardiac ECHO; abdominal ultrasound to include kidneys, bladder; eye examination. Other triazoles are alternatives. Echinocandins are not renally eliminated and should not be used to treat neonatal UTI.

B. ANTIMICROBIAL DOSAGES FOR NEONATES

Lead author Jason Sauberan, assisted by the Editors and by John van den Anker

NOTE: This table contains empiric dosage recommendations for each agent listed. Please see Table A (Recommended Therapy for Selected Newborn Conditions) in this chapter for more precise details of optimal dosages for specific pathogens, in specific tissue sites. Given the complexities of maturing organ function and drug elimination during the first few months of life, together with the wide variation in "compartments" for drug diffusion from very premature infants to term infants over the first months of life, these dosing recommendations represent our best estimates, but each infant should be independently evaluated for the appropriate dose. See also Table A for information on anti-influenza and antiretroviral drug dosages.

Antibiotic	Route	Chronologic Age ≤28 days				Chronologic Age 29–60 days
		Body Weight ≤2,000 g		Body Weight >2,000 g		
		0–7 days old	8–28 days old[a]	0–7 days old	8–28 days old	
Acyclovir	IV	40 div q12h	60 div q8h	60 div q8h	60 div q8h	60 div q8h
	PO[b]	-	900/m² div q8h	-	900/m² div q8h	900/m² div q8h
Amoxicillin/clavulanate	PO	-	-	30 div q12h	30 div q12h	30 div q12h
Amphotericin B						
– deoxycholate	IV	1 q24h	1 q24h	1 q24h	1 q24h	1 q24h
– lipid complex	IV	5 q24h	5 q24h	5 q24h	5 q24h	5 q24h
– liposomal	IV	5 q24h	5 q24h	5 q24h	5 q24h	5 q24h
Ampicillin[c]	IV, IM	100 div q12h	150 div q8h	150 div q8h	200 div q6h	200 div q6h
Anidulafungin[d]	IV	1.5 q24h[d]	1.5 q24h[d]	1.5 q24h[d]	1.5 q24h[d]	1.5 q24h[d]
Azithromycin[e]	PO	10 q24h	10 q24h	10 q24h	10 q24h	10 q24h
	IV	10 q24h	10 q24h	10 q24h	10 q24h	10 q24h
Aztreonam	IV, IM	60 div q12h	90 div q8h	60 div q12h	90 div q8h	120 div q6h

B. ANTIMICROBIAL DOSAGES FOR NEONATES (cont)

		Dosages (mg/kg/day) and Intervals of Administration				
		Chronologic Age ≤28 days				Chronologic Age 29–60 days
		Body Weight ≤2,000 g		Body Weight >2,000 g		
Antibiotic	Route	0–7 days old	8–28 days old[a]	0–7 days old	8–28 days old	
Caspofungin[f]	IV	25/m² q24h	25/m² q24h	25/m² q24h	25/m² q24h	25/m² q24h
Cefazolin	IV, IM	50 div q12h	50 div q12h	50 div q12h	75 div q8h	75 div q8h
Cefepime[g]	IV, IM	100 div q12h	150 div q8h	150 div q8h	150 div q8h	150 div q8h
Cefotaxime	IV, IM	100 div q12h	150 div q8h	100 div q12h	150 div q8h	200 div q6h
Cefoxitin	IV, IM	70 div q12h	100 div q8h	100 div q8h	100 div q8h	120 div q6h
Ceftazidime	IV, IM	100 div q12h	150 div q8h	100 div q12h	150 div q8h	150 div q8h
Ceftriaxone[h]	IV, IM	–	–	50 q24h	50 q24h	50 q24h
Cefuroxime	IV, IM	100 div q12h	150 div q8h	100 div q12h	150 div q8h	150 div q8h
Chloramphenicol[i]	IV, IM	25 q24h	50 div q12h	25 q24h	50 div q12h	50–100 div q6h
Clindamycin	IV, IM, PO	10 div q12h	15 div q8h	15 div q8h	20 div q6h	30 div q6h
Daptomycin	IV	12 div q12h	12 div q12h	12 div q12h	12 div q12h	12 div q12h
Erythromycin	PO	20 div q12h	30 div q8h	20 div q12h	30 div q8h	40 div q6h
Fluconazole						
– treatment (start with initial loading dose)[j]	IV, PO	12 q24h[i]	12 q24h[i]	12 q24h[i]	12 q24h[i]	12 q24h[i]
– prophylaxis	IV, PO	6 mg/kg/dose twice wkly	6 mg/kg/dose twice wkly	6 mg/kg/dose twice wkly	6 mg/kg/dose twice wkly	6 mg/kg/dose twice wkly

Drug	Route					
Flucytosine[k]	PO	75 div q8h	75 div q6h	75 div q6h	75 div q6h	75 div q6h
Ganciclovir	IV	See text: CMV	See text: CMV	12 div q12h	12 div q12h	12 div q12h
Linezolid	IV, PO	20 div q12h	30 div q8h	30 div q8h	30 div q8h	30 div q8h
Meropenem						
– sepsis[l]	IV	40 div q12h[l]	60 div q8h[l]	60 div q8h[l]	90 div q8h[l]	90 div q8h
– meningitis	IV	120 div q8h	120 div q8h	120 div q8h	120 div q8h	120 div q8h
Metronidazole (start with initial loading dose)[m]	IV, PO	15 div q12h	see footnote[m]	22.5 div q8h	30 div q6h	30 div q6h
Micafungin	IV	10 q24h	10 q24h	10 q24h	10 q24h	10 q24h
Nafcillin,[n] oxacillin[n]	IV, IM	50 div q12h	75 div q8h	75 div q8h	100 div q6h	150 div q6h
Penicillin G benzathine	IM	50,000 U	50,000 U	50,000 U	50,000 U	50,000 U
Penicillin G crystalline (GBS meningitis)	IV	200,000 U div q12h	300,000 U div q8h	300,000 U div q8h	400,000 U div q6h	400,000 U div q6h
Penicillin G crystalline (congenital syphilis)	IV	100,000 U div q12h	150,000 U div q8h	100,000 U div q12h	150,000 U div q8h	200,000 U div q6h
Penicillin G procaine	IM	50,000 U q24h	50,000 U q24h	50,000 U q24h	50,000 U q24h	50,000 U q24h
Piperacillin/tazobactam	IV	240 div q8h	240 div q8h	240 div q8h	320 div q6h	400 div q6h

B. ANTIMICROBIAL DOSAGES FOR NEONATES (cont)

Antibiotic	Route	Dosages (mg/kg/day) and Intervals of Administration				Chronologic Age 29–60 days
		Chronologic Age ≤28 days				
		Body Weight ≤2,000 g		Body Weight >2,000 g		
		0–7 days old	8–28 days old[a]	0–7 days old	8–28 days old	
Rifampin	IV, PO	10 q24h	10 q24h	10 q24h	10 q24h	10 q24h
Ticarcillin/clavulanate	IV	150 div q12h	225 div q8h	150 div q12h	225 div q8h	300 div q6h
Valganciclovir	PO	insufficient data	insufficient data	32 div q12h	32 div q12h	32 div q12h
Voriconazole	IV, PO	16 div q12h	16 div q12h	16 div q12h	16 div q12h	16 div q12h
Zidovudine	IV	3 div q12h[o]	3 div q12h[o]	6 div q12h	6 div q12h	See text: HIV
Zidovudine	PO	4 div q12h[o]	4 div q12h[o]	8 div q12h	8 div q12h	See text: HIV

[a] Use 0–7 days of age frequency until 14 days of age if birth weight <1,000 g.
[b] Oral suppression therapy for 6 months after initial neonatal HSV treatment. Dosing units are mg/m²/day.
[c] 300 mg/kg/day for GBS meningitis; div q8h for all neonates ≤7 days of age and q6h >7 days of age.
[d] Loading dose 3 mg/kg followed 24 hours later by maintenance dose listed.
[e] Azithromycin oral dose for pertussis should be 10 mg/kg once daily for the entire 5-day treatment course, while for other upper respiratory tract infections, 10 mg/kg is given on the first day, followed by 5 mg/kg once daily for 4 days. For CNS disease, 10 mg/kg once daily for entire course.
[f] Dosing units are mg/m². Higher dosage of 50 mg/m² may be needed for Aspergillus.
[g] Doses listed are for meningitis or Pseudomonas infections. Can give 60 mg/kg/day div q12h for treatment of non-CNS infections caused by enteric bacilli (eg, E coli, Klebsiella, Enterobacter, Serratia) as they are more susceptible to cefepime than Pseudomonas.
[h] Usually avoided in neonates. Can be considered for transitioning to outpatient treatment of GBS bacteremia in well-appearing neonates at low risk for hyperbilirubinemia.
[i] Desired serum concentration 15–25 mg/mL.
[j] Loading dose 25 mg/kg followed 24 hours later by maintenance dose listed.
[k] Desired serum concentrations peak 50–100 mg/L, trough 25–50 mg/L.
[l] Adjust dosage after 14 days of age instead of after 7 days of age.
[m] Loading dose 15 mg/kg. Maintenance dosage for PMA <34 weeks, 15 mg/kg/day div q12h; for 34–40 weeks, 22.5 mg/kg/day div q8h.
[n] Increase to 50 mg/kg/dose for meningitis.
[o] Starting dose if GA <35–0 wk and PNA ≤14 days. See Table A HIV for zidovudine dosage after 2 weeks of age.

C. AMINOGLYCOSIDES

Empiric Dosage (mg/kg/dose) by Gestational and Postnatal Age

Medication	Route	<32 wk		32–36 wk		≥37 wk (term)	
		0–14 days	>14 days	0–7 days	>7 days[a]	0–7 days	>7 days[a]
Amikacin[b]	IV, IM	15 q48h	15 q24h	15 q24h	15 q24h	15 q24h	17.5 q24h
Gentamicin[c]	IV, IM	5 q48h	5 q36h	4 q36h	4 q24h	4 q24h	4 q24h
Tobramycin[c]	IV, IM	5 q48h	5 q36h	4 q36h	4 q24h	4 q24h	4 q24h

[a] At >60 days of age can consider amikacin 15–20 mg/kg q24h and gentamicin/tobramycin 4.5–7.5 mg/kg q24h (see Chapter 11).
[b] Desired serum concentrations: 20–30 mg/L (peak), <5 mg/L (trough).
[c] Desired serum concentrations: 5–10 mg/L (peak), <2 mg/L (trough).

D. VANCOMYCIN[a]

Empiric Dosage[b,c] (mg/kg/dose) by Gestational Age and Serum Creatinine

Serum Creatinine	≤28 wk		>28 wk		
	Dose	Frequency	Serum Creatinine	Dose	Frequency
<0.5	15	q12h	<0.7	15	q12h
0.5–0.7	20	q24h	0.7–0.9	20	q24h
0.8–1	15	q24h	1–1.2	15	q24h
1.1–1.4	10	q24h	1.3–1.6	10	q24h
>1.4	15	q48h	>1.6	15	q48h

[a] Serum creatinine concentrations normally fluctuate and are partly influenced by transplacental maternal creatinine in the first week of age. Cautious use of the creatinine-based dosing strategy with frequent reassessment of renal function and vancomycin serum concentrations are recommended in neonates ≤5 days old.
[b] Up through 60 days of age. Can consider 45–60 mg/kg/day div q6-8h if >60 days of age (see Chapter 11).
[c] Desired serum concentrations vary by pathogen, site of infection, degree of illness: For MRSA and MSSA, aim for a target based on AUC/MIC of ~400. Lower targets are likely to be as effective for coagulase negative staphylococci, based on experience with dosing to obtain peaks of 20–40 mg/L (1 h post-infusion), and troughs of 5–15 mg/L.

5

Antimicrobial Therapy for Newborns

E. Use of Antimicrobials During Pregnancy or Breastfeeding

The use of antimicrobials during pregnancy should be balanced by the risk of fetal toxicity, including anatomical anomalies. A number of factors determine the degree of transfer of antibiotics across the placenta: lipid solubility, degree of ionization, molecular weight, protein binding, placental maturation, and placental and fetal blood flow. The FDA provides 5 categories to indicate the level of risk to the fetus: (1) Category A: fetal harm seems remote since controlled studies have not demonstrated a risk to the fetus; (2) Category B: animal reproduction studies have not shown a fetal risk but no controlled studies in pregnant women have been done, or animal studies have shown an adverse effect that has not been confirmed in human studies (penicillin, amoxicillin, ampicillin, cephalexin/cefazolin, azithromycin, clindamycin, vancomycin, zanamivir); (3) Category C: studies in animals have shown an adverse effect on the fetus but there are no studies in women and no animal data are available; the potential benefit of the drug may justify the possible risk to the fetus (chloramphenicol, ciprofloxacin, gentamicin, levofloxacin, oseltamivir, rifampin); (4) Category D: evidence exists of human fetal risk but the benefits may outweigh such risk (doxycycline); (5) Category X: The drug is contraindicated since animal or human studies have shown fetal abnormalities or fetal risk (ribavirin).

Fetal serum concentrations of the following commonly used drugs are equal to, or only slightly less than, those in the mother: penicillin G, amoxicillin, ampicillin, sulfonamides, trimethoprim, tetracyclines, and nitrofurantoin. The aminoglycoside concentrations in fetal serum are 20% to 50% of those in maternal serum. Cephalosporins, nafcillin, oxacillin, and clindamycin penetrate poorly (10%–15%), and fetal concentrations of erythromycin and azithromycin are less than 10% of those in the mother.

The most current, updated information on the safety of antimicrobials and other agents in human milk can be found at the National Library of Medicine LactMed Web site (www.toxnet.nlm.nih.gov/cgi-bin/sis/htmlgen?LACT, accessed November 11, 2013).[93]

In general, neonatal exposure to antimicrobials in human milk is minimal or insignificant. Aminoglycosides, β-lactams, ciprofloxacin, clindamycin, macrolides, fluconazole, and agents for tuberculosis are considered safe for the mother to take during breastfeeding.[94] The most common reported neonatal side effect of maternal antimicrobial use during breastfeeding is increased stool output. Clinicians should recommend mothers alert their pediatric provider if stool output changes occur. Maternal treatment with sulfa-containing antibiotics should be approached with caution in the breastfed infant who is jaundiced or ill.

6. Antimicrobial Therapy According to Clinical Syndromes

NOTES

- This chapter should be considered a rough guideline for a typical patient. Dosage recommendations are for patients with relatively normal hydration, renal function, and hepatic function. See Chapter 13 for information on patients with impaired renal function. Higher dosages may be necessary if the antibiotic does not penetrate well into the infected tissue (eg, meningitis) or if the child is immunocompromised.

- Duration of treatment should be individualized. Those recommended are based on the literature, common practice, and general experience. Critical evaluations of duration of therapy have been carried out in very few infectious diseases. In general, a longer duration of therapy should be used (1) for tissues in which antibiotic concentrations may be relatively low (eg, undrained abscess, central nervous system [CNS] infection); (2) for tissues in which repair following infection-mediated damage is slow (eg, bone); (3) when the organisms are less susceptible; (4) when a relapse of infection is unacceptable (eg, CNS infections); or (5) when the host is immunocompromised in some way. An assessment after therapy will ensure that your selection of antibiotic, dose, and duration of therapy was appropriate.

- Diseases in this chapter are arranged by body systems. Consult the index for the alphabetized listing of diseases and chapters 7 through 10 for the alphabetized listing of pathogens and for uncommon organisms not included in this chapter.

- **Abbreviations:** ADH, antidiuretic hormone; AFB, acid-fast bacilli; amox/clav, amoxicillin/clavulanate; amp/sulbactam, ampicillin/sulbactam; AOM, acute otitis media; AST, aspartate transaminase; ALT, alanine transaminase; bid, twice daily; CA-MRSA, community-associated methicillin-resistant *Staphylococcus aureus;* CDC, Centers for Disease Control and Prevention; CMV, cytomegalovirus; CNS, central nervous system; CSD, cat-scratch disease; CSF, cerebrospinal fluid; CT, computed tomography; div, divided; DOT, directly observed therapy; EBV, Epstein-Barr virus; ESBL, extended spectrum beta-lactamase; ESR, erythrocyte sedimentation rate; FDA, US Food and Drug Administration; GI, gastrointestinal; HIV, human immunodeficiency virus; HSV, herpes simplex virus; HUS, hemolytic uremic syndrome; I&D, incision and drainage; IDSA, Infectious Diseases Society of America; IM, intramuscular; INH, isoniazid; IV, intravenous; IVIG, intravenous immune globulin; LFT, liver function test; LP, lumbar puncture; MRSE, methicillin-resistant *Staphylococcus epidermidis;* MSSA, methicillin-susceptible *S aureus;* MSSE, methicillin-sensitive *S epidermidis;* NIH, National Institutes of Health; ophth, ophthalmic; PCV7, Prevnar 7-valent pneumococcal conjugate vaccine; PCV13, Prevnar 13-valent pneumococcal conjugate vaccine; pen-R, penicillin-resistant; pen-S, penicillin-susceptible; pip/tazo, piperacillin/tazobactam; PO, oral; PPD, purified protein derivative; PZA, pyrazinamide; qd, once daily; qid, 4 times daily; qod, every other day; RSV, respiratory syncytial virus; SPAG-2, small particle aerosol generator-2; STI, sexually transmitted infection; soln, solution; ticar/clav, ticarcillin/clavulanate; tid, 3 times daily; TB, tuberculosis; TMP/SMX, trimethoprim/sulfamethoxazole; ULN, upper limit of normal; USP-NF, US Pharmacopeia–National Formulary; UTI, urinary tract infection; VDRL, Venereal Disease Research Laboratories; WBC, white blood cell.

A. SKIN AND SOFT TISSUE INFECTIONS

Clinical Diagnosis	Therapy (evidence grade)	Comments
NOTE: CA-MRSA (see Chapter 4 on CA-MRSA) is increasingly prevalent in most areas of the world. Recommendations below are given for 2 scenarios, "standard" and "CA-MRSA." Antibiotic recommendations for CA-MRSA should be used for empiric therapy in regions with greater than 5% to 10% of serious staphylococcal infections caused by MRSA, in situations where CA-MRSA is suspected, and for documented CA-MRSA infections, while "standard" recommendations refer to treatment of MSSA. During the past few years, clindamycin resistance in MRSA has increased to 40% in some areas but remained stable at 5% in others. Please check your local susceptibility data for *S aureus* before using clindamycin for empiric therapy. For MSSA, oxacillin/nafcillin are considered equivalent agents.		
Adenitis, acute bacterial[1–7] (*S aureus*, including CA-MRSA, and group A streptococcus; consider *Bartonella* [cat-scratch disease] for subacute adenitis)[8]	Empiric therapy: Standard: oxacillin/nafcillin 150 mg/kg/day IV div q6h OR cefazolin 100 mg/kg/day IV div q8h (AI), OR cephalexin 50–75 mg/kg/day PO div tid CA-MRSA: clindamycin 30 mg/kg/day IV or PO div q8h OR vancomycin 40 mg/kg/day IV q8h (BII) CSD: azithromycin 12 mg/kg once daily (max 500 mg) for 5 days (BIII)	May need surgical drainage for staph/strep infection; not usually needed for CSD. For oral therapy for MSSA: cephalexin or cloxacillin; for CA-MRSA: clindamycin, TMP/SMX, or linezolid. For oral therapy of group A strep: amoxicillin or penicillin V. Total IV plus PO therapy for 7–10 days. For CSD: this is the same high dose that is recommended for strep pharyngitis.
Adenitis, nontuberculous (atypical) mycobacterial[9–12]	Excision usually curative (BII); azithromycin PO OR clarithromycin PO for 6–12 wk (with or without rifampin) if susceptible (BII)	Antibiotic susceptibility patterns are quite variable; cultures should guide therapy; medical therapy 60%–70% effective. Newer data suggest toxicity of antimicrobials may not be worth the small clinical benefit.
Adenitis, tuberculous[13,14] (*M tuberculosis* and *M bovis*)	Isoniazid 10–15 mg/kg/day (max 300 mg) PO qd, IV for 6 mo AND rifampin 10–20 mg/kg/day (max 600 mg) PO qd, IV for 6 mo AND PZA 20–40 mg/kg/day PO qd for first 2 mo therapy (BII); if suspected multidrug resistance, add ethambutol 20 mg/kg/day PO qd	Surgical excision usually not indicated as organisms are treatable. Adenitis caused by *Mycobacterium bovis* (unpasteurized dairy product ingestion) is uniformly resistant to PZA. Treat 9–12 mo with isoniazid and rifampin (BII).
Anthrax, cutaneous[15]	Empiric therapy: ciprofloxacin 20–30 mg/kg/day PO div bid OR doxycycline 4 mg/kg/day (max 200 mg) PO div bid (regardless of age) (AIII)	If susceptible, amoxicillin or clindamycin (BII). Ciprofloxacin and levofloxacin are FDA approved for inhalation anthrax (BII).

Condition	Therapy	Comments
Bites, animal and human[1,16-19] *Pasteurella multocida* (animal), *Eikenella corrodens* (human), *Staphylococcus* spp and *Streptococcus* spp	Amox/clav 45 mg/kg/day PO div tid (amox/clav 7:1; see Chapter 1, Aminopenicillins) for 5–10 days (AII); for hospitalized children, use ticar/clav 200 mg ticarcillin/kg/day div q6h OR ampicillin and clindamycin (BIII). For penicillin allergy, ciprofloxacin (for *Pasteurella*) plus clindamycin (BIII).	Consider rabies prophylaxis[20] for bites from at-risk animals (observe animal for 10 days, if possible) (AI); consider tetanus prophylaxis. Human bites have a very high rate of infection (do not close open wounds). *S aureus* coverage is only fair with amox/clav, ticar/clav, pip/tazo. For penicillin allergy, ciprofloxacin (for *Pasteurella*) plus clindamycin (BIII).
Bullous impetigo[1–3,5–7] (usually *S aureus*, including CA-MRSA)	Standard: cephalexin 50–75 mg/kg/day PO div tid OR amox/clav 45 mg/kg/day PO div tid (CII) CA-MRSA: clindamycin 30 mg/kg/day PO div tid OR TMP/SMX 8 mg/kg/day of TMP PO div bid; for 5–7 days (CIII)	For topical therapy if mild infection: mupirocin or retapamulin ointment
Cellulitis of unknown etiology (usually *S aureus*, including CA-MRSA, or group A streptococcus)[1–7,21]	Empiric IV therapy: Standard: oxacillin/nafcillin 150 mg/kg/day IV div q6h OR cefazolin 100 mg/kg/day IV div q8h (BII) CA-MRSA: clindamycin 30 mg/kg/day IV div q8h OR vancomycin 40 mg/kg/day IV q8h (BII) For oral therapy for MSSA: cephalexin (AII) OR amox/clav 45 mg/kg/day PO div tid (BII); for CA-MRSA: clindamycin (BII), TMP/SMX (CIII), or linezolid (BII)	For periorbital or buccal cellulitis, also consider *Streptococcus pneumoniae* or *Haemophilus influenzae* type b in unimmunized infants. Total IV plus PO therapy for 7–10 days.
Cellulitis, buccal (for unimmunized infants and preschool-aged children, *H influenzae* type b)[22]	Cefotaxime 100–150 mg/kg/day IV div q8h OR ceftriaxone 50 mg/kg/day (AI) IV, IM q24h; for 2–7 days parenteral therapy before switch to oral (BII)	Rule out meningitis (larger dosages may be needed). For penicillin allergy, levofloxacin IV/PO covers pathogens, but no clinical data available; safer than chloramphenicol. Oral therapy: amoxicillin if beta-lactamase negative; amox/clav or oral 2nd- or 3rd-generation cephalosporin if beta-lactamase positive.
Cellulitis, erysipelas (streptococcal)[1,2,7]	Penicillin G 100,000–200,000 U/kg/day IV div q4–6h (BII) initially then penicillin V 100 mg/kg/day PO div qid or tid OR amoxicillin 50 mg/kg/day PO div tid for 10 days	These dosages may be unnecessarily large, but there is little clinical experience with smaller dosages.
Gas gangrene (see Necrotizing fasciitis)		

A. SKIN AND SOFT TISSUE INFECTIONS (cont)

Clinical Diagnosis	Therapy (evidence grade)	Comments
Impetigo (*S aureus*, including CA-MRSA; occasionally group A streptococcus)[1,2,6,7,23,24]	Mupirocin OR retapamulin topically (BII) to lesions tid; OR for more extensive lesions, oral therapy: Standard: cephalexin 50–75 mg/kg/day PO div tid OR amox/clav 45 mg/kg/day PO div tid (AII) CA-MRSA: clindamycin 30 mg/kg/day (CII) PO div tid OR TMP/SMX 8 mg/kg/day of TMP PO div bid (CIII); for 5–7 days	Cleanse infected area with soap and water; bathe daily.
Ludwig angina[25]	Penicillin G 200,000–250,000 U/kg/day IV div q6h AND clindamycin 40 mg/kg/day IV div q8h (CIII)	Alternatives: meropenem, imipenem, ticar/clav, pip/tazo if gram-negative aerobic bacilli also suspected (CIII); high risk of respiratory tract obstruction from inflammatory edema
Lymphadenitis (see Adenitis, acute bacterial)		
Lymphangitis, blistering dactylitis (group A streptococcus)[1,2,7]	Penicillin G 200,000 U/kg/day IV div q6h (BII) initially then penicillin V 100 mg/kg/day PO div qid OR amoxicillin 50 mg/kg/day PO div tid for 10 days	For mild disease, penicillin V 50 mg/kg/day PO div qid for 10 days
Myositis, suppurative[26] (*S aureus*, including CA-MRSA; synonyms: tropical myositis, pyomyositis)	Standard: oxacillin/nafcillin 150 mg/kg/day IV div q6h OR cefazolin 100 mg/kg/day IV div q8h (CII) CA-MRSA: clindamycin 40 mg/kg/day IV div q8h OR vancomycin 40 mg/kg/day IV q8h (CIII)	Aggressive, emergent debridement; consider IVIG to bind bacterial toxins for life-threatening disease; use clindamycin to help decrease toxin production; abscesses may develop with CA-MRSA while on therapy.

Necrotizing fasciitis (pathogens vary, depending on the age of the child and location of infection: Single pathogen: group A streptococcus; *S aureus* [including CA-MRSA], *Pseudomonas aeruginosa*, *Vibrio* spp, *Aeromonas*; multiple pathogen, mixed aerobic/anaerobic synergistic fasciitis: any organism[s] above, plus gram-negative bacilli, plus *Bacteroides* spp, and other anaerobes)[1,27,28,29,30]	Empiric therapy: ceftazidime 150 mg/kg/day IV div q8h, or cefepime 150 mg/kg/day IV div q8h or cefotaxime 200 mg/kg/day IV div q6h AND clindamycin 40 mg/kg/day IV div q8h (BIII); OR meropenem 60 mg/kg/day IV div q8h; OR pip/tazo 400 mg/kg/day pip component IV div q6h (AIII) ADD vancomycin for suspect CA-MRSA, pending culture results (AIII) Group A streptococcal: penicillin G 200,000–250,000 U/kg/day div q6h AND clindamycin 40 mg/kg/day div q8h (AIII) Mixed aerobic/anaerobic/gram-negative: meropenem or pip/tazo AND clindamycin (AIII)	Aggressive emergent wound debridement (AII). Add clindamycin to inhibit synthesis of toxins at the ribosomal level (AIII). If CA-MRSA identified and susceptible to clindamycin, additional vancomycin is not required. Consider IVIG to bind bacterial toxins for life-threatening disease (BIII). Value of hyperbaric oxygen is not established (CIII). Focus definitive antimicrobial therapy based on culture results.
Pyoderma, cutaneous abscesses (*S aureus*, including CA-MRSA; group A streptococcus)[2,5–7,31–33]	Standard: cephalexin 50–75 mg/kg/day PO div tid OR amox/clav 45 mg/kg/day PO div tid (BII) CA-MRSA: clindamycin 30 mg/kg/day PO div tid (BII) OR TMP/SMX 8 mg/kg/day of TMP PO div bid (CIII)	I&D when indicated; IV for serious infections. For prevention of recurrent CA-MRSA infection, use bleach baths daily (½ cup of bleach per full bathtub) (BII), OR bathe with chlorhexidine soap daily, or qod. Decolonization with mupirocin may also be helpful.
Rat-bite fever (*Streptobacillus moniliformis*, *Spirillum minus*)[34]	Penicillin G 100,000–200,000 U/kg/day IV div q6h (BII) for 7–10 days; for endocarditis, ADD gentamicin for 4–6 wk (CIII) For mild disease, oral therapy with amox/clav (CIII)	Organisms are normal oral flora for rodents. High rate of associated endocarditis. Alternatives: doxycycline; 2nd- and 3rd-generation cephalosporins (CIII).
Staphylococcal scalded skin syndrome[6,35]	Standard: oxacillin 150 mg/kg/day IV div q6h OR cefazolin 100 mg/kg/day IV div q8h (CII) CA-MRSA: clindamycin 30 mg/kg/day IV div q8h (CIII) OR vancomycin 40 mg/kg/day IV q8h (CIII)	Burow or Zephiran compresses for oozing skin and intertriginous areas. Corticosteroids are contraindicated.

B. SKELETAL INFECTIONS

Clinical Diagnosis	Therapy (evidence grade)	Comments
NOTE: CA-MRSA (see Chapter 4 on CA-MRSA) is increasingly prevalent in most areas of the world. Recommendations below are given for CA-MRSA and MSSA. Antibiotic recommendations for empiric therapy should include CA-MRSA when it is suspected or documented, while treatment for MSSA with beta-lactam antibiotics (like cephalexin) is preferred over clindamycin. During the past 2 years, clindamycin resistance in MRSA has increased to 40% in some areas but remained stable at 5% in others. Please check your local susceptibility data for S aureus before using clindamycin for empiric therapy. For MSSA, oxacillin/nafcillin and cefazolin are considered equivalent agents.		
Arthritis, bacterial[36–40]	Switch to appropriate high-dose oral therapy when clinically improved, CRP decreasing (see Chapter 15).[41]	
– Newborns	See Chapter 5.	
– Infants (S aureus, including CA-MRSA; group A streptococcus; Kingella kingae; in unimmunized or immunocompromised children: pneumococcus, H influenzae type b)	Empiric therapy: clindamycin (to cover CA-MRSA unless clindamycin resistance locally is >10%, then use vancomycin) For serious infections, ADD cefazolin to provide better MSSA coverage and add Kingella coverage For CA-MRSA: clindamycin 30 mg/kg/day IV div q8h OR vancomycin 40 mg/kg/day IV q8h For MSSA: oxacillin/nafcillin 150 mg/kg/day IV div q6h OR cefazolin 100 mg/kg/day IV div q8h	Oral therapy options: For CA-MRSA: clindamycin OR linezolid.[40] For MSSA: cephalexin OR cloxacillin caps for older children. For Kingella, most penicillins or cephalosporins (but not clindamycin). Total therapy (IV plus PO) for 3 wk with normal ESR; low-risk, non-hip MSSA arthritis may respond to a 10-day course.[37,38]
– Children (S aureus, including CA-MRSA; group A streptococcus; K kingae)	For Kingella: cefazolin 100 mg/kg/day IV div q8h OR ampicillin 150 mg/kg/day IV div q6h, OR ceftriaxone 50 mg/kg/day IV, IM q24h For pen-S pneumococci or group A streptococcus: penicillin G 200,000 U/kg/day IV div q6h For pen-R pneumococci or Haemophilus: ceftriaxone 50–75 mg/kg/day IV, IM q24h, OR cefotaxime (BII)	
– Gonococcal arthritis or tenosynovitis[42,43]	Ceftriaxone 50 mg/kg IV, IM q24h (BII); for 7 days	Cefixime 8 mg/kg/day PO as a single daily dose has not yet been studied in children but is recommended as step-down therapy in adults, to complete a 7-day treatment course.
– Other bacteria	See Chapter 7 for preferred antibiotics.	

Osteomyelitis[36,39,40,44–49]	Step down to appropriate high-dose oral therapy when clinically improved (See Chapter 15.)[40,47]
– Newborn	See Chapter 5.
– Infants and children, acute infection (usually S aureus, including CA-MRSA; group A streptococcus; K kingae)	Empiric therapy: clindamycin. For serious infections, ADD cefazolin to provide better MSSA coverage and add Kingella coverage (CIII). For CA-MRSA: clindamycin 30 mg/kg/day IV div q8h or vancomycin 40 mg/kg/day IV q8h (BII). For MSSA: oxacillin/nafcillin 150 mg/kg/day IV div q6h OR cefazolin 100 mg/kg/day IV div q8h (AII). For Kingella: cefazolin 100 mg/kg/day IV div q8h OR ampicillin 150 mg/kg/day IV div q6h, OR ceftriaxone 50 mg/kg/day IV, IM q24h (BIII). Total therapy (IV plus PO) usually 4–6 wk (with end-of-therapy normal ESR, x-ray to document healing) for MSSA. May need longer for CA-MRSA (BII). Follow closely for clinical response to empiric therapy. In children with open fractures secondary to trauma, add ceftazidime for extended aerobic gram-negative activity. Kingella is often resistant to clindamycin. For MSSA (BI) and Kingella (BIII), step-down oral therapy with cephalexin 100 mg/kg/day PO tid. Oral step-down therapy alternatives for CA-MRSA include clindamycin and linezolid.[50]
– Acute, other organisms	See Chapter 7 for preferred antibiotics.
– Chronic (staphylococcal)[48]	For MSSA: cephalexin 100 mg/kg/day PO tid OR dicloxacillin caps 75–100 mg/kg/day PO div qid for 3–6 mo or longer (CIII) For CA-MRSA: clindamycin or linezolid (CIII)	Surgery to debride sequestrum is usually required for cure. For prosthetic joint infection caused by staphylococci, add rifampin (CIII). Watch for beta-lactam–associated neutropenia with high-dose, long-term therapy, and linezolid-associated neutropenia/thrombocytopenia with long-term (>2 wk) therapy.
Osteomyelitis of the foot[51] (osteochondritis after a puncture wound) P aeruginosa (occasionally S aureus, including CA-MRSA)	Ceftazidime 150 mg/kg/day IV, IM q8h AND tobramycin 6–7.5 mg/kg/day IM, IV div q8h (BIII); OR cefepime 150 mg/kg/day IV div q8h (BIII); OR meropenem 60 mg/kg/day IV div q8h (BIII); ADD vancomycin 40 mg/kg/day IV q8h for serious infection (for CA-MRSA), pending culture results	Thorough surgical debridement required (2nd drainage procedure needed in at least 20% of children); oral convalescent therapy with ciprofloxacin (BIII)[52] Treatment course 7–10 days after surgery

6

Antimicrobial Therapy According to Clinical Syndromes

C. EYE INFECTIONS

Clinical Diagnosis	Therapy (evidence grade)	Comments
Cellulitis, periorbital[57] (preseptal infection)		
– Associated with entry site lesion on skin (S aureus, including CA-MRSA, group A streptococcus)	Standard: oxacillin/nafcillin 150 mg/kg/day IV div q6h OR cefazolin 100 mg/kg/day IV div q8h (BII) CA-MRSA: clindamycin 30 mg/kg/day IV div q8h or vancomycin 40 mg/kg/day IV q8h (BIII)	Oral antistaphylococcal antibiotic for less severe infection; treatment course for 7–10 days
– Idiopathic (no entry site) in unimmunized infants: pneumococcal or H influenzae type b	Ceftriaxone 50 mg/kg/day q24h OR cefotaxime 100–150 mg/kg/day IV, IM div q8h OR cefuroxime 150 mg/kg/day IV div q8h (AII)	Treatment course for 7–10 days; rule out meningitis; alternative: other 2nd-, 3rd-, or 4th-generation cephalosporins or chloramphenicol
– Periorbital swelling (not true cellulitis), non-tender (usually associated with sinusitis), sinus pathogens rarely may erode anteriorly causing cellulitis	Ceftriaxone 50 mg/kg/day q24h OR cefotaxime 100–150 mg/kg/day IV, IM div q8h OR cefuroxime 150 mg/kg/day IV div q8h (BIII) ADD clindamycin 30 mg/kg/day IV div q8h for more severe infection with suspect S aureus including CA-MRSA or for chronic sinusitis (covers anaerobes (AIII)	For oral convalescent antibiotic therapy, see Sinusitis, acute; total treatment course of 14-21 days or 7 days after resolution of symptoms.
Conjunctivitis, acute (Haemophilus and pneumococcus predominantly)[58-60]	Polymyxin/trimethoprim ophth soln OR polymyxin/bacitracin ophth ointment OR ciprofloxacin ophth soln (BII), for 7–10 days. For neonatal infection, see Chapter 5. Steroid-containing therapy only if HSV ruled out.	Other topical antibiotics (gentamicin, tobramycin ophth soln erythromycin, besifloxacin, moxifloxacin, norfloxacin, ofloxacin, levofloxacin) may offer advantages for particular pathogens (CII). High rates of resistance to sulfacetamide.
Conjunctivitis, herpetic[61-63]	1% trifluridine, 0.1% iododeoxyuridine, or 0.15% ganciclovir ophthalmic gel (AII) AND Acyclovir PO (60–80 mg/kg/day div qid) has been effective in limited studies (BIII).	Refer to ophthalmologist. Recurrences common; corneal scars may form. Topical steroids for keratitis while using topical antiviral solution. Long-term prophylaxis for suppression of recurrent infection with oral acyclovir 300 mg/m²/dose PO TID (max 400 mg/dose) (little long-term safety data in children). Assess for neutropenia on long-term therapy; potential risks must balance potential benefits to vision (BII).

Condition	Therapy	Notes
Dacryocystitis	No antibiotic usually needed; oral therapy for more symptomatic infection, based on Gram stain and culture of pus; topical therapy as for conjunctivitis may be helpful.	Warm compresses; may require surgical probing of nasolacrimal duct
Endophthalmitis[64,65]	**NOTE:** Subconjunctival/subtenon antibiotics may be required (vancomycin/ceftazidime or clindamycin/gentamicin); steroids commonly used; requires anterior chamber and vitreous tap for microbiological diagnosis.	Refer to ophthalmologist; vitrectomy may be necessary for advanced endophthalmitis.
– Empiric therapy following open globe injury	Vancomycin 40 mg/kg/day IV div q8h AND ceftazidime 150 mg/kg/day IV div q8h (AIII)	
– Staphylococcal	Vancomycin 40 mg/kg/day IV div q8h pending susceptibility testing; oxacillin/nafcillin 150 mg/kg/day IV div q6h if susceptible (AIII)	
– Pneumococcal, meningococcal, Haemophilus	Ceftriaxone 100 mg/kg/day IV q24h; penicillin G 250,000 U/kg/day IV div q4h if susceptible (AIII)	Rule out meningitis; treatment course for 10–14 days
– Gonococcal	Ceftriaxone 50 mg/kg q24h IV, IM (AIII)	Treatment course 7 days or longer
– Pseudomonas	Ceftazidime 150 mg/kg/day IV div q8h AND tobramycin 6–7.5 mg/kg/day IM, IV, or amikacin 15–20 mg/kg/day IM, IV div q8h for 10–14 days (AIII)	Cefepime IV, meropenem IV, or imipenem IV are alternatives (no clinical data). Very poor outcomes.
– Candida	Intravitreal amphotericin AND fluconazole 12 mg/kg/day IV (AIII)	Echinocandins, usually only at higher than usual doses, can achieve antifungal activity in the eye.[66]
Hordeolum (sty) or chalazion	None (topical antibiotic not necessary)	Warm compresses; I&D when necessary
Retinitis		
– CMV[67-69] For neonatal: See Chapter 5. For HIV-infected children: visit NIH Web site at http://aidsinfo.nih.gov/guidelines/html/5/pediatric-oi-prevention-and-treatment-guidelines/0#.	Ganciclovir 10 mg/kg/day IV div q12h for 2 wk (BIII); if needed, continue at 5 mg/kg/day q24h to complete 6 wk total (BIII)	Neutropenia risk increases with duration of therapy. Foscarnet IV and cidofovir IV are alternatives but demonstrate significant nephrotoxicity. Insufficient data available to recommend valganciclovir extemporaneous suspension. Intravitreal ganciclovir and combination therapy for non-responding, immunocompromised hosts.

D. EAR AND SINUS INFECTIONS

Clinical Diagnosis	Therapy (evidence grade)	Comments
Bullous myringitis (see Otitis media, acute)	Believed to be a clinical presentation of acute bacterial otitis media	
Otitis externa		
– Bacterial, swimmer's ear (*P aeruginosa, S aureus,* including CA-MRSA)[70–73]	Topical antibiotics: fluoroquinolone (ciprofloxacin or ofloxacin) with steroid, OR neomycin/polymyxin B/hydrocortisone (BII) Irrigation and cleaning canal of detritus important	Wick moistened with Burow solution, used for marked swelling of canal; to prevent swimmer's ear, 2% acetic acid to canal after water exposure will restore acid pH.
– Bacterial, malignant otitis externa (*P aeruginosa*)[72]	Ceftazidime 150 mg/kg/day IV div q8h AND tobramycin 6–7.5 mg/kg/day IV (AIII)	Other antipseudomonal antibiotics should also be effective: cefepime IV, meropenem IV or imipenem IV, pip/tazo IV, or for more mild infection, ciprofloxacin PO.
– Bacterial furuncle of canal (*S aureus,* including CA-MRSA)	Standard: oxacillin/nafcillin 150 mg/kg/day IV div q6h OR cefazolin 100 mg/kg/day IV div q8h (BII) CA-MRSA: clindamycin 30 mg/kg/day IV div q8h or vancomycin 40 mg/kg/day IV q8h (BIII)	I&D; antibiotics for cellulitis Oral therapy for mild disease, convalescent therapy: for MSSA: cephalexin; for CA-MRSA: clindamycin, TMP/SMX, OR linezolid (BIII)
– *Candida*	Fluconazole 6–12 mg/kg PO qd for 5–7 days (CIII)	May occur following antibiotic therapy of bacterial external otitis; debride canal
Otitis media, acute		

A note on AOM: The natural history of AOM in different age groups by specific pathogens has not been well defined; therefore, the actual contribution of antibiotic therapy on resolution of disease has also been poorly defined until 2 recent, amoxicillin/clavulanate vs placebo, blinded, prospective studies were published (Hoberman A et al 2011[74] and Tähtinen P et al 2011[75]), although neither study required tympanocentesis to define a pathogen. The benefits and risks (including development of antibiotic resistance) of antibiotic therapy for AOM need to be further evaluated before the most accurate advice on the "best" antibiotic can be provided. However, based on available data, for most children, amoxicillin or amoxicillin/clavulanate can be used initially. Considerations for the need for extended antimicrobial activity of amoxicillin/clavulanate include severity of disease, age of child, previous antibiotics, child care attendance, in vitro antibacterial spectrum of antibiotic, and palatability of suspensions. With universal PCV13 immunization, preliminary data suggest that the risk of antibiotic-resistant pneumococcal otitis has decreased, and the percent of *Haemophilus* responsible for AOM has increased, which may soon result in a recommendation for the use of amox/clav as first line therapy for well-documented AOM. The most current American Academy of Pediatrics guidelines[76] and meta-analyses[77] suggest the greatest benefit with therapy occurs in children with bilateral AOM who are younger than 2 years; for other children, close observation is also an option. American Academy of Pediatrics guidelines provide an option to treatment in non-severe cases, particularly unilateral disease and disease in older children, to provide a prescription to parents, but have them only fill the prescription if the child deteriorates.[76] Although prophylaxis is only rarely indicated, amoxicillin or other antibiotics can be used in one-half the therapeutic dose once or twice daily to prevent infections if the benefits outweigh the risks of development of resistant organisms for that child.[78]

– Newborns	See Chapter 5.	
– Infants and children (pneumococcus, *H influenzae* non–type b, *Moraxella* most common)[78–80]	Usual therapy: amoxicillin 90 mg/kg/day PO bid, with or without clavulanate; failures will be caused by highly pen-R pneumococcus, or if amoxicillin is used alone, by beta-lactamase–producing *Haemophilus* (or *Moraxella*). a) For *Haemophilus* strains that are beta-lactamase–positive, the following oral antibiotics offer better in vitro activity than amoxicillin: amox/clav, cefdinir, cefpodoxime, cefuroxime, ceftriaxone IM, levofloxacin. b) For pen-R pneumococci: high-dosage amoxicillin achieves greater middle ear activity than oral cephalosporins. Options include: ceftriaxone IM 50 mg/kg/day q24h for 1–3 doses; OR levofloxacin 20 mg/kg PO div bid for children ≤5 y, and 10 mg/kg PO qd for children >5 y; OR a macrolide-class antibiotic: azithromycin PO at 1 of 3 dosages: (1) 10 mg/kg on day 1, followed by 5 mg/kg qd on days 2–5; (2) 10 mg/kg qd for 3 days; or (3) 30 mg/kg once. Caution: up to 40% of pen-R pneumococci are also macrolide-resistant.	See Chapter 11 for dosages. Until published data document the lack of penicillin-resistance in pneumococci isolated from infants with AOM,[79] high-dosage amoxicillin (90 mg/kg/day) should be used for empiric therapy. The high serum and middle ear fluid concentrations achieved with 45 mg/kg/dose of amoxicillin, combined with a long half-life in middle ear fluid, allow for a therapeutic antibiotic exposure in the middle ear with only twice-daily dosing; high-dosage amoxicillin (90 mg/kg/day) with clavulanate (Augmentin-ES) is also available. As published data document decreasing resistance to amoxicillin, standard dosage (45 mg/kg/day) can again be recommended. Tympanocentesis should be performed in children who fail second-line therapy.
Otitis, chronic suppurative (*P aeruginosa*, *S aureus*, including CA-MRSA, and other respiratory tract/skin flora)[81,82]	Topical antibiotics: fluoroquinolone (ciprofloxacin, ofloxacin, besifloxacin) with or without steroid (BIII) Cleaning of canal, view of tympanic membrane (TM), for patency; cultures important	Presumed middle ear drainage through open TM; possible aminoglycoside toxicity if neomycin-containing topical therapy used[83] Other topical fluoroquinolones with/without steroids available

6

D. EAR AND SINUS INFECTIONS (cont)

Clinical Diagnosis	Therapy (evidence grade)	Comments
Mastoiditis, acute (pneumococcus, *S aureus*, including CA-MRSA; group A streptococcus; increasing *Pseudomonas* in adolescents, *Haemophilus* rare)[84-86]	Cefotaxime 150 mg/kg/day IV div q8h or ceftriaxone 50 mg/kg/day q24h AND clindamycin 40 mg/kg/day IV div q8h (BIII) For adolescents: ceftazidime 150 mg/kg/day IV div q8h AND clindamycin 40 mg/kg/day IV div q8h (BIII)	Rule out meningitis; surgery as needed for mastoid and middle ear drainage. Change to appropriate oral therapy after clinical improvement.
Sinusitis, acute (*H influenzae* non–type b, pneumococcus, group A streptococcus, *Moraxella*)[87-90]	Same antibiotic therapy as for AOM as pathogens similar: amoxicillin 90 mg/kg/day PO div bid, OR for children at higher risk of *Haemophilus*, amox/clav 14:1 ratio, with amoxicillin component at 90 mg/kg/day PO div bid (BIII). Therapy of 14 days may be necessary while mucosal swelling resolves and ventilation is restored.	IDSA sinusitis guidelines recommend amox/clav as first-line therapy,[90] while AAP guidelines (same pediatric authors) recommend amoxicillin.[88] Lack of data prevents a definitive evidence-based recommendation. Sinus irrigations for severe disease or failure to respond.

E. OROPHARYNGEAL INFECTIONS

Clinical Diagnosis	Therapy (evidence grade)	Comments
Dental abscess[91,92]	Clindamycin 30 mg/kg/day PO, IV, IM div q6–8h OR penicillin G 100–200,000 U/kg/day IV div q6h (AIII)	Amox/clav PO; amoxicillin PO; ampicillin AND metronidazole IV are other options. Tooth extraction usually necessary. Erosion of abscess may occur into facial, sinusitis, deep head, and neck compartments.
Diphtheria[93]	Erythromycin 40–50 mg/kg/day PO div qid for 14 days OR penicillin G 150,000 U/kg/day IV div q6h; PLUS antitoxin (AIII)	Diphtheria antitoxin (DAT), a horse antisera, is investigational and only available from CDC Emergency Operations Center at 770/488-7100. The investigational protocol and dosages of DAT are provided on the CDC Web site (protocol version February 2012) at www.cdc.gov/diphtheria/downloads/protocol.pdf, accessed November 11, 2013.

Condition	Therapy	Comments
Epiglottitis (aryepiglottitis, supraglottitis; *H influenzae* type b in an unimmunized child); rarely pneumococcus, *S aureus*[94,95]	Ceftriaxone 50 mg/kg/day IV, IM q24h OR cefotaxime 150 mg/kg/day IV div q8h for 7–10 days	Emergency: provide airway. For *S aureus* (causes only 5% of epiglottitis), consider adding clindamycin 40 mg/kg/day IV div q8h.
Gingivostomatitis, herpetic[96–98]	Acyclovir 80 mg/kg/day PO div qid for 7 days (for severe disease, use IV therapy at 30 mg/kg/day div q8h) (BIII); OR for infants ≥3 mo of age, valacyclovir 20 mg/kg/dose PO bid (instructions for preparing liquid formulation with 28-day shelf life included in package insert) (CIII)[98]	Early treatment is likely to be the most effective. Start treatment as soon as oral intake compromised. This oral ACV dose is safe and effective for varicella; 75 mg/kg/day div into 5 equal doses has been studied for HSV.[97] Limited pediatric valacyclovir pharmacokinetics and preparation of an extemporaneous suspension are included in the valacyclovir FDA-approved package label. Consider adding amox/clav or clindamycin for severe disease with oral flora superinfection.
Lemierre syndrome (*Fusobacterium necrophorum*)[99,100] pharyngitis with internal jugular vein septic thrombosis, postanginal sepsis, necrobacillosis	Empiric: meropenem 60 mg/kg/day div q8h (or 120 mg/kg/day div q8h for CNS metastatic foci) (AIII) OR ceftriaxone 100 mg/kg/day q24h AND metronidazole 40 mg/kg/day div q8h or clindamycin 40 mg/kg/day div q6h (BIII)	Anecdotal reports suggest metronidazole may be effective for apparent failures with other agents. Often requires anticoagulation. Metastatic and recurrent abscesses often develop while on active, appropriate therapy, requiring multiple debridements and prolonged antibiotic therapy. Treat until CRP and ESR are normal (AIII).
Peritonsillar cellulitis or abscess (group A streptococcus with mixed oral flora)[101]	Clindamycin 30 mg/kg/day PO, IV, IM div q8h AND cefotaxime 150 mg/kg/day IV div q8h (BIII)	Consider incision and drainage for abscess. Alternatives: meropenem or imipenem; pip/tazo; amox/clav for convalescent oral therapy (BIII). No useful data on benefits of steroids.

E. OROPHARYNGEAL INFECTIONS (cont)

Clinical Diagnosis	Therapy (evidence grade)	Comments
Pharyngitis (group A streptococcus) tonsillopharyngitis[7,102-104]	Amoxicillin 50–75 mg/kg/day PO, either qd, bid, or tid for 10 days OR penicillin V 50–75 mg/kg/day PO bid or tid, OR benzathine penicillin 600,000 units IM for children <27 kg, 1.2 million units IM if >27 kg, as a single dose (AII) For penicillin-allergic children: erythromycin (estolate at 20–40 mg/kg/day PO bid to qid; or ethylsuccinate at 40 mg/kg/day PO div bid to qid) for 10 days; OR azithromycin 12 mg/kg qd for 5 days (AII)	Amoxicillin displays better gastrointestinal absorption than oral phenoxymethyl penicillin; the suspension is better tolerated. These advantages should be balanced by the unnecessary increased spectrum of activity. Once daily amoxicillin dosage: for children 50 mg/kg (max 1,000–1,200 mg).[7] Meta-analysis suggests that oral cephalosporins are more effective than penicillin for treatment of strep.[105] Clindamycin is also effective. A 5-day treatment course is FDA approved for some oral cephalosporins (cefdinir, cefpodoxime), but longer follow-up for rheumatic fever is important before short-course therapy can be recommended for all streptococcal pharyngitis (CIII).[106]
Retropharyngeal, parapharyngeal, or lateral pharyngeal cellulitis or abscess (mixed aerobic/anaerobic flora, now including CA-MRSA)[101,107,108]	Clindamycin 40 mg/kg/day IV div q8H AND cefotaxime 150 mg/kg/day IV div q8h or ceftriaxone 50 mg/kg/day IV q24h	Consider I&D; possible airway compromise, mediastinitis Alternatives: meropenem or imipenem (BIII)
Tracheitis, bacterial (*S aureus*, including CA-MRSA; group A streptococcus; pneumococcus; *H influenzae* type b, rarely *Pseudomonas*)[109,110]	Vancomycin 40 mg/kg/day IV div q8h or clindamycin 40 mg/kg/day IV div q8H AND cefotaxime 50 mg/kg/day q24h or cefotaxime 150 mg/kg/day div q8h	For susceptible *S aureus*, oxacillin/nafcillin or cefazolin May represent bacterial superinfection of viral laryngotracheobronchitis

F. LOWER RESPIRATORY TRACT INFECTIONS

Clinical Diagnosis	Therapy (evidence grade)	Comments
Abscess, lung		
– Primary (severe, necrotizing community-acquired pneumonia caused by pneumococcus, S aureus, including CA-MRSA, group A streptococcus)[111,112]	Empiric therapy with ceftriaxone 50–75 mg/kg/day q24h or cefotaxime 150 mg/kg/day div q8h AND clindamycin 40 mg/kg/day div q8h or vancomycin 45 mg/kg/day IV div q8h for 14–21 days or longer (AIII)	For severe CA-MRSA infections, see Chapter 4. Bronchoscopy may be necessary if abscess fails to drain; surgical excision rarely necessary for pneumococcus but more important for CA-MRSA and MSSA. Focus antibiotic coverage based on culture results. For susceptible staph: oxacillin/nafcillin or cefazolin.
– Primary, putrid (ie, foul-smelling; polymicrobial infection with oral aerobes and anaerobes)[113]	Clindamycin 40 mg/kg/day IV div q8h or meropenem 60 mg/kg/day IV div q8h for 10 days or longer (AIII)	Alternatives: imipenem IV or pip/tazo IV or ticar/clav IV (BIII) Oral step-down therapy with clindamycin or amox/clav (BIII)
Allergic bronchopulmonary aspergillosis	Prednisone 0.5 mg/kg every other day AND voriconazole (18 mg/kg/day div q12h load followed by 16 mg/kg/day div q12h) or itraconazole (10 mg/kg/day div q12h)	Larger steroid dosages may lead to tissue invasion by *Aspergillus*.
Aspiration pneumonia (polymicrobial infection with oral aerobes and anaerobes)[113]	Clindamycin 40 mg/kg/day IV div q8h; ADD ceftriaxone 50–75 mg/kg/day q24h or cefotaxime 150 mg/kg/day div q8h for additional *Haemophilus* activity[114] OR meropenem 60 mg/kg/day IV div q8h; for 10 days or longer (BIII)	Alternatives: imipenem IV or pip/tazo IV or ticar/clav IV (BIII) Oral step-down therapy with clindamycin or amox/clav (BIII)
Atypical pneumonia (see *Mycoplasma*, Legionnaires disease)		
Bronchitis (bronchiolitis), acute[115]	For bronchitis/bronchiolitis in children, no antibiotic needed for most cases, as disease is usually viral	
Community-acquired pneumonia (see Pneumonia: Community-acquired)		

Antimicrobial Therapy According to Clinical Syndromes

F. LOWER RESPIRATORY TRACT INFECTIONS (cont)

Clinical Diagnosis	Therapy (evidence grade)	Comments
Cystic fibrosis: Seek advice from those expert in acute and chronic management.		
– Acute exacerbation (*P aeruginosa* primarily; also *Burkholderia cepacia*, *Stenotrophomonas maltophilia*, *S aureus*, including CA-MRSA, nontuberculous mycobacteria)[116-119]	Ceftazidime 150–200 mg/kg/day div q6–8h or meropenem 120 mg/kg/day div q6h[120] AND tobramycin 6–10 mg/kg/day IM, IV div q6–8h for treatment of acute infection (AII); Alternatives: imipenem, cefepime or ciprofloxacin 30 mg/kg/day PO, IV div tid Duration of therapy not well defined: 2–3 wk (BIII)[117]	Larger than normal dosages of antibiotics required in most patients with cystic fibrosis; monitor peak serum concentrations of aminoglycosides. Insufficient evidence to recommend routine use of inhaled antibiotics for acute exacerbations.[121] Cultures with susceptibility testing and synergy testing will help select antibiotics as multidrug resistance is common.[122,123] Combination therapy may provide synergistic killing and delay the emergence of resistance (CIII).
– Chronic inflammation (minimize long-term damage to lung)	Inhaled tobramycin 300 mg bid, cycling 28 days on therapy, 28 days off therapy, is effective adjunctive therapy between exacerbation[116,124] (AI). Inhaled aztreonam[125] provides an alternative to inhaled tobramycin (AI). Azithromycin adjunctive chronic therapy, greatest benefit for those colonized with *Pseudomonas* (AII).[116,126,127]	Alternative inhaled antibiotics: aztreonam[127]; colistin[121,128] (BII)
Pertussis[129,130]	Azithromycin (10 mg/kg/day for 5 days) or clarithromycin (15 mg/kg/day div bid for 7 days) or erythromycin (estolate preferable) 40 mg/kg/day PO div qid; for 14 days (AII) Alternative: TMP/SMX (8 mg/kg/day TMP) div bid for 14 days (BII)	Azithromycin and clarithromycin are better tolerated than erythromycin; azithromycin is preferred in young infants to reduce pyloric stenosis risk (see Chapter 5). The azithromycin dosage that is recommended for very young infants <1 mo (12 mg/kg/day for 5 days) with the highest risk of mortality, is FDA approved for streptococcal pharyngitis and is well tolerated and safe for older children. Alternatively, 10 mg/kg on day 1, followed by 5 mg/kg on days 2–5 should also be effective.[129] Provide prophylaxis to family members.

2014 Nelson's Pediatric Antimicrobial Therapy — 53

Pneumonia: Community-acquired, bronchopneumonia		
– Mild to moderate illness (overwhelmingly viral, especially in preschool children)[131]	No antibiotic therapy unless epidemiologic, clinical, or laboratory reasons to suspect bacteria or *Mycoplasma*	Broad-spectrum antibiotics may increase risk of subsequent infection with antibiotic-resistant pathogens.
– Moderate to severe illness (pneumococcus; group A streptococcus; *S aureus*, including CA-MRSA; or *Mycoplasma pneumoniae*[11,112,132-134]; or for those with aspiration due to underlying comorbidities, *Haemophilus influenzae*, nontypable[114])	Empiric therapy: For regions with high PCV13 vaccine use or low pneumococcal resistance to penicillin: ampicillin 200 mg/kg/day div q6h. For regions with low rates of PCV13 use or high pneumococcal resistance to penicillin: ceftriaxone 50–75 mg/kg/day q24h or cefotaxime 150 mg/kg/day div q8h (AI). For suspected CA-MRSA, use vancomycin 40–60 mg/kg/day (AIII).[2] For suspect *Mycoplasma*/atypical pneumonia agents, particularly in school-aged children, ADD azithromycin 10 mg/kg IV, PO once, then decrease dose to 5 mg/kg qd for days 2–5 of treatment (AII).	Tracheal aspirate or bronchoalveolar lavage for Gram stain/culture for severe infection in intubated children. Check vancomycin serum concentrations and renal function, particularly at the higher dosage for CA-MRSA. Alternatives to azithromycin for atypical pneumonia include erythromycin IV, PO or clarithromycin PO, or doxycycline IV, PO for children >7 y, or levofloxacin for postpubertal older children. New data suggest that combination empiric therapy with a beta-lactam and a macrolide result in shorter hospitalization compared with a beta-lactam alone, but we are not ready to recommend routine empiric combination therapy yet.[135]

Antimicrobial Therapy According to Clinical Syndromes

F. LOWER RESPIRATORY TRACT INFECTIONS (cont)

Clinical Diagnosis	Therapy (evidence grade)	Comments
Pneumonia: Community-acquired, lobar consolidation		
Pneumococcus (even if immunized), S aureus, including CA-MRSA (can cause necrotizing pneumonia) and group A streptococcus,[111,112,132–134] Consider H influenzae type b in the unimmunized child. M pneumoniae may cause lobar pneumonia.	Empiric therapy: For regions with high PCV13 vaccine use or low pneumococcal resistance to penicillin: ampicillin 200 mg/kg/day div q6h. For regions with low rates of PCV13 use or high pneumococcal resistance to penicillin: ceftriaxone 50–75 mg/kg/day q24h or cefotaxime 150 mg/kg/day div q8h (AI); for more severe disease ADD clindamycin 40 mg/kg/day div q8h or vancomycin 40–60 mg/kg/day div q6h for S aureus (AIII).[2] For suspect Mycoplasma/atypical pneumonia agents, particularly in school-aged children, ADD azithromycin 10 mg/kg IV, PO once, then decrease dose to 5 mg/kg qd for days 2–5 of treatment (AII). Empiric oral outpatient therapy for less severe illness: high-dosage amoxicillin 80–100 mg/kg/day PO div q8h (NOT q12h); for Mycoplasma, ADD a macrolide as above (BII).	Change to PO after improvement (decreased fever, no oxygen needed); treat until clinically asymptomatic and chest radiography significantly improved (7–21 days) (BII). No reported failures of ceftriaxone/cefotaxime for pen-R pneumococcus: no need to add empiric vancomycin for this reason (CIII). Oral therapy for pneumococcus and Haemophilus may also be successful with amox/clav, cefdinir, cefpodoxime, or cefuroxime. Levofloxacin is an alternative, particularly those with severe allergy to beta-lactam antibiotics (BI)[136] but due to cartilage toxicity concerns, should not be first-line therapy.
– Pneumococcal, pen-S	Penicillin G 250,000–400,000 U/kg/day IV div q4–6h for 10 days (BII) or ampicillin 200 mg/kg/day IV divided q6h	After improvement, change to PO amoxicillin 50–75 mg/kg/day PO div tid, or penicillin V 50–75 mg/kg/day div qid.
– Pneumococcal, pen-R	Ceftriaxone 75 mg/kg/day q24h, or cefotaxime 150 mg/kg/day div q8h for 10–14 d (BII)	Addition of vancomycin has not been required for eradication of pen-R strains. For oral convalescent therapy, high-dosage amoxicillin (100–150 mg/kg/day PO div tid), or clindamycin (30 mg/kg/day PO div tid), or linezolid (30 mg/kg/day PO div tid).

S aureus (including CA-MRSA)[2,6,111,132,137,138]	For MSSA: oxacillin/nafcillin 150 mg/kg/day IV div q6h or cefazolin 100 mg/kg/day IV div q8h (AII) For CA-MRSA: vancomycin 60 mg/kg/day; may need addition of rifampin, clindamycin, or gentamicin (AIII) (see Chapter 4)	Check vancomycin serum concentrations and renal function, particularly at the higher dosage (serum trough concentrations of 15 μg/mL) needed for invasive CA-MRSA disease. For life-threatening disease, optimal therapy of CA-MRSA is not defined: add gentamicin and/or rifampin. Linezolid 30 mg/kg/day IV, PO div q8h is another option (follow platelets and WBC weekly).
Pneumonia: with pleural fluid/empyema (same pathogens as for community-associated bronchopneumonia) Based on extent of fluid and symptoms, may benefit from chest tube drainage with fibrinolysis or video-assisted thoracoscopic surgery[132,139-142]	Empiric therapy: ceftriaxone 50–75 mg/kg/day q24h or cefotaxime 150 mg/kg/day div q8h AND vancomycin 40–60 mg/kg/day IV div q8h (BIII)	Initial therapy based on Gram stain of empyema fluid; typically clinical improvement is slow, with persisting but decreasing "spiking" fever for 2–3 wk. Broad spectrum empiric therapy recommended due to need to provide initial effective therapy for best outcomes.[114]
– Group A streptococcal	Penicillin G 250,000 U/kg/day IV div q4–6h for 10 days (BII)	Change to PO amoxicillin 75 mg/kg/day div tid or penicillin V 50–75 mg/kg/day, div qid to tid after clinical improvement (BIII)
– Pneumococcal	(See Pneumonia: Community-acquired, lobar consolidation, Pneumococcal)	
– S aureus (including CA-MRSA)[2,6,111,137]	For MSSA: oxacillin/nafcillin or cefazolin (AII) For CA-MRSA: use vancomycin 60 mg/kg/day (AIII) (follow serum concentrations and renal function); may need additional antibiotics (see Chapter 4)	For life-threatening disease, optimal therapy of CA-MRSA is not defined: add gentamicin and/or rifampin. Oral convalescent therapy for MSSA: cephalexin PO; for CA-MRSA: clindamycin PO. Total course for 21 days or longer (AIII). Linezolid 30 mg/kg/day IV, PO div q8h is another option (follow platelets and WBC weekly).

F. LOWER RESPIRATORY TRACT INFECTIONS (cont)

Clinical Diagnosis	Therapy (evidence grade)	Comments
Pneumonia: immunosuppressed, neutropenic host[143] *P aeruginosa*, other community-associated or nosocomial gram-negative bacilli, *S aureus*, fungi, AFB, *Pneumocystis*, viral (adenovirus, CMV, EBV, influenza, RSV, others)	Ceftazidime 150 mg/kg/day IV div q8h and tobramycin 6.0–7.5 mg/kg/day IM, IV div q8h (AII), OR cefepime 150 mg/kg/day div q8h, or meropenem 60 mg/kg/day div q8h (AII) ± tobramycin (BIII); AND if *S aureus* suspected clinically, ADD vancomycin 40–60 mg/kg/day IV div q8h (AIII)	Biopsy or bronchoalveolar lavage usually needed to determine need for antifungal, antiviral, antimycobacterial treatment. Antifungal therapy usually started if no response to antibiotics in 48–72h (amphotericin B, voriconazole, or caspofungin/micafungin—see Chapter 8). Amikacin 15–22.5 mg/kg/day is alternative aminoglycoside. Use 2 active agents for possible bacterial synergy and decreased risk of emergence of resistance (BII).
– Pneumonia: Interstitial pneumonia syndrome of early infancy	If *Chlamydia trachomatis* suspected, azithromycin 10 mg/kg on day 1, followed by 5 mg/kg/day qd days 2–5 OR erythromycin 40 mg/kg/day PO qid for 14 days (BII)	Most often respiratory viral pathogens, CMV, or chlamydial; role of *Ureaplasma* uncertain
– Pneumonia, Nosocomial (health care–associated/ ventilator-associated) *P aeruginosa*, gram-negative enteric bacilli (*Enterobacter, Klebsiella, Serratia, Escherichia coli*), *Acinetobacter, Stenotrophomonas*, and gram-positive organisms including CA-MRSA and *Enterococcus*[144-147]	Commonly used regimens: Meropenem 60 mg/kg/day div q8h, OR pip/tazo 240–300 mg/kg/day div q6–8h, OR cefepime 150 mg/kg/day div q8h; ± gentamicin 6.0–7.5 mg/kg/day div q8h (AIII); ADD vancomycin 40–60 mg/kg/day IV div q8h for suspect CA-MRSA (AIII)	For multidrug-resistant gram-negative bacilli, colistin may be required.[130] Empiric therapy should be institution-specific, based on your hospital's nosocomial pathogens and susceptibilities. Pathogens that cause nosocomial pneumonia often have multidrug resistance. Cultures are critical. Empiric therapy also based on child's prior colonization/infection. Aminoglycosides may not achieve therapeutic concentrations in airways.[147] Aerosol delivery of antibiotics may be required for multidrug-resistant pathogens.[148]

Pneumonias of other established etiologies
(see Chapter 7 for treatment by pathogen)

– *Chlamydophila*[149] (formerly *Chlamydia*) *pneumoniae, C psittaci,* or *Chlamydia trachomatis*[149]	Azithromycin 10 mg/kg on day 1, followed by 5 mg/kg/day qd days 2–5 or erythromycin 40 mg/kg/day PO div qid; for 14 days	Doxycycline (patients >7 y)

– CMV (immunocompromised host)[150]	Ganciclovir IV 10 mg/kg/day IV div q12h for 2 wk (BIII); if needed, continue at 5 mg/kg/day q24h to complete 4–6 wk total (BIII)	Add IVIG or CMV immune globulin to provide a small incremental benefit (BII). For older children, oral valganciclovir may be used for convalescent therapy (BIII).
– E coli	Ceftriaxone 50–75 mg/kg/day q24h or cefotaxime 150 mg/kg/day div q8h (AII)	For resistant strains (ESBL-producers), use meropenem, imipenem, or ertapenem (AIII).
– Enterobacter spp	Cefepime 100 mg/kg/day div q12h or meropenem 60 mg/kg/day div q8h; OR ceftriaxone 50–75 mg/kg/day q24h or cefotaxime 150 mg/kg/day div q8h AND gentamicin 6.0–7.5 mg/kg/day IM, IV div q8h (AIII)	Addition of aminoglycoside to 3rd-generation cephalosporins may retard the emergence of constitutive high-level resistance, but concern for inadequate concentration in airways[147], not needed with cefepime, meropenem, or imipenem.
– Francisella tularensis[151,152]	Gentamicin 6.0–7.5 mg/kg/day IM, IV div q8h for 10 days or longer for more severe disease (AIII); for less severe disease, doxycycline PO for 14–21 days (AII)	Alternatives for oral therapy of mild disease: ciprofloxacin or levofloxacin (BIII)
– Fungi (see Chapter 8) – Community-associated pathogens vary by region (eg, coccidioides,[153,154] histoplasma[155,156]) – Aspergillus, mucor, others in immunocompromised hosts	For pathogen-specific recommendations, see Chapter 8. For suspected endemic fungi or mucormycosis in immunocompromised host, treat empirically with a lipid amphotericin B; biopsy needed to guide therapy. For suspected invasive aspergillosis, treat with voriconazole (AI) (load 18 mg/kg/day div q12h on day 1, then continue 16 mg/kg/day div q12h).	For normal hosts, triazoles (fluconazole, itraconazole, voriconazole, posaconazole) are better tolerated than amphotericin B and equally effective for many community-associated pathogens (see Chapter 2). For dosage, see Chapter 8. Check voriconazole trough concentrations; need to be at least >1 µg/ml.

6

Antimicrobial Therapy According to Clinical Syndromes

6

F. LOWER RESPIRATORY TRACT INFECTIONS (cont)

Clinical Diagnosis	Therapy (evidence grade)	Comments
– Influenza virus[157,158] – Recent seasonal FluA and FluB strains continue to be resistant to adamantanes.	Empiric therapy, or documented FluA or FluB: Oseltamivir[159] (AII): <12 mo: Term infants 0 to ≤8 mo: 3 mg/kg/dose bid 9 to ≤11 mo: 3.5 mg/kg/dose bid ≥12 mo ≤15 kg: 30 mg PO bid >15 to 23 kg: 45 mg PO bid >23 to 40 kg: 60 mg PO bid >40 kg: 75 mg PO bid Zanamivir inhaled (AII): for those ≥7 y 10 mg (two 5-mg inhalations) bid	Check for susceptibility each season at www.cdc.gov/flu/professionals/antivirals/index.htm. Adamantanes are amantadine and rimantadine. FluB is intrinsically resistant to adamantanes. Limited data for premature infants: <38 wk postmenstrual age (gestational plus chronologic age): 1.0 mg/kg/dose, PO bid 38–40 wk postmenstrual age: 1.5 mg/kg/dose, PO bid
– Klebsiella pneumoniae[160]	Ceftriaxone 50–75 mg/kg/day IV, IM q24h OR cefotaxime 150 mg/kg/day IV, IM div q8h (AIII); for ceftriaxone-resistant strains (ESBL strains), use meropenem 60 mg/kg/day IV div q8h (AIII)	For K pneumoniae carbapenemase-producing strains: alternatives include fluoroquinolones or colistin (BIII).
– Legionnaires disease (Legionella pneumophila)[161]	Azithromycin 10 mg/kg IV, PO q24h for 5 days (AIII)	Alternatives: clarithromycin, erythromycin, ciprofloxacin, levofloxacin, doxycycline
– Mycobacteria, nontuberculous (M avium complex most common)[11]	In a normal host: azithromycin PO or clarithromycin PO for 6–12 wk if susceptible For more extensive disease: a macrolide AND rifampin AND ethambutol; ± amikacin or streptomycin (AIII)	Highly variable susceptibilities of different nontuberculous mycobacterial species Check for immunocompromise: HIV or gamma-interferon receptor deficiency
– Mycobacterium tuberculosis (see Tuberculosis)		
– M pneumoniae[132,162]	Azithromycin 10 mg/kg on day 1, followed by 5 mg/kg/day qd days 2–5, or clarithromycin 15 mg/kg/day div bid for 7–14 days, or erythromycin 40 mg/kg/day PO div qid for 14 days	Mycoplasma often causes self-limited infection and does not require treatment (AIII). For older children, doxycycline. Macrolide-resistant strains have recently appeared worldwide.[163]

Organism	Therapy
– *Paragonimus westermani*	See Chapter 10.
– *Pneumocystis jiroveci* (formerly *Pneumocystis carinii*)[164,165]	Mild-moderate disease: TMP/SMX 20 mg of TMP/kg/day PO div qid for 14–21 days (AII). Moderate-severe disease: same dosage of TMP/SMX given IV, each dose over 1h (AI). Use steroid adjunctive treatment for more severe disease (AII).	Alternatives: pentamidine 3–4 mg IV qd, infused over 60–90 min (AII); TMP AND dapsone; OR primaquine AND clindamycin; OR atovaquone Prophylaxis: TMP/SMX as 5 mg TMP/kg/day PO, divided in 2 doses, q12h, either daily or 3 times/wk (AII); OR TMP/SMX 5 mg TMP/kg/day PO as a single dose, once daily, given 3 times/wk (AII); OR dapsone 2 mg/kg (max 100 mg) PO once daily, or 4 mg/kg (max 200 mg) once weekly
– *P aeruginosa*[144,147,166,167]	Ceftazidime 150 mg/kg/day IV div q8h AND tobramycin 6.0–7.5 mg/kg/day IM, IV div q8h (AII). Alternatives: cefepime 150 mg/kg/day div q8h or meropenem 60 mg/kg/day div q8h, OR pip/tazo 240–300 mg/kg/day div q6–8h (AII) ± tobramycin (BIII).	Ciprofloxacin IV, or colistin IV for multidrug-resistant strains
– RSV infection (bronchiolitis, pneumonia)[168]	For immunocompromised hosts: ribavirin aerosol: 6-g vial (20 mg/mL in sterile water), by SPAG-2 generator, over 18–20 h daily for 3–5 days	Treat only for severe disease, immunocompromise, severe underlying cardiopulmonary disease. Efficacy data are limited, however, and benefit is not likely to be robust. Ribavirin may also be given systemically, PO, or IV but has not been systemically studied for RSV. Palivizumab is not effective for treatment, only prevention.

Tuberculosis

– Primary pulmonary disease[13,14]	Isoniazid (INH) 10–15 mg/kg/day (max 300 mg) PO qd for 6 mo AND rifampin 10–20 mg/kg/day (max 600 mg) PO qd for 6 mo AND PZA 20–40 mg/kg/day PO qd for first 2 mo therapy only (AII). If risk factors present for multidrug resistance, ADD ethambutol 20 mg/kg/day PO qd OR streptomycin 30 mg/kg/day IV, IM q12h initially.	Contact TB specialist for therapy of drug-resistant TB. Fluoroquinolones may play a role in treating multidrug-resistant strains. Directly observed therapy preferred; after 2 wk of daily therapy, can change to twice-weekly dosing double dosage of INH (max 900 mg), PZA (max 2 g), and ethambutol (max 2.5 g); rifampin remains same dosage (10–20 mg/kg/day, max 600 mg) (AII). LP ± CT of head for children ≤2 y to rule out occult, concurrent CNS infection; consider testing for HIV infection (AIII).

F. LOWER RESPIRATORY TRACT INFECTIONS (cont)

Clinical Diagnosis	Therapy (evidence grade)	Comments
– Latent TB infection (skin test conversion)	INH 10–15 mg/kg/day (max 300 mg) PO daily for 9 mo (12 mo for immunocompromised patients) (AIII); treatment with INH at 20–30 mg/kg twice weekly for 9 mo is also effective (AIII). Alternative[169] (BII): For children ≥12 years, once weekly DOT for 12 weeks: INH (15 mg/kg/dose, max 900 mg), AND rifapentine: 10.0–14.0 kg: 300 mg 14.1–25.0 kg: 450 mg 25.1–32.0 kg: 600 mg 32.1–49.9 kg: 750 mg ≥50.0 kg: 900 mg (max)	Obtain baseline LFTs. Consider monthly LFTs or as needed for symptoms. Stop INH-rifapentine if AST or ALT ≥5 times the ULN even in the absence of symptoms or ≥3 times the ULN in the presence of symptoms. For children ≥2 years, 12 weeks of INH and rifapentine may be used, but less data on safety and efficacy. Insufficient data for children <2 years. For exposure to known INH-R but rifampin-S strains, use rifampin 6 mo (AIII).
– Exposed infant <4 y, or immunocompromised patient (high risk of dissemination)	INH 10–15 mg/kg PO daily for 2–3 mo after last exposure with repeat skin test or interferon-gamma release assay test negative (AIII)	If PPD remains negative at 2–3 mo and child well, consider stopping empiric therapy. PPD may not be reliable in immunocompromised patients.

G. CARDIOVASCULAR INFECTIONS

Clinical Diagnosis	Therapy (evidence grade)	Comments
– **Bacteremia**		
– Occult bacteremia (late-onset neonatal sepsis; fever without focus), infants <2 mo (group B streptococcus, E coli, Listeria, pneumococcus, meningococcus)[170–172]	In general, hospitalization with cultures of blood, urine, and CSF; start ampicillin 200 mg/kg/day IV div q6h AND cefotaxime 150 mg/kg/day IV div q8h (AII)	For a nontoxic, febrile infant with good access to medical care: cultures may be obtained of blood, urine, and CSF; ceftriaxone 50 mg/kg IM (lacks Listeria activity) given with outpatient follow-up the next day (Boston criteria) (BII); alternative is home without antibiotics if evaluation is negative (Rochester; Philadelphia criteria)[170] (BI).

– Occult bacteremia (fever without focus) in ages 2–3 mo–36 mo (*H influenzae*, pneumococcus, meningococcus; increasingly *S aureus*)[173-175]	Empiric therapy: If unimmunized, febrile, mild-moderate toxic: after blood culture: ceftriaxone 50 mg/kg IM (BII). If fully immunized (*Haemophilus* and *Pneumococcus*) and nontoxic, no routine antibiotic therapy recommended, but follow closely in case of vaccine failure or meningococcal bacteremia (BIII).	Oral convalescent therapy is selected by susceptibility of blood isolate, following response to IM/IV treatment, with CNS and other foci ruled out by examination ± laboratory tests ± imaging.
– *H influenzae* type b, non-CNS infections	Ceftriaxone IM/IV OR if beta-lactamase negative, ampicillin IV, followed by oral convalescent therapy (AII)	If beta-lactamase negative: amoxicillin 75–100 mg/kg/day PO div tid (AII) If pos: high-dosage cefixime, ceftibuten, cefdinir PO, or levofloxacin PO (CIII)
– Meningococcus	Ceftriaxone IM/IV or penicillin G IV, followed by oral convalescent therapy (AII)	Amoxicillin 75–100 mg/kg/day PO div tid (AIII)
– Pneumococcus, non-CNS infections	Ceftriaxone IM/IV or penicillin G IV (if pen-S), followed by oral convalescent therapy (AII)	If pen-S: amoxicillin 75–100 mg/kg/day PO tid (AII). If pen-R: continue ceftriaxone IM, or switch to clindamycin if susceptible (CIII); linezolid or levofloxacin may also be effective (CIII).
– *S aureus*[2, 6,176–179] usually associated with focal infection	MSSA: nafcillin or oxacillin/nafcillin IV (150–200 mg/kg/day div q6h) ± gentamicin (6 mg/kg/day div q8h) MRSA: vancomycin (40–60 mg/kg/day IV div q8h) ± gentamicin (6 mg/kg/day div q8h) ± rifampin (20 mg/kg/day div q12h)	For persisting bacteremia caused by MRSA, consider daptomycin 6–8 mg/kg qd (but will not treat pneumonia) or ceftaroline. For toxic shock syndrome, clindamycin should be added for the initial 48–72h of therapy to decrease toxin production; IVIG may be added to bind circulating toxin (linezolid may also act in this way). Watch for the development of metastatic foci of infection, including endocarditis. If catheter-related, remove catheter.[179]

Endocarditis: Surgical indications: intractable heart failure; persistent uncontrollable infection; large mobile vegetations; peripheral embolism; and valve dehiscence, perforation, rupture or fistula, or a large perivalvular abscess[179]

G. CARDIOVASCULAR INFECTIONS (cont)

Clinical Diagnosis	Therapy (evidence grade)	Comments
— Native valve[180,181]		
— Empiric therapy for presumed endocarditis	Ceftriaxone IV (100 mg/kg q24h) AND gentamicin IV, IM (6 mg/kg/day div q8h) (AII) For severe infection, ADD vancomycin (40–60 mg/kg/day IV div q8h) to cover *S aureus* (AIII)	Combination (ceftriaxone + gentamicin) provides bactericidal activity against most strains of viridans streptococci, the most common pathogens in infective endocarditis. May administer gentamicin with a qd regimen (CIII). For beta-lactam allergy, use vancomycin 40 mg/kg/day IV div q8h AND gentamicin 6 mg/kg/day IV div q8h.
— Viridans streptococci: Follow echocardiogram for resolution of vegetation (BIII); for beta-lactam allergy: vancomycin.		
Fully susceptible to penicillin	Ceftriaxone 50 mg/kg IV, IM q24h for 4 wk OR penicillin G 200,000 U/kg/day IV div q4–6h for 4 wk (BII); OR penicillin G or ceftriaxone AND gentamicin 6 mg/kg IM, IV div q8h for 14 days (AII)	
Relatively resistant to penicillin	Penicillin G 300,000 U/kg/day IV div q4–6h for 4 wk, or ceftriaxone 100 mg/kg IV q24h for 4 wk; AND gentamicin 6 mg/kg/day IM, IV div q8h for 2 wk (AIII)	Gentamicin is used for the first 2 wk of a total of 4 wk of therapy for relatively resistant strains.
— Enterococcus (dosages for both native or prosthetic valve infections)		
Ampicillin-susceptible (gentamicin-S) Ampicillin-resistant (gentamicin-S) Vancomycin-resistant (gentamicin-S)	Ampicillin 300 mg/kg/day IV, IM div q6h or penicillin G 300,000 U/kg/day IV div q4–6h; AND gentamicin 6 mg/kg/day IV div q8h; for 4–6 wk (AII) Vancomycin 40 mg/kg/day IV div q8h AND gentamicin 6 mg/kg/day IV div q8h; for 4–6 wk (AIII) Daptomycin 6–8 mg/kg/day q24h AND gentamicin 6 mg/kg/day IV div q8h; for 4–6 wk (AIII)	Combined treatment with cell-wall active antibiotic plus aminoglycoside used to achieve bactericidal activity. For beta-lactam allergy: vancomycin. Little data exist in children. Linezolid and quinopristin/dalfopristin are alternatives. For gentamicin-R strains, use streptomycin if susceptible.
— Staphylococci: *S aureus*, including CA-MRSA; *S epidermidis*;[6,177] Consider continuing therapy at end of 6 wk if vegetations persist on echocardiogram.	MSSA or MSSE: nafcillin or oxacillin/nafcillin 150–200 mg/kg/day IV div q6h for 6 wk AND gentamicin 6 mg/kg/day div q8h for 14 days CA-MRSA or MRSE: vancomycin 40–60 mg/kg/day IV div q8h AND gentamicin; ADD rifampin 20 mg/kg/day IV div q8–12h	Surgery may be necessary in acute phase; avoid cephalosporins (conflicting data on efficacy). For failures on vancomycin, consider daptomycin 6–8 mg/kg/day q24h AND gentamicin 6 mg/kg/day IV div q8h.

Condition	Therapy	Notes
– Pneumococcus, gonococcus, group A streptococcus	Penicillin G 200,000 U/kg/day IV div q4–6h for 4 wk; alternatives: ceftriaxone or vancomycin	Ceftriaxone for gonococcus until susceptibilities known. For penicillin non-susceptible strains of pneumococcus, use high-dosage penicillin G 300,000 U/kg/day IV div q4–6h or high-dosage ceftriaxone 100 mg/kg IV div q24h for 4 wk.
– Prosthetic valve/material[180,181]		
– Viridans streptococci		Follow echocardiogram for resolution of vegetation. For beta-lactam allergy: vancomycin.
Fully susceptible to penicillin	Ceftriaxone 100 mg/kg IV, IM q24h for 6 wk OR penicillin G 300,000 U/kg/day IV div q4–6h for 6 wk (AII); OR penicillin G or ceftriaxone AND gentamicin 6.0 mg/kg/day IM, IV div q8h for 14 days (AII)	Gentamicin is used for the first 2 wk of a total of 6 wk of therapy for prosthetic valve/material endocarditis.
Relatively resistant to penicillin	Penicillin G 300,000 U/kg/day IV div q4–6h for 6 wk, or ceftriaxone 100 mg/kg IV q24h for 6 wk; AND gentamicin 6.0 mg/kg/day IM, IV div q8h for 6 wk (AIII)	Gentamicin is used for all 6 wk of therapy for prosthetic valve/material endocarditis caused by relatively resistant strains.
– Enterococcus (see dosages under Native valve)		
– Staphylococci: S aureus, including CA-MRSA; S epidermidis. Consider continuing therapy at end of 6 wk if vegetations persist on echocardiogram.	MSSA or MSSE: nafcillin or oxacillin/nafcillin 150–200 mg/kg/day IV div q6h AND gentamicin 6 mg/kg/day div q8h AND rifampin 20 mg/kg/day IV div q8–12h IV (AIII) CA-MRSA or MRSE: vancomycin 40–60 mg/kg/day IV div q8h AND gentamicin 6 mg/kg/day div q8h AND rifampin 20 mg/kg/day IV div q8–12h IV (AIII)	Surgery may be necessary in acute phase; avoid cephalosporins (conflicting data on efficacy). For failure to respond in CA-MRSA, consider daptomycin 6–8 mg/kg/day q24h AND gentamicin 6 mg/kg/day div q8h (CIII).
– In highest risk patients: dental procedures that involve manipulation of the gingival or periodontal region of teeth	Amoxicillin 50 mg/kg PO 1 h before procedure OR ampicillin or ceftriaxone or cefazolin, all at 50 mg/kg IM/IV 30–60 min before procedure	If penicillin allergy: clindamycin 20 mg/kg PO (60 min before) or IV (30 min before); OR azithromycin 15 mg/kg or clarithromycin 15 mg/kg, 1 h before
– Genitourinary and gastrointestinal procedures	None	No longer recommended

G. CARDIOVASCULAR INFECTIONS (cont)

Clinical Diagnosis	Therapy (evidence grade)	Comments
Purulent pericarditis		
– Empiric (acute, bacterial: S aureus, group A streptococcus, pneumococcus, meningococcus, H influenzae type b)[187,188]	Vancomycin 40 mg/kg/day IV div q8h AND ceftriaxone 50–75 mg/kg/day q24h (AIII). For presumed staphylococcal infection, ADD gentamicin (AIII).	Increasingly uncommon with immunization against pneumococcus and H influenzae type b).[187] Pericardiocentesis is essential to establish diagnosis. Surgical drainage of pus with pericardial window or pericardiectomy is important to prevent tamponade.
– S aureus	For MSSA: oxacillin/nafcillin 150–200 mg/kg/day IV div q6h OR cefazolin 100 mg/kg/day IV div q8h For CA-MRSA: continue vancomycin	Continue therapy with gentamicin; consider use of rifampin in severe cases. Treatment for 3–4 wk.
– H influenzae type b in unimmunized children	Ceftriaxone 50 mg/kg/day q24h or cefotaxime 150 mg/kg/day div q8h; for 10–14 days (AIII)	Ampicillin for beta-lactamase–negative strains
– Pneumococcus, meningococcus, group A streptococcus	Penicillin G 200,000 U/kg/day IV, IM div q6h for 10–14 days OR ceftriaxone 50 mg/kg qd for 10–14 days (AIII)	Ceftriaxone or cefotaxime for penicillin-nonsusceptible pneumococci
– Coliform bacilli	Ceftriaxone 50–75 mg/kg/day q24h or cefotaxime 150 mg/kg/day div q8h for 3 wk or longer (AIII)	Alternative drugs depending on susceptibilities; for Enterobacter, Serratia, or Citrobacter use cefepime or meropenem.
– Tuberculous[13]	Isoniazid 10–15 mg/kg/day (max 300 mg) PO qd, IV for 6 mo AND rifampin 10–20 mg/kg/day (max 600 mg) PO qd, IV for 6 mo. ADD PZA 20–40 mg/kg/day PO qd for first 2 mo therapy; if suspected multidrug resistance, also add ethambutol 20 mg/kg/day PO qd (AIII).	Corticosteroids improve survival in adults: prednisone 1 mg/kg/day for 4 wk, then 0.5 mg/kg/day for 4 wk, then 0.25 mg/kg/day for 2 wk, then 0.1 mg/kg/day for 1 wk (AIII)[13]

H. GASTROINTESTINAL INFECTIONS (see Chapter 10 for parasitic infections)

Clinical Diagnosis	Therapy (evidence grade)	Comments
Diarrhea/Gastroenteritis		

Note on E coli and diarrheal disease: Antibiotic susceptibility of *E coli* varies considerably from region to region. For mild to moderate disease, TMP/SMX may be started as initial therapy, but for more severe disease, and for locations with rates of TMP/SMX resistance greater than 10% to 20%, oral 3rd-generation cephalosporins (eg, cefixime, cefdinir, ceftibuten), azithromycin, or ciprofloxacin should be used (AIII). Cultures and antibiotic susceptibility testing are recommended for significant disease (AIII).

Clinical Diagnosis	Therapy (evidence grade)	Comments
– Empiric therapy of community-associated diarrhea in the US (*E coli* [including O157:H7 strains], *Salmonella, Campylobacter,* and *Shigella* predominate; *Yersinia,* and parasites causing <5%; however, viral pathogens are far more common, especially for children <3 y)[189,190]	Cefixime 8 mg/kg/day PO qd (BII); OR azithromycin 10 mg/kg qd for 3 days (BII)	Alternatives: other oral 3rd-generation cephalosporins (eg, cefdinir, ceftibuten); or ciprofloxacin 30 mg/kg/day PO div bid; for 5 days; or rifaximin 600 mg/day div tid for 3 days (for nonfebrile, nonbloody diarrhea for children >11 y). Controversy exists regarding treatment of O157:H7 strains, with retrospective data to support treatment or withholding treatment.[191–193]
– Traveler's diarrhea: empiric therapy (*E coli, Campylobacter, Salmonella, Shigella,* plus many other pathogens including protozoa)[194–201]	Azithromycin 10 mg/kg qd for 3 days (AII); OR rifaximin 600 mg/day div tid for 3 days (for nonfebrile, nonbloody diarrhea for children ≥12 y) (BII); OR cefixime 8–10 mg/kg qd for 5 days (CII); OR ciprofloxacin 30 mg/kg/day div bid for 5 days (CII)	Susceptibility patterns of *E coli, Campylobacter, Salmonella,* and *Shigella* vary widely by country; check country-specific data for departing or returning travelers. Azithromycin preferable to ciprofloxacin for travelers to SE Asia given high prevalence of quinolone-resistant *Campylobacter.* Rifaximin is less effective than ciprofloxacin for invasive bloody bacterial enteritis; rifaximin may not be as efficacious for *Shigella* and other enterics in patients with dysentery. Adjunctive therapy with loperamide (antimotility) is not recommended for children <2 y and should be used only in nonfebrile, non-bloody diarrhea.[202,203] May shorten symptomatic illness by about 24 h.
– Traveler's diarrhea: prophylaxis[195,196]	– Prophylaxis: Early self-treatment with agents listed above is preferred over long-term prophylaxis, but may use prophylaxis for a short-term (<14 days) visit to very high-risk region: rifaximin (for older children), azithromycin, or bismuth subsalicylate (BIII).	

H. GASTROINTESTINAL INFECTIONS (see Chapter 10 for parasitic infections) (cont)

Clinical Diagnosis	Therapy (evidence grade)	Comments
– Campylobacter jejuni[205–207]	Azithromycin 10 mg/kg/day for 3 days (BII) or erythromycin 40 mg/kg/day PO div qid for 5 days (BII)	Alternatives: doxycycline or ciprofloxacin (high rate of fluoroquinolone resistance in Thailand and India). Single-dose azithromycin (1 g, once) is effective in adults.
– Cholera[200,208]	Azithromycin 20 mg/kg once; OR doxycycline 4 mg/kg/day (max 200 mg/day) PO div bid, for all ages	Ciprofloxacin or TMP/SMX (if susceptible)
– Clostridium difficile (antibiotic-associated colitis)[209,210]	Metronidazole 30 mg/kg/day PO div qid OR vancomycin 40 mg/kg/day PO div qid for 7 days; for relapsing C difficile enteritis, consider pulse therapy (1 wk on/1 wk off for 3–4 cycles) or prolonged tapering therapy[209]	Vancomycin is more effective for severe infection.[211] Fidaxomicin approved for adults; pediatric studies underway. Many infants and children may have asymptomatic colonization with C difficile.[211] Higher risk of relapse in children with multiple comorbidities.
– E coli		
Enterotoxigenic (etiology of most traveler's diarrhea)[197,199,212]	Azithromycin 10 mg/kg qd for 3 days; OR cefixime 8 mg/kg/day PO qd for 5 days	Most illnesses brief and self-limited Alternatives: ciprofloxacin or TMP/SMX Resistance increasing worldwide[199]
Enterohemorrhagic (O157:H7; shiga toxin–producing E coli; etiology of HUS)[191–193]	Controversy on whether treatment of O157:H7 diarrhea results in more or less toxin-mediated renal damage.[191–193] For severe infection, therapy as for enterotoxigenic strains above.	Injury to colonic mucosa may lead to invasive bacterial colitis.
Enteropathogenic	Neomycin 100 mg/kg/day PO div q6–8h for 5 days	Most traditional "enteropathogenic" strains are not toxigenic or invasive. Postinfection diarrhea may be problematic.
– Gastritis, peptic ulcer disease (Helicobacter pylori)[213–216]	Triple agent therapy: clarithromycin 7.5 mg/kg/dose 2–3 times each day, AND amoxicillin 40 mg/kg/dose (max 1 g) PO bid AND omeprazole 0.5 mg/kg/dose PO bid 2 wk (BII)	Most data from studies in adults; of effective regimens, no one combination has been shown superior. New, current regimens use 4 drugs (with metronidazole) initially, or with relapse, due to concerns for clarithromycin resistance.[213,215] Other regimens include bismuth, metronidazole instead of amoxicillin, and other proton pump inhibitors.

– Salmonellosis		
Non-typhoid strains[217,218]	Usually none for self-limited diarrhea (eg, diarrhea is much improved by the time culture results are available) For persisting symptomatic infection: azithromycin 10 mg/kg PO qd for 5 days (AII); OR ceftriaxone 75 mg/kg/day IV, IM q24h for 5 days (AII); OR cefixime 20–30 mg/kg/day PO for 5 days (BII); OR for susceptible strains: TMP/SMX (8 mg/kg/day of TMP) PO div bid for 5 days (AI)	Alternatives: ciprofloxacin 30 mg/kg/day PO div bid for 5 days (AI). Carriage of strains is prolonged in treated children.
Typhoid fever[219–222]	Azithromycin 10 mg/kg qd for 5–7 days (AII); OR ceftriaxone 75 mg/kg/day IV, IM q24h for 5 days (AII); OR cefixime 20–30 mg/kg/day PO, div q12h for 14 days (BII); OR for susceptible strains: TMP/SMX (8 mg/kg/day of TMP) PO div bid for 10 days (AI)	Watch for relapse if ceftriaxone used. Alternatives: ciprofloxacin 30 mg/kg/day PO div bid for 5–7 days (AI).
– Shigellosis[207,223–226]	Cefixime 8 mg/kg/day PO qd for 5 days (AII); OR azithromycin 10 mg/kg/day PO for 3 days (AII); OR ciprofloxacin 30 mg/kg/day PO div bid for 3–5 days (BII)	Alternatives for susceptible strains: TMP/SMX (8 mg/kg/day of TMP) PO div bid for 5 days; OR ampicillin (not amoxicillin). Ceftriaxone 50 mg/kg/day IM, IV if parenteral therapy necessary, for 2–5 days. Avoid antiperistaltic drugs. Treat to decrease communicability, even if symptoms resolving.
– *Yersinia enterocolitica*[227,228]	Antimicrobial therapy probably not of value for mild disease in normal hosts TMP/SMX PO, IV; OR ciprofloxacin PO, IV (BIII)	Alternatives: ceftriaxone or gentamicin May mimic appendicitis. Limited clinical data exist on oral therapy.

H. GASTROINTESTINAL INFECTIONS *(see Chapter 10 for parasitic infections)* (cont)

Clinical Diagnosis	Therapy (evidence grade)	Comments
– Appendicitis; bowel-associated (enteric gram-negative bacilli, *Bacteroides* spp, *Enterococcus* spp, increasingly *Pseudomonas*)[229–233]	Meropenem 60 mg/kg/day IV div q8h or imipenem 60 mg/kg/day IV div q6h; OR pip/tazo 240 mg piperacillin/kg/day div q6h; for 7–10 days or longer if suspicion of persisting intra-abdominal abscess (AII) Data support IV outpatient therapy[232] or oral step-down therapy[232] when clinically improved	Many other regimens may be effective, including ampicillin 150 mg/kg/day div q6h AND gentamicin 6–7.5 mg/kg/day IV, IM div q8h AND metronidazole 40 mg/kg/day IV div q8h; OR ceftriaxone 50 mg/kg q24h AND metronidazole 40 mg/kg/day IV div q8h. Gentamicin demonstrates poor activity at low pH; surgical source control is critical to achieve cure.
– Tuberculosis, abdominal (*Mycobacterium bovis*, from unpasteurized dairy products)[13,14,234,235]	INH 10–15 mg/kg/day (max 300 mg) PO qd for 6 mo AND rifampin 10–20 mg/kg/day (max 600 mg) PO qd for 6 mo. *M bovis* is resistant to PZA. If risk factors are present for multidrug resistance (eg, poor adherence to previous therapy), ADD ethambutol 20 mg/kg/day PO qd OR a fluoroquinolone (moxifloxacin or levofloxacin).	Directly observed therapy preferred; after 2+ wk of daily therapy, can change to twice-weekly dosing double dosage of INH (max 900 mg); rifampin remains same dosage (10–20 mg/kg/day, max 600 mg) (AII) LP ± CT of head for children ≤2 y with active disease to rule out occult, concurrent CNS infection (AIII)
Perirectal abscess (*Bacteroides* spp other anaerobes, enteric bacilli, and *S aureus* predominate)[236]	Clindamycin 30–40 mg/kg/day IV div q8h AND cefotaxime or ceftriaxone or gentamicin (BIII)	Surgical drainage alone may be curative.
Peritonitis – Peritoneal dialysis indwelling catheter infection (staphylococcal; enteric gram-negatives; yeast)[237,238]	Antibiotic added to dialysate in concentrations approximating those attained in serum for systemic disease (eg, 4 µg/mL for gentamicin; 25 µg/mL for vancomycin, 125 µg/mL for cefazolin, 25 µg/mL for ciprofloxacin) after a larger loading dose (AII)[238]	Selection of antibiotic based on organism isolated from peritoneal fluid; systemic antibiotics if there is accompanying bacteremia/fungemia
– Primary (pneumococcus or group A streptococcus)[239]	Ceftriaxone 50 mg/kg/day q24h, or cefotaxime 150 mg/kg/day div q8h; if penicillin-S, then penicillin G 150,000 U/kg/day IV div q6h; for 7–10 days (AII)	Other antibiotics according to culture and susceptibility tests

I. GENITAL AND SEXUALLY TRANSMITTED INFECTIONS

Clinical Diagnosis	Therapy (evidence grade)	Comments
Consider testing for HIV and other STIs in a child with one documented STI; consider sexual abuse in prepubertal children. The most recent CDC STI treatment guidelines are posted online at www.cdc.gov/std/treatment.		
Chancroid (*Haemophilus ducreyi*)[162]	Azithromycin 1 g PO as single dose OR ceftriaxone 250 mg IM as single dose	Alternative: erythromycin 1.5 g/day PO tid for 7 days OR ciprofloxacin 1,000 mg PO qd, div bid for 3 days
C trachomatis (cervicitis, urethritis)[42,240]	Azithromycin 20 mg/kg (max 1 g) PO for 1 dose; OR doxycycline (patients >7 y) 40 mg/kg/day (max 200 mg/day) PO div bid for 7 days	Alternatives: erythromycin 2 g/day PO div qid for 7 days; OR levofloxacin 500 mg PO q24h for 7 days
Epididymitis (associated with positive urine cultures and STIs)[42,241,242]	Ceftriaxone 50 mg/kg/day q24h for 7–10 days AND (for older children) doxycycline 200 mg/day div bid	Microbiology not well studied in children; in infants, also associated with urogenital tract anomalies. Treat infants for *S aureus* and *E coli*; may resolve spontaneously; in STI, caused by *Chlamydia* and gonococcus.
Gonorrhea		
– Newborns	See Chapter 5.	
– Genital infections (uncomplicated vulvovaginitis, cervicitis, urethritis, or proctitis)[42,240,243]	Ceftriaxone 250 mg IM for 1 dose (regardless of weight); AND azithromycin 1 g PO for 1 dose or doxycycline 200 mg/day div q12h x 7 days	Cefixime no longer recommended due to increasing cephalosporin resistance.[244] Fluoroquinolones are no longer recommended due to resistance.
– Pharyngitis[42,245]	Ceftriaxone 250 mg IM for 1 dose (regardless of weight); AND azithromycin 1 g PO for 1 dose or doxycycline 200 mg/day div q12h x 7 days	
– Disseminated gonococcal infection[42,245]	Ceftriaxone 50 mg/kg/day IM, IV q24h (max: 1 g); total course for 7 days	No studies in children: increase dosage for meningitis.

I. GENITAL AND SEXUALLY TRANSMITTED INFECTIONS (cont)

Clinical Diagnosis	Therapy (evidence grade)	Comments
Herpes simplex virus, genital infection[42,246,247]	Acyclovir 20–25 mg/kg/dose (max 400 mg) PO tid for 7–10 days (first episode) (AI); OR valacyclovir 20 mg/kg/dose of extemporaneous suspension (directions on package label), max 1.0 g PO BID for 7–10 days (first episode) (AI); OR famciclovir 250 mg PO TID for 7–10 days (AI); for more severe infection: acyclovir 15 mg/kg/day IV div q8h as 1 h infusion for 7–10 days (AII) For recurrent episodes: treat as above with acyclovir PO, valacyclovir PO, or famciclovir PO, immediately when symptoms begin, for 5 days For suppression: acyclovir 20–25 mg/kg/dose (max 400 mg) PO bid; OR valacyclovir 20 mg/kg/dose PO qd (little long-term safety data in children; no efficacy data in children)	
Lymphogranuloma venereum (C trachomatis)[42]	Doxycycline 4 mg/kg/day (max 200 mg/day) PO (patients >7 y) div bid for 21 days; OR erythromycin 2 g/day PO div qid; for 21 days	Azithromycin 1.0 g PO once weekly for 3 wk
Pelvic inflammatory disease (Chlamydia, gonococcus, plus anaerobes)[42,248]	Cefoxitin 2 g IV q6h; AND doxycycline 200 mg/day PO or IV div bid; OR clindamycin 900 mg IV q8h and gentamicin 1.5 mg/kg IV, IM q8h for 14 days	Drugs given IV until clinical improvement for 24 h, followed by doxycycline 200 mg/day PO div bid AND clindamycin 1,800 mg/day PO div qid to complete 14 days of therapy Optional regimen: ceftriaxone 250 mg IM for 1 dose AND doxycycline 200 mg/day PO div bid; WITH/WITHOUT metronidazole 1 g/day PO div bid; for 14 days
Syphilis[42,249] (test for HIV)		
– Congenital	See Chapter 5.	

– Neurosyphilis (positive CSF VDRL or CSF pleocytosis with serologic diagnosis of syphilis)	Crystalline penicillin G 200–300,000 U/kg/day (max 24 mill U/day) div q6h for 10–14 days (AIII)	
– Primary, secondary	Benzathine penicillin G 50,000 U/kg (max 2,400,000 U) IM as a single dose (AIII); do not use benzathine-procaine penicillin mixtures.	Follow-up serologic tests at 6, 12, and 24 mo; 15% may remain seropositive despite adequate treatment. If allergy to penicillin: doxycycline (patients >7 y) 4 mg/kg/day (max 200 mg) PO div bid for 14 days. CSF examination should be obtained for children being treated for primary or secondary syphilis to rule out asymptomatic neurosyphilis. Test for HIV.
– Syphilis of <1 y duration, without clinical symptoms (early latent syphilis)	Benzathine penicillin G 50,000 U/kg (max 2,400,000 U) IM as a single dose (AIII)	Alternative if allergy to penicillin: doxycycline (patients >7 y) 4 mg/kg/day (max 200 mg/day) PO bid for 14 days
– Syphilis of >1 y duration, without clinical symptoms (late latent syphilis) or syphilis of unknown duration	Benzathine penicillin G 50,000 U/kg (max 2,400,000 U) IM weekly for 3 doses (AIII)	Alternative if allergy to penicillin: doxycycline (patients >7 y) 4 mg/kg/day (max 200 mg/day) PO bid for 28 days. Look for neurologic, eye, and aortic complications of tertiary syphilis.
Trichomoniasis[42]	Metronidazole 2 g PO as a single dose, OR 500 mg PO bid for 7 days	Tinidazole 50 mg/kg (max 2 g) PO for 1 dose twice daily for 7 days
Urethritis, nongonococcal (see page 69 for gonorrhea therapy)[42]	Azithromycin 20 mg/kg (max 1 g) PO for 1 dose, OR doxycycline (patients >7 y) 40 mg/kg/day (max 200 mg/day) PO bid for 7 days (AII)	Erythromycin, levofloxacin, or ofloxacin

6

Antimicrobial Therapy According to Clinical Syndromes

I. GENITAL AND SEXUALLY TRANSMITTED INFECTIONS (cont)

Clinical Diagnosis	Therapy (evidence grade)	Comments
– Bacterial vaginosis[250]	Metronidazole 500 mg PO twice daily for 7 days or metronidazole vaginal gel (0.75%) qd for 5 days	Alternative: tinidazole 1 g PO qd for 5 days, OR clindamycin 300 mg PO bid for 7 days or clindamycin vaginal cream for 7 days Relapse common Caused by synergy of *Gardnerella* with anaerobes
– Candidiasis, vulvovaginal[42,251]	Fluconazole 5 mg/kg PO (max 150 mg) for 1 dose; topical treatment with azole creams (see Comments).	Many topical vaginal azole agents are available without prescription (eg, butoconazole, clotrimazole, miconazole, ticonazole) and some require a prescription for unique agents or unique dosing regimens (terconazole, butoconazole).
– *Shigella*[252]	Cefixime 8 mg/kg PO qd for 5 days; OR ciprofloxacin 30 mg/kg/day PO div bid for 5 days	50% have bloody discharge; usually not associated with diarrhea.
– *Streptococcus*, group A[253]	Penicillin V 50–75 mg/kg/day PO div tid for 10 days	Amoxicillin 50–75 mg/kg/day PO div tid

J. CENTRAL NERVOUS SYSTEM INFECTIONS

Clinical Diagnosis	Therapy (evidence grade)	Comments
Abscess, brain (respiratory tract flora, skin flora, or bowel flora, depending on the pathogenesis of infection based on underlying comorbid disease and origin of bacteremia)[254-256]	Until etiology established, cover normal flora of respiratory tract, skin, and/or bowel, based on individual patient evaluation: meropenem 120 mg/kg/day div q8h (AIII); OR nafcillin 150–200 mg/kg/day IV div q6h AND cefotaxime 200–300 mg/kg/day IV div q6h or ceftriaxone 100 mg/kg/day IV q24h AND metronidazole 30 mg/kg/day IV div q8h (BIII); for 2–3 wk after successful drainage (depending on pathogen, size of abscess, and response to therapy); longer course if no surgery (3–6 wk) (BIII)	Surgery for abscesses ≥2 cm diameter. If CA-MRSA suspected, ADD vancomycin 60 mg/kg/day IV div q8h ± rifampin 20 mg/kg/day IV div q12h, pending culture results. If secondary to chronic otitis, include meropenem or cefepime in regimen for anti-*Pseudomonas* activity. Follow abscess size by CT. For treatment of rare and unusual pathogens that present with symptoms of encephalitis, see IDSA guidelines on encephalitis (2008).[257]

Encephalitis[257,258]	
— Amebic (*Naegleria fowleri, Balamuthia mandrillaris,* and *Acanthamoeba*)	See Chapter 10 (parasitic pathogens), Amebiasis.
— CMV[257]	Not studied in children. Consider ganciclovir (10–20 mg/kg/day IV div q12h); for severe immunocompromise, ADD foscarnet. (180 mg/kg/day IV div q 8 h) for 3 weeks. High-dose ganciclovir[259] IV (20 mg/kg/day div q12h) not well studied. Reduce dose for renal insufficiency. Watch for neutropenia.
— Enterovirus	Supportive therapy; no antivirals currently available
— EBV[260]	Not studied. Consider ganciclovir (10–20 mg/kg/day IV div q12h) or acyclovir (60 mg/kg/day IV div q8h). Efficacy and toxicity of high-dose ganciclovir and acyclovir are not well defined; some experts recommend against antiviral treatment.[257]
— Herpes simplex virus[257,261]	Acyclovir 60 mg/kg/day IV as 1–2 h infusion div q8h; for 21 days for infants ≤ 4 mo. For older infants and children, 45–60 mg/kg/day IV for 21 days (AIII). (See Chapter 5 for neonatal infection.) Safety of high-dose acyclovir (60 mg/kg/day) not well defined beyond the neonatal period; can be used, but monitor for neurotoxicity and nephrotoxicity; FDA has approved acyclovir at this dosage for encephalitis for children up to 12 y.
— Toxoplasma	See Chapter 10.
— Arbovirus (flavivirus—West Nile, St Louis encephalitis, tickborne encephalitis; togavirus—Western equine encephalitis, Eastern equine encephalitis; bunyavirus—LaCrosse encephalitis, California encephalitis)[257,258]	Supportive therapy Investigational only (antiviral, interferon, immune globulins)

J. CENTRAL NERVOUS SYSTEM INFECTIONS (cont)

Clinical Diagnosis	Therapy (evidence grade)	Comments
Meningitis, bacterial, community-associated		
NOTES		
— In areas where pen-R pneumococci exist (>5% of invasive strains), initial empiric therapy for suspect pneumococcal meningitis should be with vancomycin AND cefotaxime or ceftriaxone until susceptibility test results are available.		
— Dexamethasone (0.6 mg/kg/day IV div q6h for 2 days) as an adjunct to antibiotic therapy decreases hearing deficits and other neurologic sequelae in adults and children (for *Haemophilus* and pneumococcus; not studied in children for meningococcus or *E coli*). The first dose of dexamethasone is given before or concurrent with the first dose of antibiotic; probably little benefit if given ≥1 h after the antibiotic.[262,263]		
— We hope to see more data on osmotic therapy before we recommend it, based on early data suggesting that oral glycerol (85% solution, 1 mL to contain 1 g of glycerol) given at 1.5 g (1.5 mL) per kg (max 25 mL) every 6 h for 48 h, may decrease neurologic sequelae.[264,265]		
— Empiric therapy[266]	Cefotaxime 200–300 mg/kg/day IV div q6h, or ceftriaxone 100 mg/kg/day IV q24h; AND vancomycin 60 mg/kg/day IV div q8h (AII)	If Gram stain or cultures demonstrate a pathogen other than pneumococcus, vancomycin is not needed; vancomycin used empirically only for possible pen-R pneumococcus.
— H influenzae type b[266]	Cefotaxime 200–300 mg/kg/day IV div q6h, or ceftriaxone 100 mg/kg/day IV q24h; for 10 days (AI)	Alternative: ampicillin 200–400 mg/kg/day IV div q6h (for beta-lactamase–negative strains) OR chloramphenicol 100 mg/kg/day IV div q6h
— Meningococcus (*Neisseria meningitidis*)[266]	Penicillin G 250,000 U/kg/day IV div q4h; or ceftriaxone 100 mg/kg/day IV q24h, or cefotaxime 200 mg/kg/day IV div q6h; treatment course for 7 days (AI)	Meningococcal prophylaxis: rifampin 10 mg/kg PO q12h for 4 doses OR ceftriaxone 125–250 mg IM once OR ciprofloxacin 500 mg PO once (adolescents and adults)
— Neonatal	See Chapter 5.	
— Pneumococcus (*S pneumoniae*)[266]	For penicillin- and cephalosporin-susceptible strains: penicillin G 250,000 U/kg/day IV div q4–6h, OR ceftriaxone 100 mg/kg/day IV q24h or cefotaxime 200–300 mg/kg/day IV div q6h; for 10 days (AI) For pen-R pneumococci: continue the combination of vancomycin and cephalosporin IV for total course (AIII)	Some pneumococci may be resistant to penicillin but susceptible to cefotaxime and ceftriaxone and may be treated with the cephalosporin alone. Test-of-cure LP helpful in those with pen-R pneumococci.

Meningitis, TB
(M tuberculosis; M bovis)[13,14]

For non-immunocompromised children:
INH 15 mg/kg/day PO, IV div q12–24h AND rifampin 15 mg/kg/day PO, IV, div q12–24h for 12 mo AND PZA 30 mg/kg/day PO div q12–24h for first 2 mo of therapy, AND streptomycin 30 mg/kg/day IV, IM div q12h for first 4–8 wk of therapy until susceptibility test results available. For recommendations for drug-resistant strains and treatment of TB in HIV-infected patients, visit the CDC Web site for TB: www.cdc.gov/tb.

Hyponatremia from inappropriate ADH secretion is common; ventricular drainage may be necessary for obstructive hydrocephalus.
Corticosteroids (can use the same dexamethasone dose as for bacterial meningitis, 0.6 mg/kg/day div q6h) for 2–4 wk until neurologically stable, then taper dose for 1–3 mo to decrease neurologic complications and improve prognosis by decreasing the incidence of infarction.[267]

Shunt infections: The use of antibiotic-impregnated shunts has decreased the frequency of this infection.[268] Shunt removal usually necessary for cure.[269]

– Empiric therapy pending Gram stain and culture[266,269]

Vancomycin 60 mg/kg/day IV div q8h, AND ceftriaxone 100 mg/kg/day IV q24h (AII)

If Gram stain shows only gram-positive cocci, can use vancomycin alone.
Ceftazidime, cefepime, or meropenem should be used instead of ceftriaxone if *Pseudomonas* is suspected.

– *S epidermidis* or *S aureus*[266,269]

Vancomycin (for *S epidermidis* and for CA-MRSA) 60 mg/kg/day IV div q8h; OR nafcillin (if organisms susceptible) 150–200 mg/kg/day AND (if severe infection or slow response) gentamicin or rifampin; for 10–14 days (AIII)

Shunt removal usually necessary; may need to treat with ventriculostomy until ventricular CSF cultures negative; obtain CSF cultures at time of shunt replacement, continue therapy an additional 48–72 h pending cultures.

– Gram-negative bacilli[266,269]

Empiric therapy with meropenem 120 mg/kg/day IV div q8h OR cefepime 150 mg/kg/day IV div q8h (AIII) For *E coli*: ceftriaxone 100 mg/kg/day IV q12h OR cefotaxime 200–300 mg/kg/day IV div q6h; ADD gentamicin 6–7.5 mg/kg/day IV until CSF sterile; for 21 days or longer

Remove shunt. Select appropriate therapy based on in vitro susceptibilities.
Intrathecal therapy with aminoglycosides not routinely necessary with highly active beta-lactam therapy and shunt removal.

K. URINARY TRACT INFECTIONS

Clinical Diagnosis	Therapy (evidence grade)	Comments
NOTE: Antibiotic susceptibility profiles of *E coli*, the most common cause of urinary tract infection, vary considerably. For mild disease, TMP/SMX may be started as initial therapy if local susceptibility ≥80% and a 20% failure rate is acceptable. For moderate to severe disease (possible pyelonephritis), obtain cultures and begin oral 2nd- or 3rd-generation cephalosporins (cefuroxime, cefaclor, cefprozil, cefixime, ceftibuten, cefdinir, cefpodoxime), ciprofloxacin PO, or ceftriaxone IM. Antibiotic susceptibility testing will help direct your therapy to the most narrow spectrum agent.		
Cystitis, acute (*E coli*)[270,271]	For mild disease: TMP/SMX (8 mg/kg/day of TMP) PO div bid for 3 days For moderate to severe disease: cefixime 8 mg/kg/day PO qd; OR ceftriaxone 50 mg/kg IM q24h for 3–5 days (with normal anatomy) (BIII); follow-up culture after 36–48 h treatment ONLY if still symptomatic	Alternative: amoxicillin 30 mg/kg/day PO div tid if susceptible (BIII); ciprofloxacin 15–20 mg/kg/day PO div bid for otherwise resistant organisms
Nephronia, lobar *E coli* and other enteric rods (also called focal bacterial nephritis)[272,273]	Ceftriaxone 50 mg/kg/day IM/IV q24h. Duration depends on resolution of cellulitis vs development of abscess (10–21 days) (AIII).	Invasive, consolidative parenchymal infection; complication of pyelonephritis, can evolve into renal abscess.
Pyelonephritis, acute (*E coli*)[270,271,274–276]	Ceftriaxone 50 mg/kg/day IV, IM q24h OR gentamicin 5–6 mg/kg/day IV, IM q24h; OR use meropenem IV, imipenem IV, or ertapenem IV for ESBL-positive strains. Switch to oral therapy following clinical response (BII). If organisms resistant to amoxicillin and TMP/SMX, use an oral 2nd- or 3rd-generation cephalosporin (BII); if cephalosporin-R, can use ciprofloxacin PO 30 mg/kg/day div q12h (BII); for 7–10 days total (depending on response to therapy).	For mild to moderate infection, oral therapy is likely to be as effective as IV/IM therapy for susceptible strains, down to 3 months of age. If bacteremia documented, and infant is <2–3 mo, rule out meningitis and treat 14 days IV or IM (AIII). Aminoglycosides at any dose are more nephrotoxic than beta-lactams (AI).
Recurrent urinary tract infection, prophylaxis[270,277–279]	Only for those with grade III–V reflux or with recurrent febrile UTI: TMP/SMX (2 mg/kg/dose of TMP) PO qd OR nitrofurantoin 1–2 mg/kg PO qd at bedtime; more rapid resistance may develop using beta-lactams (BII).	Prophylaxis no longer recommended for patients with grade I–II reflux and no evidence of renal damage. Early treatment of new infections is recommended for these children. Resistance eventually develops to every antibiotic; follow resistance patterns for each patient.

L. MISCELLANEOUS SYSTEMIC INFECTIONS

Clinical Diagnosis	Therapy (evidence grade)	Comments
Actinomycosis[280,281]	Penicillin G 250,000 U/kg/day IV div q6h, or ampicillin 150 mg/kg/day IV div q8h until improved (often up to 6 wk); then long-term convalescent therapy with penicillin V 100 mg/kg/day (up to 4 g/day) PO for 6–12 mo (AII)	Surgery as indicated Alternatives: amoxicillin, clindamycin, erythromycin; ceftriaxone IM/IV, doxycycline for children >7 y
Anaplasmosis (human granulocytotropic anaplasmosis), *Anaplasma phagocytophilum*	Doxycycline 4 mg/kg/day IV, PO (max 200 mg/day) div bid for 7–10 days (regardless of age) (AIII)	For mild disease, consider rifampin 20 mg/kg/day PO div bid for 7–10 days (BII).
Anthrax, sepsis/pneumonia (inhalation), cutaneous, gastrointestinal[15,282,283]	For bioterror-associated infection (regardless of age): ciprofloxacin 20–30 mg/kg/day IV div q12h, OR levofloxacin 16 mg/kg/day IV div q12h not to exceed 250 mg/dose (AIII)	For oral step-down therapy, can use oral ciprofloxacin or doxycycline; if susceptible, can use penicillin, amoxicillin, or clindamycin. For community-associated anthrax infection, amoxicillin (75 mg/kg/day div q8h) or doxycycline for children >7 y should be effective.
Appendicitis (see Peritonitis)		
Brucellosis[284–287]	Doxycycline 4 mg/kg/day PO (max 200 mg/day) div bid (for children >7 y) AND rifampin (15–20 mg/kg/day div q12h) (BIII); OR (for children <8 y) TMP/SMX (10 mg/kg/day of TMP) IV, PO div q12h AND rifampin (15–20 mg/kg/day div q12h) (BIII); for 4–8 wk	Combination therapy with rifampin will decrease the risk of relapse. ADD gentamicin 6–7.5 mg/kg/day IV, IM div q8h for the first 1–2 wk of therapy to further decrease risk of relapse[286] (BIII), particularly for endocarditis, osteomyelitis, or meningitis. Prolonged treatment for 4–6 mo and surgical debridement may be necessary for deep infections (AIII).

L. MISCELLANEOUS SYSTEMIC INFECTIONS (cont)

Clinical Diagnosis	Therapy (evidence grade)	Comments
Chickenpox/Shingles (varicella-zoster virus)[290,291]	Acyclovir 30 mg/kg/day IV as 1–2 h infusion div q8h; for 10 days (acyclovir doses of 45–60 mg/kg/day in 3 divided doses IV should be used for disseminated or central nervous system infection). Dosing can also be provided as 1,500 mg/m²/day IV div q8h. Duration in immunocompromised children: 7–14 days, based on clinical response (AI). For treatment in normal immunocompetent children, acyclovir 80 mg/kg/day PO div qid, for 5 days (AI). Valacyclovir pharmacokinetics have been assessed in an extemporaneously[291] compounded suspension of crushed tablets and simple syrup (60 mg/kg/day div tid) for children 3 mo to 12 y; instructions for preparation provided in package insert, and shelf life is 28 days.	See Chapter 9; therapy for 10 days in immunocompromised children. Famciclovir can be made into a suspension with 25-mg and 100-mg sprinkle capsules.[292] See Chapter 9 for dosages by body weight. No treatment data in children (CIII).
Ehrlichiosis (human monocytic ehrlichiosis, caused by *Ehrlichia chaffeensis*, and *Ehrlichia ewingii*)[293–296]	Doxycycline 4 mg/kg/day IV, PO div bid (max 100 mg/dose) for 7–10 days (regardless of age) (AII)	For mild disease, consider rifampin 20 mg/kg/day PO div bid (max 300 mg/dose) for 7–10 days (BII)
Febrile neutropenic patient (empiric therapy of invasive infection: *Pseudomonas*, enteric gram-negative bacilli, staphylococci, streptococci, yeast, fungi)[297]	Cefepime 150 mg/kg/day IV div q8h (AI); or meropenem 60 mg/kg/day div q8h (AII); OR ceftazidime 150 mg/kg/day IV div q8h AND tobramycin 6 mg/kg/day IV q8h (AII) ADD vancomycin 40 mg/kg/day IV q8h if methicillin-resistant *S aureus* or coag-negative staph suspected (eg, central catheter infection) (AII) ADD metronidazole to ceftazidime or cefepime if colitis or other deep anaerobic infection suspected (AII)	Alternatives: other anti-*Pseudomonas* beta-lactams (imipenem, pip/tazo) AND anti-staphylococcal antibiotics. If no response in 4–7 days and no bacterial etiology demonstrated, consider additional empiric therapy with antifungals (BII); dosages and formulations outlined in Chapter 8. For low-risk patients with close follow-up, oral therapy with amox/clav and ciprofloxacin may be used.[285]
Human immunodeficiency virus infection	See Chapter 9.	

Infant botulism[298]	Botulism immune globulin for infants (BabyBIG) 50 mg/kg IV for 1 dose (AI); BabyBIG can be obtained from the California Department of Public Health at www.infantbotulism.org.	www.infantbotulism.org provides information for physicians and parents. Web site organized by the California Department of Public Health (accessed November 11, 2013). Aminoglycosides should be avoided as they potentiate the neuromuscular effect of botulinum toxin.
Kawasaki syndrome[299-301]	No antibiotics; IVIG 2 g/kg as single dose (AI); may need to repeat dose in up to 15% of children for persisting fever that lasts 24 hours after completion of the IVIG infusion (AII). For subsequent relapse, consult an infectious disease physician or pediatric cardiologist.	Aspirin 80–100 mg/kg/day div qid in acute, febrile phase; once afebrile for 24–48 h, initiate low dosage (3–5 mg/kg/day) aspirin therapy for 6–8 wk (assuming echocardiogram is normal). Role of corticosteroids[300,301] and infliximab[302] for IVIG-resistant Kawasaki syndrome under investigation but may improve outcome in severe cases.
Leprosy (Hansen disease)[304]	Dapsone 1 mg/kg/day PO qd AND rifampin 10 mg/kg/day PO qd; ADD (for multibacillary disease) clofazimine 1 mg/kg/day PO qd; for 12 mo for paucibacillary disease; for 24 mo for multibacillary disease (AII)	Consult HRSA (National Hansen's Disease Program) at www.hrsa.gov/hansensdisease (accessed November 11, 2013) for advice about treatment and free antibiotics: 800/642-2477.
Leptospirosis[305,306]	Penicillin G 250,000 U/kg/day IV, IM div q6h, or ceftriaxone 50 mg/kg/day q24h; for 7 days (BII) For mild disease, doxycycline (>7 years) 4 mg/kg/day (max 200 mg/day) PO bid for 7–10 days and for those ≤7 years or intolerant of doxycycline, azithromycin 20 mg/kg on day one, 10 mg/kg on days 2 and 3 (BII)	Alternative: amoxicillin for children ≤7 y of age with mild disease
Lyme disease (*Borrelia burgdorferi*)[295-307]	Neurologic evaluation, including LP, if there is clinical suspicion of CNS involvement	
– Early localized disease	>7 y of age: doxycycline 4 mg/kg/day (max 200 mg/day) PO bid for 14–21 days (AII) ≤7 y of age: amoxicillin 50 mg/kg/day (max 1.5 g/day) PO tid for 14–21 days (AII)	Alternative: erythromycin 30 mg/kg/day PO tid

Antimicrobial Therapy According to Clinical Syndromes

L. MISCELLANEOUS SYSTEMIC INFECTIONS (cont)

Clinical Diagnosis	Therapy (evidence grade)	Comments
Arthritis (no CNS disease)	Oral therapy as outlined above; for 28 days (AIII)	Persistent or recurrent joint swelling after treatment: repeat a 4-wk course of oral antibiotics or give ceftriaxone 75–100 mg/kg IV q24h IV OR penicillin 300,000 U/kg/day IV div q4h; either for 14–28 days
Erythema migrans	Oral therapy as outlined above; for 21 days (AIII)	
Isolated facial (Bell) palsy	Oral therapy as outlined above; for 21–28 days (AIII)	LP is not routinely required unless CNS symptoms present. Treatment to prevent late sequelae; will not provide a quick response for palsy.
Carditis	Ceftriaxone 75–100 mg/kg IV q24h IV OR penicillin 300,000 U/kg/day IV div q4h; for 14–21 days (AIII)	
Neuroborreliosis	Ceftriaxone 75–100 mg/kg IV q24h, or penicillin G 300,000 U/kg/day IV div q4h; for 14–28 days (AIII)	
Melioidosis (Burkholderia pseudomallei)[308-310]	Acute sepsis: meropenem 75 mg/kg/day div q8h; OR ceftazidime 150 mg/kg/day IV div q8h; followed by TMP/SMX (10 mg/kg/day of TMP) PO div bid for 3–6 mo	Alternative convalescent therapy: amox/clav (90 mg/kg/day amox div tid, not bid) for children ≤7 y, or doxycycline for children >7 y; for 20 wk (AII)
Mycobacteria, nontuberculous[8-12,311]		
– Adenitis in normal host (see Adenitis under Skin and Soft Tissue Infections)	Excision usually curative (BII); azithromycin PO OR clarithromycin PO for 6–12 wk (with or without rifampin) if susceptible (BII)	Antibiotic susceptibility patterns are quite variable; cultures should guide therapy; medical therapy 60%–70% effective. Newer data suggest toxicity of antimicrobials may not be worth the small clinical benefit.
– Pneumonia or disseminated infection in compromised hosts (HIV or gamma interferon receptor deficiency)	Usually treated with 3 or 4 active drugs (eg, clarithromycin OR azithromycin, AND amikacin, cefoxitin, meropenem). Also test for ciprofloxacin, TMP/SMX, ethambutol, rifampin, linezolid, clofazimine, and doxycycline (BII)	See Chapter 11 for dosages; cultures are essential, as the susceptibility patterns of nontuberculous mycobacteria are varied.

Condition (organism)	Therapy	Comments
Nocardiosis (*Nocardia asteroides* and *Nocardia brasiliensis*)[312,313]	TMP/SMX (8 mg/kg/day of TMP) div bid or sulfisoxazole 120–150 mg/kg/day PO div qid for 6–12 wk or longer. For severe infection, particularly in immuno-compromised hosts, use ceftriaxone or imipenem AND amikacin 15–20 mg/kg/day IM, IV div q8h (AIII).	Wide spectrum of disease from skin lesions to brain abscess Surgery when indicated Alternatives: doxycycline (for children >7 y of age), amox/clav, or linezolid
Plague (*Yersinia pestis*)[314–316]	Gentamicin 7.5 mg/kg/day IV div q8h (AII)	Doxycycline 4 mg/kg/day (max 200 mg/day) PO div bid; or ciprofloxacin 30 mg/kg/day PO div bid
Q fever (*Coxiella burnetii*)[317,318]	Acute stage: doxycycline 4.4 mg/kg/day (max 200 mg/day) PO bid for 14 days (AII) for children of any age Endocarditis and chronic disease (ongoing symptoms for 6–12 mo): doxycycline for children >7 y AND hydroxychloroquine for 18–36 mo (AIII) Seek advice from pediatric ID specialist for children ≤7 y: May require TMP-SMX, 8–10 mg TMP/kg/day div q12h with doxycycline; or levofloxacin with rifampin for 18 mo	Follow doxycycline and hydroxychloroquine serum concentrations during endocarditis/chronic disease therapy. CNS: Use fluoroquinolone (no prospective data) (BII). Clarithromycin may be an alternative based on limited data (CIII).
Rocky Mountain spotted fever (fever, petechial rash with centripetal spread; *Rickettsia rickettsii*)[319,320]	Doxycycline 4.4 mg/kg/day (max 200 mg/day) PO div bid for 7–10 days (AI) for children of any age	Start empiric therapy early.
Tetanus (*Clostridium tetani*)[321,322]	Metronidazole 30 mg/kg/day IV, PO div q8h or penicillin G 100,000 U/kg/day IV div q6h for 10–14 days AND tetanus immune globulin (TIG) 3,000–6,000 U IM (AII)	Wound debridement essential; IVIG may provide antibody to toxin if TIG not available. Immunize with Td or Tdap. See Chapter 14 for prophylaxis recommendations.
Toxic shock syndrome (toxin-producing strains of *S aureus* [including MRSA] or group A streptococcus)[6,7,323,324]	Empiric: Vancomycin 45 mg/kg/day IV div q8h AND oxacillin/nafcillin 150 mg/kg/day IV div q6h, AND clindamycin 30–40 mg/kg/day div q8h ± gentamicin for 7–10 days (AIII)	Clindamycin added for the initial 48–72 h of therapy to decrease toxin production; IVIG has a theoretical benefit and may bind circulating toxin (CIII). For MSSA: oxacillin/nafcillin AND clindamycin ± gentamicin. For CA-MRSA: vancomycin AND clindamycin ± gentamicin. For group A streptococcus: penicillin G AND clindamycin.
Tularemia (*Francisella tularensis*)[151,152]	Gentamicin 6–7.5 mg/kg/day IM, IV div q8h; for 10–14 days (AII)	Alternatives: doxycycline (for 14–21 days) or ciprofloxacin (for 10 days)

7. Preferred Therapy for Specific Bacterial and Mycobacterial Pathogens

NOTES

- For fungal, viral, and parasitic infections see chapters 8, 9, and 10, respectively.

- Limitations of space do not permit listing of all possible alternative antimicrobials.

- **Abbreviations:** amox/clav, amoxicillin/clavulanate (Augmentin); amp/sul, ampicillin/sulbactam (Unasyn); CA-MRSA, community-associated methicillin-resistant *Staphylococcus aureus;* CDC, Centers for Disease Control and Prevention; CNS, central nervous system; ESBL, extended spectrum beta-lactamase; HRSA, Health Resources and Services Administration; IM, intramuscular; IV, intravenous; KPC, *Klebsiella pneumoniae* carbapenemase; MRSA, methicillin-resistant *S aureus;* MSSA, methicillin-susceptible *S aureus;* NDM, New Delhi Metallo-beta-lactamase; pen-S, penicillin-susceptible; pip/tazo, piperacillin/tazobactam (Zosyn); PO, oral; PZA, pyrazinamide; qd, once daily; ticar/clav, ticarcillin/clavulanate (Timentin); TMP/SMX, trimethoprim/ sulfamethoxazole; UTI, urinary tract infection.

Organism	Clinical Illness	Drug of Choice (evidence grade)	Alternatives
Acinetobacter baumanii[1-3]	Sepsis, meningitis, nosocomial pneumonia	Meropenem (BIII) or other carbapenem	Use culture results to guide therapy; ceftazidime, amp/sul; pip/tazo; TMP/SMX; ciprofloxacin; tigecycline; colistin. Watch for emergence of resistance on therapy. Consider combination therapy for life-threatening infection.
Actinomyces israelii[4]	Actinomycosis (cervicofacial, thoracic, abdominal)	Penicillin G; ampicillin (CIII)	Amoxicillin; doxycycline; clindamycin; ceftriaxone; imipenem
Aeromonas hydrophila[5,6]	Diarrhea	Ciprofloxacin (CIII)	Azithromycin, cefepime, TMP/SMX
	Sepsis, cellulitis, necrotizing fasciitis	Ceftazidime (BIII)	Cefepime; ceftriaxone, meropenem; ciprofloxacin
Aggregatibacter (formerly Actinobacillus) actinomycetemcomitans[7]	Periodontitis, abscesses (including brain), endocarditis	Ampicillin (amoxicillin) ± gentamicin (CIII)	Doxycycline; TMP/SMX; ciprofloxacin; ceftriaxone
Anaplasma (formerly Ehrlichia) phagocytophilum[8,9]	Human granulocytic anaplasmosis	Doxycycline (all ages) (AII)	Rifampin
Arcanobacterium haemolyticum[10]	Pharyngitis, cellulitis, Lemierre syndrome	Erythromycin; penicillin (BIII)	Azithromycin, amoxicillin, clindamycin; doxycycline; vancomycin
Bacillus anthracis[11]	Anthrax (cutaneous, gastrointestinal, inhalational, meningoencephalitis)	Ciprofloxacin (regardless of age) (AIII). For invasive, systemic infection, use combination therapy.	Doxycycline; amoxicillin, levofloxacin, clindamycin; penicillin G; vancomycin, meropenem
Bacillus cereus or subtilis[12,13]	Sepsis; toxin-mediated gastroenteritis	Vancomycin (BIII)	Ciprofloxacin, linezolid, daptomycin

Bacteroides fragilis[14,15]	Peritonitis, sepsis, abscesses	Metronidazole (AI)	Meropenem or imipenem (AI); ticar/clav; pip/tazo (AI); clindamycin (AI), although recent surveillance suggests resistance up to 25%; amox/clav (BII)
Bacteroides, other spp[14,15]	Pneumonia, sepsis, abscesses	Metronidazole (BII)	Meropenem or imipenem; penicillin G or ampicillin if beta-lactamase negative
Bartonella henselae[16,17]	Cat-scratch disease	Azithromycin for lymph node disease (BII); gentamicin in combination with TMP/SMX AND rifampin for invasive disease (BII)	Cefotaxime; ciprofloxacin; doxycycline
Bartonella quintana[18]	Bacillary angiomatosis, peliosis hepatis	Gentamicin plus doxycycline (BIII); erythromycin; ciprofloxacin (BIII)	Azithromycin; doxycycline
Bordetella pertussis, parapertussis[19,20]	Pertussis	Azithromycin (AIII); erythromycin (BII)	Clarithromycin; TMP/SMX; ampicillin
Borrelia burgdorferi, Lyme disease[21-23]	Treatment based on stage of infection (see Lyme disease in Chapter 6)	Doxycycline if >8 y (AII); amoxicillin or erythromycin in children ≤7 y (AIII); ceftriaxone IV for meningitis (AII)	
Borrelia recurrentis, louse-borne relapsing fever[24,25]	Relapsing fever	Single-dose doxycycline if >8 y (AIII); penicillin or erythromycin in children ≤7 y (BII)	
Borrelia hermsii, turicatae, parkeri, tickborne relapsing fever[24,25]	Relapsing fever	Doxycycline if >8 y (AIII); penicillin or erythromycin in children ≤7 y (BII)	
Brucella spp[26-28]	Brucellosis (see Chapter 6)	Doxycycline AND rifampin (BII); OR, for children <8 y: TMP/SMX AND rifampin (BII)	For serious infection: doxycycline AND gentamicin; or TMP/SMX AND gentamicin (AIII)

7

Preferred Therapy for Specific Bacterial and Mycobacterial Pathogens

Organism	Clinical Illness	Drug of Choice (evidence grade)	Alternatives
Burkholderia cepacia complex[29–31]	Pneumonia, sepsis in immunocompromised children; pneumonia in children with cystic fibrosis[32]	Meropenem (BIII); for severe disease, ADD tobramycin AND TMP/SMX (AIII)	Imipenem, doxycycline; ceftazidime; ciprofloxacin. Aerosolized antibiotics may provide higher concentrations in lung[31]
Burkholderia pseudomallei[33–35]	Melioidosis	Meropenem (AIII) or ceftazidime (BIII); followed by prolonged TMP/SMX and doxycycline (AIII)	TMP/SMX, doxycycline, or amox/clav for chronic disease
Campylobacter fetus[36]	Sepsis, meningitis in the neonate	Meropenem (BIII)	Cefotaxime; gentamicin; erythromycin
Campylobacter jejuni[37–39]	Diarrhea	Azithromycin (BII); erythromycin (BII)	Doxycycline; ciprofloxacin (very high rates of cipro-R strains in Thailand, Hong Kong, and Spain)
Capnocytophaga canimorsus[42]	Sepsis after dog bite	Pip/tazo OR meropenem; amox/clav (BIII); (BII)	Clindamycin; linezolid penicillin G, ciprofloxacin
Capnocytophaga ochracea[42]	Sepsis, abscesses	Clindamycin (BIII); amox/clav (BIII)	Meropenem; pip/tazo
Chlamydophila (formerly Chlamydia) pneumoniae[43,44]	Pneumonia	Azithromycin (AII); erythromycin (AII)	Doxycycline; ciprofloxacin
Chlamydophila (formerly Chlamydia) psittaci[45]	Psittacosis	Azithromycin (AIII); erythromycin (AIII)	Doxycycline
Chlamydia trachomatis[46–48]	Lymphogranuloma venereum	Doxycycline (AII)	Azithromycin; erythromycin
	Urethritis, vaginitis	Doxycycline (AII)	Azithromycin; erythromycin; ofloxacin
	Inclusion conjunctivitis of newborn	Azithromycin (AIII)	Erythromycin
	Pneumonia of infancy	Azithromycin (AIII)	Erythromycin; ampicillin
	Trachoma	Azithromycin (AI)	Doxycycline; erythromycin

Chromobacterium violaceum[49,50]	Sepsis, pneumonia, abscesses	Meropenem AND ciprofloxacin (AIII)	Imipenem, TMP/SMX
Citrobacter koseri (diversus) and *freundii*[51-53]	Meningitis, sepsis	Meropenem (AIII)	Cefepime; ciprofloxacin; ceftriaxone AND gentamicin; TMP/SMX Carbapenem-resistant strains now reported
Clostridium botulinum[54-56]	Botulism: foodborne; wound; potentially bioterror-related	Botulism antitoxin heptavalent (equine) types A–G (HBAT) is now FDA approved (www.fda.gov/downloads/ BiologicsBloodVaccines/ BloodBloodProducts/ApprovedProducts/ LicensedProductsBLAs/ FractionatedPlasmaProducts/ UCM345147.pdf). No antibiotic treatment.	For more information, call your state health department or the CDC Emergency Operations Center, 770/488-7100.
	Infant botulism	Human botulism immune globulin for infants (BabyBIG) (AII) No antibiotic treatment	BabyBIG available nationally from the California Department of Public Health at 510/231-7600 (www.infantbotulism.org) (accessed November 11, 2013).
Clostridium difficile[57,58]	Antibiotic-associated colitis (see Chapter 6, Gastrointestinal Infections, *C difficile*)	Metronidazole PO (AI)	Vancomycin PO for metronidazole failures; stop the predisposing antimicrobial therapy, if possible. No pediatric data on fidaxomicin PO.
Clostridium perfringens[59,60]	Gas gangrene/necrotizing fasciitis/sepsis (also caused by *C sordellii*, *C septicum*, *C novyi*) Food poisoning	Penicillin G AND clindamycin for invasive infection (BII); no antimicrobials indicated for foodborne illness	Meropenem, metronidazole, clindamycin monotherapy

Preferred Therapy for Specific Bacterial and Mycobacterial Pathogens

7

Preferred Therapy for Specific Bacterial and Mycobacterial Pathogens

Organism	Clinical Illness	Drug of Choice (evidence grade)	Alternatives
Clostridium tetani[61,62]	Tetanus	Metronidazole (AIII); penicillin G (BIII)	Treatment: tetanus immune globulin (TIG) 3,000 to 6,000 U IM, with part injected directly into the wound. Prophylaxis for contaminated wounds: 250 U IM for those with <3 tetanus immunizations. Start/continue immunization for tetanus. Alternative antibiotics: meropenem; doxycycline, clindamycin.
Corynebacterium diphtheriae[63]	Diphtheria	Diphtheria equine antitoxin (available through CDC, under an investigational protocol [www.cdc.gov/diphtheria/dat.html]) AND erythromycin or penicillin G (AIII)	Antitoxin from the CDC at the Emergency Operations Center, 770/488-7100 (accessed November 11, 2013)
Corynebacterium jeikeium[64]	Sepsis, endocarditis	Vancomycin (AIII)	Penicillin G AND gentamicin, tigecycline, linezolid, daptomycin
Corynebacterium minutissimum[65,66]	Erythrasma; bacteremia in compromised hosts	Erythromycin PO for erythrasma (BIII); vancomycin IV for bacteremia (BIII)	Topical clindamycin for cutaneous infection
Coxiella burnetii[67,68]	Q fever	Acute infection: Doxycycline (all ages) (AII) Chronic infection: TMP/SMX AND doxycycline; OR levofloxacin AND rifampin	Alternative for acute infection: TMP/SMX
Ehrlichia chafeensis[8,9] Ehrlichia muris-like[69]	Human monocytic ehrlichiosis	Doxycycline (all ages) (AII)	Rifampin
Ehrlichia ewingii[8,9]	E ewingii ehrlichiosis	Doxycycline (all ages) (AII)	Rifampin
Eikenella corrodens[70]	Human bite wounds; abscesses, meningitis, endocarditis	Ampicillin; penicillin G (BII)	Amox/clav; ticar/clav; pip/tazo; amp/sul; ceftriaxone; ciprofloxacin; imipenem Resistant to clindamycin, cephalexin, erythromycin

Organism	Infection	Preferred therapy	Alternative
Elizabethkingia (formerly *Chryseobacterium*) *meningosepticum*[71,72]	Sepsis, meningitis	Levofloxacin; TMP/SMX (BIII)	Add rifampin to another active drug; pip/tazo.
Enterobacter spp[53,73,74]	Sepsis, pneumonia, wound infection, UTI	Cefepime; meropenem (BII)	Ertapenem; imipenem; cefotaxime or ceftriaxone AND gentamicin; TMP/SMX; ciprofloxacin. Newly emerging carbapenem-R strains worldwide[75]
Enterococcus spp[74-78]	Endocarditis, UTI	Ampicillin AND gentamicin (AI)	Vancomycin AND gentamicin. For vancomycin-resistant strains that are also amp-R: linezolid, daptomycin, tigecycline
Erysipelothrix rhusiopathiae[79]	Sepsis, cellulitis, abscesses, endocarditis	Ampicillin (BIII); penicillin G (BIII)	Ceftriaxone; clindamycin, meropenem; ciprofloxacin. Resistant to vancomycin, daptomycin, TMP/SMX
Escherichia coli[80] See Chapter 6 for specific infection entities with *E. coli*. Increasing resistance to 3rd-generation cephalosporins due to ESBLs.	UTI, not hospital acquired	A 2nd- or 3rd-generation cephalosporin PO, IM (BI)	Amoxicillin; TMP/SMX if susceptible. For hospital-acquired UTI, review hospital antibiogram for choices.
	Traveler's diarrhea	Azithromycin (AII)	Rifaximin (for nonfebrile, nonbloody diarrhea for children >11 y); cefixime
	Sepsis, pneumonia, hospital-acquired UTI	A 2nd- or 3rd-generation cephalosporin IV (BI)	For ESBL-producing strains: meropenem (AIII) or other carbapenem. Ciprofloxacin if resistant to other antibiotics
	Meningitis	Ceftriaxone; cefotaxime (AIII)	For ESBL-producing strains: meropenem (AIII)
Francisella tularensis[81]	Tularemia	Gentamicin (AII)	Doxycycline; ciprofloxacin
Fusobacterium spp[82,83]	Sepsis, soft tissue infection, Lemierre syndrome	Metronidazole (AIII); clindamycin (BIII)	Penicillin G; meropenem

Preferred Therapy for Specific Bacterial and Mycobacterial Pathogens

7

7

Preferred Therapy for Specific Bacterial and Mycobacterial Pathogens

Organism	Clinical Illness	Drug of Choice (evidence grade)	Alternatives
Gardnerella vaginalis[84]	Bacterial vaginosis	Metronidazole (BII)	Clindamycin
Haemophilus (now *Aggregatibacter*) *aphrophilus*[85]	Sepsis, endocarditis, abscesses (including brain abscess)	Ceftriaxone (AII); OR ampicillin AND gentamicin (BII)	Ciprofloxacin, amox/clav
Haemophilus ducreyi[48]	Chancroid	Azithromycin (AIII); ceftriaxone (BIII)	Erythromycin; ciprofloxacin
Haemophilus influenzae[86]			
– Non-encapsulated strains	Upper respiratory tract infections	Beta-lactamase neg: ampicillin IV (AII); amoxicillin PO (AI) Beta-lactamase positive: ceftriaxone IV, IM (AI), or cefotaxime IV (AI); amox/clav (AI) OR 2nd- or 3rd-generation cephalosporins PO (AI)	Levofloxacin; azithromycin; TMP/SMX
– Type b strains	Meningitis, arthritis, cellulitis, epiglottitis, pneumonia	Beta-lactamase neg: ampicillin IV (AII); amoxicillin PO (AI) Beta-lactamase positive: ceftriaxone IV, IM (AI), or cefotaxime IV (AI); amox/clav (AI) OR 2nd- or 3rd-generation cephalosporins PO (AI)	Full IV course (10 days) for meningitis
Helicobacter pylori[87,88]	Gastritis, peptic ulcer	Clarithromycin AND amoxicillin AND omeprazole (AII)	Other regimens include metronidazole (especially for concerns of clarithro-R),[89] and other proton pump inhibitors
Klebsiella spp (*K pneumoniae*, *K oxytoca*)[73,74,90-92]	UTI	A 2nd- or 3rd-generation cephalosporin (AII)	Use most narrow spectrum agent active against pathogen: TMP/SMX; gentamicin. ESBL producers should be treated with a carbapenem (meropenem, ertapenem, imipenem), but KPC-containing carbapenem-R organisms may require ciprofloxacin or colistin.[85]

Organism	Condition	Preferred Therapy	Alternative / Comments
	Sepsis, pneumonia, meningitis	Ceftriaxone; cefotaxime, cefepime (AIII)	Carbapenem or ciprofloxacin if resistant to other routine antibiotics Meningitis caused by ESBL producer: meropenem KPC carbapenemase producers: ciprofloxacin, colistin
Klebsiella granulomatis[48]	Granuloma inguinale	Doxycycline (AII)	Azithromycin; TMP/SMX; ciprofloxacin
Kingella kingae[93,94]	Osteomyelitis, arthritis	Ampicillin; penicillin G (AII)	Ceftriaxone; TMP/SMX; cefuroxime; ciprofloxacin
Legionella spp[95]	Legionnaires disease	Azithromycin (AI) OR levofloxacin (AII)	Erythromycin
Leptospira spp[96]	Leptospirosis	Penicillin G(AIII); ceftriaxone(AII)	Amoxicillin; doxycycline; azithromycin
Leuconostoc[97]	Bacteremia	Penicillin G (AIII); ampicillin (BIII)	Clindamycin; erythromycin; doxycycline (resistant to vancomycin)
Listeria monocytogenes[98]	Sepsis, meningitis in compromised host; neonatal sepsis	Ampicillin (ADD gentamicin for severe infection) (AII)	TMP/SMX; vancomycin
Moraxella catarrhalis[99]	Otitis, sinusitis, bronchitis	Amox/clav (AI)	TMP/SMX; a 2nd- or 3rd-generation cephalosporin
Morganella morganii[100,101]	UTI, sepsis, wound infection	Cefepime (AIII); meropenem (AIII)	Pip/tazo; ceftriaxone AND gentamicin; ciprofloxacin
Mycobacterium abscessus[102,103]	Skin and soft tissue infections; pneumonia in cystic fibrosis	Clarithromycin or azithromycin (AIII); ADD amikacin ± cefoxitin for invasive disease (AIII)	Also test for susceptibility to meropenem, tigecycline, linezolid.
Mycobacterium avium complex[102,104]	Cervical adenitis, pneumonia[104]	Clarithromycin (AIII); azithromycin (AIII)	Surgical excision is more likely to lead to cure than sole medical therapy. May increase cure rate with addition of rifampin ± ethambutol.
	Disseminated disease in competent host, or disease in immunocompromised host	Clarithromycin or azithromycin AND ethambutol AND rifampin (AIII)	Depending on susceptibilities and the severity of illness, ADD amikacin ± ciprofloxacin.

7

Preferred Therapy for Specific Bacterial and Mycobacterial Pathogens

7

Preferred Therapy for Specific Bacterial and Mycobacterial Pathogens

Organism	Clinical Illness	Drug of Choice (evidence grade)	Alternatives
Mycobacterium bovis[105,106]	Tuberculosis (adenitis; abdominal tuberculosis; meningitis)	Isoniazid AND rifampin (AII); ADD ethambutol for suspected resistance (AII)	Add streptomycin for severe infection. M bovis is always resistant to PZA.
Mycobacterium chelonae[102,104,107,108]	Abscesses; catheter infection	Clarithromycin or azithromycin (AIII); ADD amikacin ± cefoxitin for invasive disease (AIII)	Also test for susceptibility to cefoxitin; TMP/SMX; doxycycline; tobramycin, imipenem; moxifloxacin, linezolid.
Mycobacterium fortuitum complex[102,108]	Skin and soft tissue infections; catheter infection	Amikacin AND meropenem (AIII) ± ciprofloxacin (AIII)	Also test for susceptibility to clarithromycin, cefoxitin; sulfonamides; doxycycline; linezolid.
Mycobacterium leprae[109]	Leprosy	Dapsone AND rifampin (for paucibacillary (1–5 patches) (AII) ADD clarithromycin (or clofazimine) for lepromatous, multibacillary (>5 patches) disease (AII)	Consult HRSA (National Hansen's Disease Program) at www.hrsa.gov/hansensdisease for advice about treatment and free antibiotics: 800/642-2477 (accessed November 12, 2013).
Mycobacterium marinum/balnei[102,110]	Papules, pustules, abscesses (swimmer's granuloma)	Clarithromycin ± rifampin (AIII)	TMP/SMX AND rifampin; doxycycline
Mycobacterium tuberculosis[105,111] See Tuberculosis in Chapter 6, Lower Respiratory Tract Infections, for detailed recommendations for active infection, latent infection, and exposures in high-risk children.	Tuberculosis (pneumonia; meningitis; cervical adenitis; mesenteric adenitis; osteomyelitis)	For active infection: isoniazid AND rifampin AND PZA (AI) For latent infection: isoniazid daily, biweekly, or in combination with rifapentine once weekly (AII)	Add ethambutol for suspect resistance; add streptomycin for severe infection. Corticosteroids should be added to regimens for meningitis, mesenteric adenitis, and endobronchial infection (AIII).
Mycoplasma hominis[48,112,113]	Nongonococcal urethritis; neonatal infection including meningitis	Clindamycin (AIII)	Fluoroquinolones; doxycycline Usually erythromycin-resistant

Organism	Indication	Preferred	Alternatives
Mycoplasma pneumoniae[114]	Pneumonia	Azithromycin (AI); erythromycin (BI); macrolide resistance emerging worldwide[115]	Doxycycline and fluoroquinolones are active against macrolide-S and macrolide-R strains.
Neisseria gonorrhoeae[48]	Gonorrhea; arthritis	Ceftriaxone AND azithromycin or doxycycline (AIII)	Oral cefixime as single drug therapy no longer recommended due to increasing resistance.[117] Spectinomycin IM.
Neisseria meningitidis[117]	Sepsis, meningitis	Ceftriaxone (AI); cefotaxime (AI)	Penicillin G or ampicillin if susceptible[119] For prophylaxis following exposure: rifampin or ciprofloxacin (cipro-resistant strains have now been reported)
Nocardia asteroides or *brasiliensis*[119,120]	Nocardiosis	TMP/SMX (AII); sulfisoxazole (BII); imipenem AND amikacin for severe infection (AII)	Ceftriaxone; minocycline; linezolid, levofloxacin, tigecycline
Oerskovia (now known as *Cellulosimicrobium cellulans*)[121]	Wound infection; catheter infection	Vancomycin ± rifampin (AIII)	Linezolid; resistant to beta-lactams, macrolides, aminoglycosides
Pasteurella multocida[122]	Sepsis, abscesses, animal bite wound	Penicillin G (AIII); ampicillin (AIII); amoxicillin (AIII)	Amox/clav; ticar/clav; pip/tazo; doxycycline; ceftriaxone; cefpodoxime; TMP/SMX
Peptostreptococcus[123]	Sepsis, deep head/neck space and intra-abdominal infection	Penicillin G (AII); ampicillin (AII)	Clindamycin; vancomycin; meropenem, imipenem, metronidazole
Plesiomonas shigelloides[124,125]	Diarrhea, neonatal sepsis, meningitis	Antibiotics may not be necessary to treat diarrhea: 2nd- and 3rd-generation cephalosporins (AIII); azithromycin (BIII); ciprofloxacin (CIII) For meningitis/sepsis: ceftriaxone	Meropenem; pip/tazo.

7

Preferred Therapy for Specific Bacterial and Mycobacterial Pathogens

Organism	Clinical Illness	Drug of Choice (evidence grade)	Alternatives
Prevotella (Bacteroides) spp[126] *melaninogenicus*[127]	Deep head/neck space abscess; dental abscess	Metronidazole (AII); meropenem or imipenem (AII)	Pip/tazo; clindamycin
Propionibacterium acnes[127,128]	In addition to acne, invasive infection: sepsis, post-op wound infection	Penicillin (AIII); vancomycin (AIII) wound infection	Cefotaxime; doxycycline; clindamycin; ciprofloxacin; linezolid
Proteus mirabilis[129]	UTI, sepsis, meningitis	Ceftriaxone (AII); cefotaxime (AII)	Aminoglycosides. Increasing resistance to ampicillin, TMP/SMX, and fluoroquinolones, particularly in nosocomial isolates. Colistin resistant.
Proteus vulgaris, other spp (indole-positive strains)[153]	UTI, sepsis, meningitis	Cefepime; ciprofloxacin, gentamicin (BIII)	Meropenem or other carbapenem; pip/tazo; TMP/SMX. Colistin resistant.
Providencia spp[53,130,131]	Sepsis	Cefepime; ciprofloxacin, gentamicin (BIII)	Meropenem or other carbapenem; pip/tazo; TMP/SMX. Colistin resistant.
Pseudomonas aeruginosa[74,132-135]	UTI	Ceftazidime (AI); other anti-pseudomonal beta-lactams	Tobramycin; amikacin; ciprofloxacin
	Nosocomial sepsis, pneumonia	Cefepime (AI) or meropenem (AI); OR pip/tazo AND tobramycin (BI); ceftazidime AND tobramycin (BI)	Ceftazidime AND tobramycin (BII); ciprofloxacin AND tobramycin
	Pneumonia in cystic fibrosis.[136-138] See Cystic Fibrosis in Chapter 6, Lower Respiratory Tract Infections.	Cefepime (AII) or meropenem (AII); OR ceftazidime AND tobramycin (BII); ADD aerosol tobramycin (AI). Azithromycin provides benefit in prolonging interval between exacerbations.	Inhalational antibiotics for prevention of acute exacerbations: tobramycin, aztreonam, colistin. Many organisms are multidrug resistant; consider ciprofloxacin or colistin parenterally; in vitro synergy testing may suggest effective combinations.[138] For multidrug-resistant organisms, colistin aerosol (AIII).

Pseudomonas cepacia, mallei, or *pseudomallei* (see *Burkholderia*)		
Rhodococcus equi[139]	Necrotizing pneumonia	Imipenem AND vancomycin (AIII)	Dual drug combination therapy with ciprofloxacin AND azithromycin or rifampin
Rickettsia[68,140,141]	Rocky Mountain spotted fever, Q fever, typhus, rickettsial pox	Doxycycline (all ages) (AII)	Chloramphenicol is less effective than doxycycline.
Salmonella, non-*typhi*[142-144]	Gastroenteritis; focal infections; bacteremia	Ceftriaxone (AII); cefixime (AIII); azithromycin (AII)	For susceptible strains: ciprofloxacin; TMP/SMX; ampicillin; resistance to fluoroquinolones detected by nalidixic acid testing
Salmonella typhi[145]	Typhoid fever	Azithromycin (AII); ceftriaxone (AII); ciprofloxacin (AII)	For susceptible strains: TMP/SMX; ampicillin
Serratia marcescens[53,74,130]	Nosocomial sepsis, pneumonia	Cefepime (AII); a carbapenem (AII)	Ceftriaxone or cefotaxime AND gentamicin; or ciprofloxacin
Shewanella spp[146]	Wound infection, nosocomial pneumonia, peritoneal-dialysis peritonitis, ventricular shunt infection	Ceftazidime (AIII); cefepime (AIII)	Ampicillin, meropenem, pip/tazo, ciprofloxacin
Shigella spp[147,148]	Enteritis, UTI, prepubertal vaginitis	Ceftriaxone (AIII); azithromycin[149] (AIII); cefixime (AIII); ciprofloxacin[150] (AII)	Resistance to azithromycin now reported. Use most narrow spectrum agent active against pathogen: ampicillin (not amoxicillin for enteritis); TMP/SMX.
Spirillum minus[151,152]	Rat-bite fever (sodoku fever)	Penicillin G IV (AII); for endocarditis, ADD gentamicin or streptomycin (AIII)	Ampicillin; doxycycline; cefotaxime, vancomycin, streptomycin

7

Preferred Therapy for Specific Bacterial and Mycobacterial Pathogens

Organism	Clinical Illness	Drug of Choice (evidence grade)	Alternatives
Staphylococcus aureus (see Chapter 4: CA-MRSA)[153,154]			
Mild-moderate infections	Skin infections, mild–moderate	MSSA: a 1st-generation cephalosporin (cefazolin IV, cephalexin PO) (AI); oxacillin/nafcillin IV (AI), dicloxacillin PO (AI) MRSA: vancomycin IV or clindamycin IV or PO (AIII)	For MSSA: amox/clav For CA-MRSA: TMP/SMX (if susceptible); linezolid IV, PO; daptomycin IV
Moderate-severe infections, treat empirically for CA-MRSA	Pneumonia, sepsis, myositis, osteomyelitis, etc	MSSA: oxacillin/nafcillin IV (AI); a 1st-generation cephalosporin (cefazolin IV) (AI) ± gentamicin (AIII) MRSA: vancomycin (AII) or clindamycin (AII); ± gentamicin ± rifampin (AIII)	For CA-MRSA: linezolid (AII); OR daptomycin for non-pulmonary infection (AII) (studies underway in children); ceftaroline IV (studies underway in children)
Staphylococcus, coagulase negative[155]	Nosocomial sepsis, infected intravascular catheters, CNS shunts,[156] UTI	Vancomycin (AII)	If susceptible: nafcillin (or other anti-staph beta-lactam); rifampin (in combination); linezolid; ceftaroline IV (studies underway in children)
Stenotrophomonas maltophilia[157,158]	Sepsis	TMP/SMX (AII)	Ceftazidime; ticar/clav; doxycycline; levofloxacin
Streptobacillus moniliformis[151,152]	Rat-bite fever (Haverhill fever)	Penicillin G (AIII); ampicillin (AIII); for endocarditis, ADD gentamicin or streptomycin (AIII)	Doxycycline; ceftriaxone; carbapenems; clindamycin; vancomycin
Streptococcus, group A[159]	Pharyngitis, impetigo, adenitis, cellulitis, necrotizing fasciitis	Penicillin (AI); amoxicillin (AI)	A 1st-generation cephalosporin (cefazolin or cephalexin) (AI); clindamycin (AI); a macrolide (AI), vancomycin (AIII) For relapsing pharyngitis, clindamycin or amox/clav (AIII)
Streptococcus, group B[160]	Neonatal sepsis, pneumonia, meningitis	Penicillin (AII) or ampicillin (AII) ± gentamicin (AIII)	Vancomycin (AIII)

Streptococcus, milleri/anginosus group (*S intermedius, anginosus,* and *constellatus*; includes some beta-hemolytic group C and group G streptococci)[161–163]	Pneumonia, sepsis, skin and soft tissue infection, sinusitis,[164] arthritis, brain abscess, meningitis	Penicillin G (AIII); ampicillin (AIII); ADD gentamicin for serious infection (AIII). Many strains may show decreased susceptibility to penicillin.	Clindamycin; a 1st-generation cephalosporin; vancomycin
Streptococcus pneumoniae[165–168] With widespread use of conjugate pneumococcal vaccines, antibiotic resistance in pneumococci has decreased substantially.[169]	Sinusitis, otitis	Amoxicillin, high-dose (90 mg/kg/day) (AII)	Amox/clav; cefdinir; cefpodoxime; cefuroxime; clindamycin; OR ceftriaxone IM
	Meningitis	Ceftriaxone (AI) or cefotaxime (AI); AND vancomycin for possible ceftriaxone-resistant strains (AIII)	Penicillin G alone for pen-S strains; ceftriaxone alone for ceftriaxone-susceptible strains
	Pneumonia,[114] osteomyelitis/arthritis, sepsis	Ampicillin (AIII); ceftriaxone (AI); cefotaxime (AI)	Penicillin G for pen-S strains (AI)
Streptococcus, viridans group (alpha-hemolytic streptococci, most commonly *S sanguis, S oralis (mitis), S salivarius, S mutans, S morbillorum*)[168]	Endocarditis	Penicillin G ± gentamicin (AII) OR ceftriaxone ± gentamicin (AII)	Vancomycin
Treponema pallidum[48,170]	Syphilis	Penicillin G (AII)	Desensitize to penicillin preferred to alternate therapies. Doxycycline; ceftriaxone.
Ureaplasma urealyticum[48,171]	Genitourinary infections Neonatal pneumonia (therapy may not be effective)	Azithromycin (AII) Azithromycin (AIII)	Erythromycin; doxycycline, ofloxacin (for adolescent genital infections)
Vibrio cholerae[172,173]	Cholera	Doxycycline (AI) or azithromycin (AII)	If susceptible: ciprofloxacin; TMP/SMX

7

Preferred Therapy for Specific Bacterial and Mycobacterial Pathogens

7

Preferred Therapy for Specific Bacterial and Mycobacterial Pathogens

Organism	Clinical Illness	Drug of Choice (evidence grade)	Alternatives
Vibrio vulnificus[174,175]	Sepsis, necrotizing fasciitis	Doxycycline AND ceftazidime (AIII)	Ciprofloxacin AND cefotaxime
Yersinia enterocolitica[176,177]	Diarrhea, mesenteric enteritis, reactive arthritis, sepsis	TMP/SMX (AIII); ciprofloxacin (AIII)	Ceftriaxone; gentamicin, doxycycline
Yersinia pestis[178,179]	Plague	Gentamicin (AIII)	Doxycycline; TMP/SMX, ciprofloxacin
Yersinia pseudotuberculosis[177,180]	Mesenteric adenitis; Far East scarlet fever; reactive arthritis	TMP/SMX (AIII); ciprofloxacin (AIII)	Ceftriaxone; gentamicin, doxycycline

8. Preferred Therapy for Specific Fungal Pathogens

NOTES

- See Chapter 2 for discussion of the differences between polyenes, azoles, and echinocandins.

- **Abbreviations:** AmB-D, amphotericin B deoxycholate, the conventional standard AmB (original trade name Fungizone); ABLC, amphotericin B lipid complex (Abelcet); ABCD, amphotericin B colloidal suspension (Amphotec); bid, twice daily; CNS, central nervous system; CSF, cerebrospinal fluid; div, divided; L-AmB, liposomal amphotericin B (AmBisome); IV, intravenous; PO, orally; qd, once daily; qid, 4 times daily; soln, solution; tab, tablet; tid, 3 times daily; TMP/SMX, trimethoprim/sulfamethoxazole.

A. OVERVIEW OF FUNGAL PATHOGENS AND USUAL PATTERN OF SUSCEPTIBILITY TO ANTIFUNGALS

Fungal Species	Amphotericin B Formulations	Fluconazole	Itraconazole	Voriconazole	Posaconazole	Flucytosine	Caspofungin, Micafungin, or Anidulafungin
Aspergillus calidoustus	++	–	+	–	–	–	++
Aspergillus fumigatus	+	–	+	++	+	–	+
Aspergillus terreus	–	–	+	++	+	–	+
Blastomyces dermatitidis	++	+	++	+	+	–	–
Candida albicans	+	++	+	+	+	+	++
Candida glabrata	+	–	–	+/–	+/–	+	+
Candida guilliermondii	+	+	+	+	+	+	+/–
Candida krusei	+	–	–	+	+	+	++
Candida lusitaniae	–	++	+	+	+	+	+
Candida parapsilosis	++	++	+	+	+	+	+/–
Candida tropicalis	+	++	+	+	+	+	++
Coccidioides immitis	++	+	++	+	+	–	–
Cryptococcus spp	++	+	+	+	+	++	–
Fusarium spp	+	–	–	++	+	–	–
Histoplasma capsulatum	++	+	++	+	+	–	–

Mucor spp	++	–	+/–	–	+	–
Paracoccidioides spp	+	+	++	+	+	–
Penicillium spp	+/–	–	++	+	+	–
Rhizopus spp	++	–	–	–	+	–
Scedosporium apiospermum	–	+	+	++	+	–
Scedosporium prolificans	–	–	+/–	+/–	+/–	–
Sporothrix spp	+	+	++	+	+	–
Trichosporon spp	–	+	+	++	+	–

NOTE: ++ = preferred therapy(ies); + = usually active; +/– =variably active; – = usually not active.

8

Preferred Therapy for Specific Fungal Pathogens

B. SYSTEMIC INFECTIONS

Infection	Therapy (evidence grade)	Comments
PROPHYLAXIS		
Prophylaxis of invasive fungal infection in patients with hematologic malignancies[1-4]	Fluconazole 6 mg/kg/day for prevention of infection (AII)	Fluconazole is not effective against molds and some strains of *Candida*. Posaconazole PO, voriconazole PO, and micafungin IV are effective in adults in preventing infection but are not well studied in children for this indication.[5]
Prophylaxis of invasive fungal infection in patients with solid organ transplants[6-8]	Fluconazole 6 mg/kg/day for prevention of infection (AII)	AmB, caspofungin, micafungin, voriconazole, or posaconazole may be effective in preventing infection.
TREATMENT		
Aspergillosis[9-11]	Voriconazole 18 mg/kg/day IV div q12h for a loading dose on the first day, then 16 mg/kg/day IV div q12h as a maintenance dose for children 2–12 y. In children >12 y, use adult dosing (load 12 mg/kg/day IV div q12h on first day, then 8 mg/kg/day div q12h as a maintenance dose) (AII). When stable, may switch from voriconazole IV to voriconazole PO at a dose of 18 mg/kg/day div bid for children 2–12 y and 400 mg/day div bid for children >12 y (AIII). Alternatives: Caspofungin 70 mg/m² IV loading dose on day 1 (max dose 70 mg), followed by 50 mg/m² IV (max dose 70 mg) on subsequent days (BII) OR L-AmB 3–5 mg/kg/day as 3–4 h infusions (in adults, higher dosages have not produced improved outcome)[12] (AII).	Voriconazole is the preferred primary antifungal therapy for all clinical forms of infection. Optimal voriconazole trough serum concentrations (generally thought to be >1–2 µg/mL) are important for success, but it is critical to monitor trough concentrations to guide therapy due to high interpatient variability.[13] Low voriconazole concentrations are a leading cause of clinical failure. Total treatment course is at least 6 wk or until disease controlled. Salvage therapy options include a change of antifungal class (using L-AmB or an echinocandin), switching to posaconazole (trough concentrations >0.7 µg/mL), or using combination antifungal therapy. The addition of anidulafungin to voriconazole as combination therapy found no clear statistical benefit to the combination over voriconazole monotherapy.[14] In vitro data suggest some synergy with 2 (but not 3) drug combinations: an azole plus an echinocandin is the most well studied.

Both voriconazole and AmB are fungicidal, while the echinocandins are fungistatic against most Aspergillus spp. Against most Aspergillus spp, micafungin[15] demonstrates equivalent activity to caspofungin.

Return of immune function is paramount to treatment success; for children receiving corticosteroids, decreasing the corticosteroid dosage or changing to steroid-sparing protocols are also important.

Itraconazole oral solution provides greater and more reliable absorption than capsules; serum concentrations of itraconazole should be determined 2 wk after start of therapy to ensure adequate drug exposure (maintain trough concentrations >0.5 μg/mL).

Alternative to itraconazole: 12 mg/kg/day fluconazole (BIII).

Patients with extrapulmonary blastomycosis should receive at least 12 mo of total therapy.

CNS blastomycosis should begin with ABLC/L-AmB for 4–6 wk, followed by an azole (fluconazole preferred, at 12 mg/kg/day) for a total therapy of at least 12 mo and until resolution of CSF abnormalities.

Lifelong itraconazole if immunosuppression cannot be reversed.

Blastomycosis
(North American)[16–18]

For moderate to severe disease: ABLC or L-AmB 3–5 mg/kg IV daily as 3–4 h infusion for 1–2 wk or until improvement noted, followed by oral solution itraconazole 10 mg/kg/day div bid (max 400 mg/day) PO for a total of 12 mo (AIII)

For mild-moderate disease: oral solution itraconazole 10 mg/kg/day div bid (max 400 mg/day) PO for a total of 6–12 mo (AIII)

B. SYSTEMIC INFECTIONS (cont)

Infection	Therapy (evidence grade)	Comments
Candidiasis[19] (See Chapter 2.)		
– Disseminated infection	**For neutropenic patients** An echinocandin is recommended. Caspofungin 70 mg/m² IV loading dose on day 1 (max dose 70 mg), followed by 50 mg/m² IV (max dose 70 mg) on subsequent days (AII); OR micafungin 2–4 mg/kg/day q24h (max dose 150 mg) (BII)²⁰; preterm neonates require 10 mg/kg/day to achieve adequate drug exposure (BIII)¹⁹ OR ABLC or L-AmB 5 mg/kg/day IV q24h (BII). For neutropenic but less critically ill patients with no recent azole exposure, fluconazole (12 mg/kg/day q24h) is an alternative. **For non-neutropenic patients** Fluconazole (12 mg/kg/day) is recommended in those patients who are less critically ill and with no recent azole exposure. An echinocandin is recommended in those non-neutropenic patients who are more critically ill, patients who have had recent azole exposure, or patients at risk for *Candida glabrata* or *Candida krusei*. L-AmB or ABLC (3–5 mg/kg/day) are alternatives, and voriconazole could be used for step-down oral therapy for voriconazole-susceptible *Candida krusei* or *Candida glabrata*, but otherwise offers little advantage over fluconazole. **For CNS infections** AmB-D 1 mg/kg/day or L-AmB/ABLC (3–5 mg/kg/day) AND flucytosine 100 mg/kg/day PO div q6h (AII) until initial clinical response, followed by step-down therapy with fluconazole (12 mg/kg/day); echinocandins do NOT achieve therapeutic concentrations in CSF.	Prompt removal of infected intravenous catheter or any infected devices is critical to success. For infections with *Candida krusei* or *Candida glabrata*, an echinocandin is preferred; however, there are increasing reports of some *C glabrata* resistance to echinocandins. Transition to an azole as step-down therapy only after confirmation of isolate susceptibility. Patients already receiving an empiric azole who are clinically improving can remain on the azole. For infections with *Candida parapsilosis*, fluconazole or ABLC/L-AmB is preferred. Patients already receiving an empiric echinocandin who are clinically improving can remain on the echinocandin. Therapy is for 2 wk after negative cultures in pediatric patients but 3 wk in neonates due to higher rate of meningitis and dissemination. Load with fluconazole at 25 mg/kg on day 1, followed by 12 mg/kg/day q24h to achieve steady-state more rapidly. For children on ECMO, 35 mg/kg load followed by 12 mg/kg/day is also likely to be beneficial.

— Oropharyngeal, esophageal[19,20]	Oropharyngeal: Mild disease; clotrimazole 10 mg troches PO 5 times daily OR nystatin (either 100,000 U/mL with 4–6 mL 4 times daily or 1–2 200,000 U pastilles 4 times daily) for 7–14 days. Moderate-severe disease: Fluconazole 3–6 mg/kg once daily PO for 7–14 days (AII). Esophageal: Oral fluconazole (6–12 mg/kg/day) for 14–21 days. If cannot tolerate oral therapy, then use fluconazole IV OR ABLC/L-AmB OR an echinocandin.	For fluconazole-refractory disease: Itraconazole OR posaconazole OR AmB IV OR an echinocandin for 14–28 days. Esophageal disease always requires systemic antifungal therapy. Suppressive therapy (3 times weekly) with fluconazole is recommended for recurrent infections.
— Neonatal candidiasis[21]	L-AmB/ABLC (5 mg/kg/day) or AmB-D (1 mg/kg/day). Theoretical risk of AmB-D less penetration, so some would NOT recommend lipid formulation if urinary tract involvement is possible. Fluconazole (12 mg/kg/day, after loading dose of 25 mg/kg) is an alternative (BIII). Therapy is for 3 wk (not 2 wk as in pediatric patients). For treatment of neonates and young infants (<120 days) on ECMO, fluconazole load with 35 mg/kg on day one, followed by 12 mg/kg/day q24h (BII).	Nurseries with high rates of candidiasis (generally thought to be >10%) should consider fluconazole prophylaxis (AI) (6 mg/kg twice weekly) in high-risk neonates (birth weight <1,000 g). Lumbar puncture and thorough retinal examination recommended (BIII). Imaging of genitourinary tract, liver, and spleen recommended if persistently positive cultures (BIII). Assume meningoencephalitis in the neonate due to the high incidence of this complication. Role of flucytosine in neonates with meningitis is questionable and not routinely recommended due to toxicity concerns. Echinocandins are generally used in cases of antifungal resistance or toxicity.
— Peritonitis (secondary to peritoneal dialysis)[22]	Fluconazole 200 mg intraperitoneal q24h (AII)	Remove peritoneal dialysis catheter; replace after 4–6 wk of treatment, if possible. High-dosage oral fluconazole may also be used. AmB should not be instilled into the peritoneal cavity.
— Vulvovaginal[23]	Topical vaginal cream/tabs/suppositories (alphabetic order): Butoconazole, clotrimazole, econazole, fenticonazole, miconazole, sertaconazole, terconazole, or tioconazole for 3–7 days OR Fluconazole 10 mg/kg (max 150 mg) as a single dose (AII)	No topical agent is clearly superior. Avoid azoles during pregnancy. For recurrent disease, consider 10–14 days of induction with topical or systemic azole followed by fluconazole once weekly for 6 mo.

B. SYSTEMIC INFECTIONS (cont)

Infection	Therapy (evidence grade)	Comments
– Cutaneous candidiasis	Topical therapy (alphabetic order): Ciclopirox, clotrimazole, econazole, haloprogin, ketoconazole, miconazole, oxiconazole, sertaconazole, sulconazole	Fluconazole 3–6 mg/kg/day PO once daily for 5–7 days
– Chronic mucocutaneous[19]	Fluconazole 3–5 mg/kg daily PO until lesions clear (AII)	Alternative: Itraconazole 5 mg/kg PO solution q24h Relapse common
Chromoblastomycosis[24,25]	Itraconazole oral solution 10 mg/kg/day div bid PO for 12–18 mo, in combination with surgical excision or repeated cryotherapy (AIII)	Alternative: Terbinafine or an AmB
Coccidioidomycosis[26–30]	For moderate infections: Fluconazole 12 mg/kg IV, PO q24h (AII). For severe pulmonary disease: AmB-D 1 mg/kg/day IV q24h; OR ABLC/ L-AmB 5 mg/kg/day IV q24h (AIII) as initial therapy until clear improvement, followed by an oral azole for total therapy of up to 12 mo, depending on genetic or immunocompromising risk factors. For meningitis: Fluconazole 12 mg/kg/day IV q24h (AII); for failures, intrathecal AmB-D (0.1–1.5 mg/dose) OR voriconazole IV (AIII). Lifelong azole suppressive therapy may be required. For extrapulmonary (nonmeningeal), particularly for osteomyelitis: Itraconazole solution 10 mg/kg/day div bid for 12 mo appears more effective than fluconazole (AIII), and AmB as an alternative if worsening.	Mild pulmonary disease does not require therapy in the normal host and only requires periodic reassessment. Posaconazole also active, but little experience in children. Treat until serum cocci complement fixation titers drop to 1:8 or 1:4, about 3–6 mo. Disease in immunocompromised hosts may need to be treated longer, including potentially lifelong azole secondary prophylaxis. Watch for relapse up to 1–2 y after therapy.

Cryptococcosis[31-34]	For mild-moderate pulmonary disease: Fluconazole 12 mg/kg/day IV, PO q24h for 6–12 mo (AIII). For meningitis or severe pulmonary disease: Induction therapy with AmB-D 1 mg/kg/day IV q24h OR ABLC or L-AmB 3–5 mg/kg/day q24h; AND flucytosine 100 mg/kg/day PO div q6h for a minimum of 2 wk until CSF cleared, FOLLOWED BY consolidation therapy with fluconazole (12 mg/kg/day) for a minimum of 8 more wk (AI).	Monitor flucytosine serum trough concentrations to keep peaks less than 80–100 µg/mL (and ideally 60–80 µg/mL) to prevent neutropenia. For HIV-positive patients, continue maintenance therapy with fluconazole (6 mg/kg/day) indefinitely. In organ transplant recipients, continue maintenance fluconazole (6 mg/kg/day) for 6–12 mo after consolidation therapy. For cryptococcal relapse, restart induction therapy and determine susceptibility of relapse isolate.
Fusarium, Scedosporium prolificans, and **Pseudallescheria boydii** (and its asexual form, **Scedosporium apiospermum**)[35,36]	Voriconazole 18 mg/kg/day IV div q12h for a loading dose on the first day, then 16 mg/kg/day IV div q12h as a maintenance dose for children 2–12 y. In children >12 y, use adult dosing (load 12 mg/kg/day IV div q12h on first day, then 8 mg/kg/day div q12h as a maintenance dose) (AIII). When stable, may switch from voriconazole IV to voriconazole PO at a dose of 18 mg/kg/day div bid for children 2–12 y and 400 mg/day div bid for children >12 y (AIII).	Optimal voriconazole trough concentrations (generally thought to be >1–2 µg/mL) are important. Resistant to AmB in vitro. Alternatives: Echinocandins have been successful at salvage therapy anecdotally; posaconazole (trough concentrations >0.7 µg/mL) likely helpful; while there are reports of combinations with terbinafine, terbinafine does not obtain good tissue concentrations for these disseminated infections. These can be very resistant infections, so highly recommend antifungal susceptibility testing.
Histoplasmosis[37,38]	For severe pulmonary disease: AmB-D 1 mg/kg/day q24h OR ABLC/L-AmB at 3–5 mg/kg/day q24h for 1–2 wk, FOLLOWED BY itraconazole 10 mg/kg/day div bid to complete a total of 12 wk (AIII). For mild-moderate acute pulmonary disease, itraconazole 10 mg/kg/day PO solution div BID for 6–12 wk (AIII).	Mild disease may not require therapy and, in most cases, resolves in 1 mo. For disease with respiratory distress, ADD corticosteroids in first 1–2 wk of antifungal therapy. Progressive disseminated or CNS disease requires AmB therapy for the initial 4–6 wk. Potential lifelong suppressive itraconazole if cannot reverse immunosuppression.
Paracoccidioidomycosis[39-41]	Itraconazole 10 mg/kg/day PO solution div bid for 6 mo (AIII) OR ketoconazole 5 mg/kg/day PO q24h for 6 mo (BII).	Alternatives: voriconazole; sulfadiazine or TMP/SMX for 3–5 y. AmB is another alternative and may be combined with sulfa or azole antifungals.

B. SYSTEMIC INFECTIONS (cont)

Infection	Therapy (evidence grade)	Comments
Pneumocystis jiroveci (carinii) pneumonia[43]	Serious disease: preferred regimen is TMP/SMX, 15–20 mg TMP component/kg/day IV div q8h (AI) OR, for TMP/SMX intolerant or TMP/SMX treatment failure, pentamidine isethionate 4 mg base/kg/day IV daily (BII); for 3 wk Mild-moderate disease: start with IV therapy, then after acute pneumonitis is resolved, TMP/SMX, 20 mg TMP component/kg/day PO div qid for 3 wk total treatment course (AII)	Alternatives: TMP AND dapsone; OR primaquine AND clindamycin; OR atovaquone. Prophylaxis: preferred regimen is TMP/SMX (5 mg TMP component/kg/day) PO div bid, 3 times/wk on consecutive days; OR same dose, given once daily, every day; OR atovaquone: 30 mg/kg/day for infants 13 months; 45 mg/kg/day for infants 4–24 months; and 30 mg/kg/day for infants >24 months; OR dapsone 2 mg/kg (max 100 mg) PO once daily, OR dapsone 4 mg/kg (max 200 mg) PO once weekly. Use steroid therapy for more severe disease.
Sporotrichosis[44]	For cutaneous/lymphocutaneous: Itraconazole 10 mg/kg/day div bid PO solution for 2–4 wk after all lesions gone (generally total of 3–6 mo) (AII). For serious pulmonary or disseminated infection or disseminated sporotrichosis: ABLC/L-AmB at 3–5 mg/kg/day q24h until stable, then step-down therapy with itraconazole PO for a total of 12 mo (AIII). For less severe disease, itraconazole for 12 mo.	If no response for cutaneous disease, treat with higher itraconazole dose, terbinafine, or saturated solution of potassium iodide. Fluconazole is less effective. Obtain serum concentrations of itraconazole after 2 wk of therapy, want serum trough concentration >0.5 µg/mL. For meningeal disease, initial AmB should be 4–6 wk before change to itraconazole for at least 12 mo of therapy. Surgery may be necessary in osteoarticular or pulmonary disease.
Zygomycosis (mucormycosis)[45–48]	Requires aggressive surgery with antifungal therapy: ABLC/L-AmB at 5 mg/kg/day q24h (AIII). For AmB failures, posaconazole may be effective against most strains (AIII).	Following clinical response with AmB, long-term oral step-down therapy with posaconazole (trough concentrations >0.7 µg/mL) can be attempted for 2–6 mo. Voriconazole has NO activity against zygomycetes.

C. LOCALIZED MUCOCUTANEOUS INFECTIONS

Infection	Therapy (evidence grade)	Comments
Dermatophytoses		
– Scalp (tinea capitis, including kerion)[49-51]	Griseofulvin ultramicrosized 10–15 mg/kg/day or microsized 20–25 mg/kg/day once daily PO for 2 mo or longer (AII) (taken with milk or fatty foods to augment absorption) For kerion, treat concurrently with prednisone (1–2 mg/kg/day for 1–2 wk) (AIII)	No need to routinely follow liver function tests in normal healthy children taking griseofulvin. 2.5% selenium sulfide shampoo, or 2% ketoconazole shampoo, 2–3 times/wk should be used concurrently to prevent recurrences. Alternatives: terbinafine PO (4 wk), itraconazole solution 5 mg/kg PO qd, or fluconazole PO; terbinafine superior for *Trichophyton tonsurans*, but griseofulvin superior for *Microsporum canis*.
– Tinea corporis (infection of trunk/limbs/face) – Tinea cruris (infection of the groin) – Tinea pedis (infection of the toes/feet)	Alphabetic order of topical agents: butenafine, ciclopirox, clotrimazole, econazole, haloprogin, ketoconazole, miconazole, naftifine, oxiconazole, sertaconazole, sulconazole, terbinafine, and tolnaftate (AII); apply daily for 4 wk	For unresponsive tinea lesions, use griseofulvin PO in dosages provided above; fluconazole PO, itraconazole PO; OR terbinafine PO. For tinea pedis: Terbinafine PO or itraconazole PO are preferred over other oral agents. Keep skin as clean and dry as possible, particularly for tinea cruris and tinea pedis.
– Tinea unguium (onychomycosis)[51,52]	Topical 8% ciclopirox nail lacquer solution applied daily for 6–12 mo (AII); OR itraconazole 5 mg/kg PO solution q24h (AII)	Recurrence or partial response common Alternative: terbinafine PO 500 mg daily (adult dosage) for 1 wk per mo for 3 mo (hands) or 6–12 mo (toes) until new nail growth; requires systemic treatment (not topical)
– Tinea versicolor (also pityriasis versicolor)[51,53]	Apply topically: selenium sulfide 2.5% lotion or 1% shampoo daily, leave on 30 min, then rinse; for 7 d, then monthly for 6 mo (AIII); OR ciclopirox 1% cream for 4 wk (BII); OR terbinafine 1% solution (BII); OR ketoconazole 2% shampoo daily for 5 days (BII) For small lesions, topical clotrimazole, econazole, haloprogin, ketoconazole, miconazole, or naftifine	For lesions that fail to clear with topical therapy or for extensive lesions: Fluconazole PO or itraconazole PO are equally effective. Recurrence common.

9. Preferred Therapy for Specific Viral Pathogens

NOTE
- **Abbreviations:** ACV, acyclovir; adamantanes, amantadine and rimantadine; ART, antiretroviral therapy; ARV, antiretroviral; bid, twice daily; CA, chronologic age; CDC, Centers for Disease Control and Prevention; CMV, cytomegalovirus; EBV, Epstein-Barr virus; FDA, US Food and Drug Administration; GA, gestational age; G-CSF, granulocyte-colony stimulating factor; HAART, highly active anti-retroviral therapy; HIV, human immunodeficiency virus; HSV, herpes simplex virus; IG, immune globulin; IFN, interferon; NAI, neuraminadase inhibitors (oseltamivir, zanamivir, peramivir); NRTI, nucleoside analog reverse transcriptase inhibitor; PO, orally; qd, once daily; postmenstrual age, weeks of gestation since last menstrual period PLUS weeks of chronologic age since birth; qid, 4 times daily; tid, 3 times daily; VZV, varicella-zoster virus.

Infection	Therapy (evidence grade)	Comments
Adenovirus (pneumonia or disseminated infection in immunocompromised hosts)[1]	Cidofovir and ribavirin are active in vitro, but no prospective clinical data exist and both have significant toxicity. Two cidofovir dosing schedules have been employed in clinical settings: (1) 5 mg/kg/dose administered intravenously once weekly; or (2) 1–1.5 mg/kg/dose administered intravenously 3 times/wk. If parenteral cidofovir is utilized, intravenous hydration and oral probenicid should be used to reduce renal toxicity.	The orally bioavailable lipophilic derivative of cidofovir, CMX001, is under investigation for the treatment of adenovirus in immunocompromised hosts. It is not yet commercially available.
Cytomegalovirus		
– Neonatal[2]	See Chapter 5.	
– Immunocompromised (HIV, chemotherapy, transplant-related)[3-15]	For induction: ganciclovir 10 mg/kg/day IV div q12h for 14–21 days (AII) (may be increased to 15 mg/kg/day IV div q12h). For maintenance: 5 mg/kg IV q24h for 5–7 days per week. Duration dependent on degree of immunosuppression (AII). CMV hyperimmune globulin may decrease morbidity in bone marrow transplant patients with CMV pneumonia (AII).	Use foscarnet or cidofovir for ganciclovir-resistant strains; for HIV-positive children on HAART, CMV may resolve without therapy. Also used for prevention of CMV disease post-transplant for 100–120 days. Data on valganciclovir dosing in young children for treatment of retinitis are unavailable, but consideration can be given to transitioning from IV ganciclovir to oral valganciclovir after improvement of retinitis is noted. Limited data on oral valganciclovir in neonates[16,17] (32 mg/kg/day PO div bid) and children dosing by body surface area (BSA) (dose [mg] = $7 \times BSA \times$ creatinine clearance).[5]

– Prophylaxis of infection in immunocompromised hosts[4,18]	Ganciclovir 5 mg/kg IV daily (or 3 times/wk) (started at engraftment for stem cell transplant patients) (BII) Valganciclovir oral solution (50 mg/mL) at total dose in milligrams = 7 x BSA x CrCl (use maximum CrCl 150 mL/min/1.73 m²) orally once daily with food for children aged 4 mo–16 y (max dose 900 mg/day) for primary prophylaxis in HIV patients[19] who are CMV antibody positive and have severe immunosuppression (CD4 count <50 cells/mm³ in children ≥6 y; CD4 percentage <5% in children <6 y) (CIII)	Neutropenia is a complication with GCV prophylaxis and may be addressed with G-CSF. Both prophylaxis and preemptive strategies are effective; neither has been shown clearly superior to the other.[9]
Epstein-Barr virus		
– Mononucleosis, encephalitis[20–22]	Limited data suggest clinical benefit of valacyclovir in adolescents for mononucleosis (3 g/day div tid for 14 days) (CIII) For EBV encephalitis: ganciclovir IV OR acyclovir IV (AIII)	No prospective data on benefits of acyclovir IV or ganciclovir IV in EBV clinical infections of normal hosts
– Post-transplant lymphoproliferative disorder (PTLD)[23,24]	Ganciclovir (AIII)	Decrease immune suppression if possible, as this has the most impact on control of EBV; rituximab, methotrexate have been used but without controlled data. Preemptive treatment with GCV may decrease PTLD in solid organ transplants.

Infection	Therapy (evidence grade)	Comments
Hepatitis B virus (chronic)[25-38]	IFN-alpha 3 million units/m²body surface area SQ 3 times/wk for 1 wk, followed by dose escalation to 6 million units/m² body surface area (max 10 million units/dose), to complete a 24-wk course for children 1–18 y; OR lamivudine 3 mg/kg/day (max 100 mg) PO q24h for 52 wk for children ≥2 y (children coinfected with HIV and hepatitis B should use the approved dose for HIV) (AII); OR adefovir for children ≥12 y (10 mg PO q24h for a minimum of 12 mo; optimum duration of therapy unknown) (BII); OR entecavir for children ≥16 y (0.5 mg qd in patients who have not received prior nucleoside therapy; 1 mg qd in patients who are previously treated (not first choice in this setting); optimum duration of therapy unknown (BII)	Indications for treatment of chronic HBV infection, with or without HIV coinfection, are: (1) evidence of ongoing HBV viral replication, as indicated by serum HBV DNA (>10,000–100,000 IU/mL) for >6 mo and persistent elevation of serum transaminase levels (at least twice the upper limit of normal for >6 mo); or (2) evidence of chronic hepatitis on liver biopsy (BII). Antiviral therapy is not warranted in children without necroinflammatory liver disease (BII). Treatment is not recommended for children with immunotolerant chronic HBV infection (ie, normal serum transaminase levels despite detectable HBV DNA) (BII). Standard interferon-alfa (IFN-2a or -2b) is recommended for treating chronic hepatitis B infection with compensated liver disease in HIV-uninfected children aged ≥2 y who warrant treatment (AII). Interferon-alfa therapy in combination with oral antiviral therapy cannot be recommended for pediatric HBV infection in HIV-uninfected children until more data are available (BII). In HIV/HBV-coinfected children who do not require ART for their HIV infection, IFN-alpha therapy is the preferred agent to treat chronic hepatitis B (BIII), whereas adefovir can be considered in children ≥12 y (BIII). Treatment options for HIV/HBV-coinfected children who meet criteria for HBV therapy and who are already receiving lamivudine- or emtricitabine-containing HIV-suppressive ART, include the standard IFN-alpha therapy to the ARV regimen (BIII), or adefovir if the child can receive adult dosing (BIII), or use of tenofovir disoproxil fumarate (TDF) in lamivudine (or emtricitabine)-containing ARV regimen in children ≥2 y (BIII). HIV/HBV-coinfected children should not be given lamivudine (or emtricitabine) without additional anti-HIV drugs for treatment of chronic hepatitis B (CIII).[19] Alternatives: Tenofovir (adult and adolescent dose [≥12 y] 300 mg qd). Telbivudine (adult dose 600 mg qd). There are not sufficient clinical data to identify the appropriate dose for use in children. Lamivudine approved for children ≥2 y, but antiviral resistance develops on therapy in 30%. Entecavir is superior to lamivudine in the treatment of chronic HBV infection and is the most potent anti-HBV agent available.

Hepatitis C virus
(chronic)[39-45]

Pegylated IFN-alpha: PEG-IFN 2a 180 μg/1.73 m² body surface area subcutaneously once per wk (maximum dose 180 μg) OR PEG-IFN 2b 60 μg/m² body surface area once per wk
PLUS

Ribavirin (oral) 7.5 mg/kg body weight twice daily (fixed dose by weight recommended):
25–36 kg: 200 mg am and pm
>36–49 kg: 200 mg in am and 400 mg in pm
>49–61 kg: 400 mg in am and pm
>61–75 kg: 400 mg in am and 600 mg in pm
>75 kg: 600 mg in am and pm
Treatment duration: 24-48 wk
(AII)

Treatment of children aged <3 y who have HCV infection usually is not recommended (BIII).

HCV-infected, HIV-uninfected children ≥3 y should be individualized because HCV usually causes mild disease in this population and few data exist to identify risk factors differentiating those at greater risk for progression of liver disease. Those who are chosen for treatment should receive combination therapy with IFN-alpha and ribavirin for 48 wk for genotype 1 and 24 wk for genotypes 2 or 3 (AI).

Treatment should be considered for all HIV/HCV-coinfected children aged >3 y who have no contraindications to treatment (BIII).

A liver biopsy to stage disease is recommended before deciding whether to initiate therapy for chronic HCV genotype 1 infection (BIII). However, some specialists would treat children infected with HCV genotypes 2 or 3 without first obtaining a liver biopsy (BIII).

Treatment of HCV-infected children, regardless of HIV status, should include IFN-alpha plus ribavirin combination therapy (AI). Duration of treatment for HIV/HCV-coinfected children should be 48 wk, regardless of HCV genotype (BIII).

IFN-alpha therapy is contraindicated for children with decompensated liver disease, substantial cytopenias, renal failure; severe cardiac or neuropsychiatric disorders, and non–HCV-related autoimmune disease (AII).[19]

The protease inhibitors telaprevir and boceprevir have been approved for use in adults for treatment of HCV genotype 1, in concert with peg-IFN-alpha and ribavirin therapy. This "triple therapy" was associated with markedly improved viral clearance, with sustained virologic responses demonstrated in up to 68% of treated patients. These agents may be tested and approved for use in children in the near future. No recommendations for use of these agents in children can be made at this time.

Infection	Therapy (evidence grade)	Comments
Herpes simplex virus		
– Third trimester maternal suppressive therapy[46,47]	Acyclovir or valacyclovir maternal suppressive therapy in pregnant women reduces HSV recurrences and viral shedding at the time of delivery but does not fully prevent neonatal HSV[48] (BIII).	
– Neonatal	See Chapter 5.	
– Mucocutaneous (normal host)	Acyclovir 60–80 mg/kg/day PO div tid–qid for 5–7 days; or 15 mg/kg/day IV as 1–2 h infusion div q8h (AII) Suppressive therapy for frequent recurrence (no pediatric data): 20 mg/kg/dose given bid or tid (up to 400 mg) for 6–12 mo; then reevaluate need (AIII) Valacyclovir 20 mg/kg/dose (max dose: 1 g) PO bid[49] for 5–7 days (BII)	Foscarnet for acyclovir-resistant strains. Immunocompromised hosts may require 10–14 days of therapy.
– Genital	Adult doses: acyclovir 400 mg PO tid, for 7–10 days; OR valacyclovir 1 g PO bid for 10 days; OR famciclovir 250 mg PO tid for 7–10 days (AI)	All 3 drugs have been used as prophylaxis to prevent recurrence.
– Encephalitis	Acyclovir 60 mg/kg/day IV as 1–2 h infusion div q8h; for 21 days for infants ≤4 mo. For older infants and children, 45–60 mg/kg/day IV (AIII).	Safety of high-dose acyclovir (60 mg/kg/day) not well defined beyond the neonatal period; can be used, but monitor for neurotoxicity and nephrotoxicity.
– Keratoconjunctivitis	1% trifluridine, 0.1% iododeoxyuridine, or 0.15% ganciclovir ophthalmic gel (AII)	Treat in consultation with an ophthalmologist. Topical steroids may be helpful when used together with antiviral agents.
Human herpesvirus 6 (HHV-6)		
– Immunocompromised children[50]	No prospective comparative data; ganciclovir 10–20 mg/kg/day IV div q12h case report (AIII)	May require high dose to control infection; safety and efficacy not defined at high doses.

Human immunodeficiency virus (HIV)

Current information on HIV treatment and opportunistic infections for children[51] is posted at http://aidsinfo.nih.gov/ContentFiles/PediatricGuidelines.pdf; other information on HIV programs is available at www.cdc.gov/hiv/policies/index.html. Consult with an HIV expert, if possible, for current recommendations.

– Therapy of HIV infection State-of-the-art therapy is rapidly evolving with introduction of new agents and combinations; currently there are 23 individual anti-retroviral agents approved for use by the FDA that have pediatric indications, as well as multiple combinations; guidelines for children and adolescents are continually updated on the AIDSINFO and CDC Web site given above.	Effective therapy (HAART) consists of ≥3 agents, including 2 nucleoside reverse transcriptase inhibitors, plus a protease inhibitor or non-nucleoside reverse transcriptase inhibitor (integrase inhibitors are currently available for 2nd-line therapy options); many different combination regimens give similar treatment outcomes; choice of agents depends on the age of the child, viral load, consideration of potential viral resistance, and extent of immune depletion, in addition to judging the child's ability to adhere to the regimen.	Assess drug toxicity (based on the agents used) and virologic/immunologic response to therapy (quantitative plasma HIV and CD4 count) initially monthly and then every 3–6 mo during the maintenance phase.
– Children of any age	Any child with AIDS or significant HIV-related symptoms (clinical category C and most B conditions) should be treated (AI).	Adherence counseling and appropriate ARV formulations are critical for successful implementation.
– First year of life[52]	HAART with ≥3 drugs is now recommended for all infants ≤12 mo, regardless of clinical status or laboratory values (AI for < 12 wk; AII for 12–52 wk).	Preferred therapy in the first year of life is zidovudine plus lamivudine plus lopinavir/ritonavir (toxicity concerns preclude its use until a postmenstrual age of 42 wk and a postnatal age of at least 14 days is reached).

Infection	Therapy (evidence grade)	Comments
– HIV-infected children ≥1 y who are asymptomatic or have mild symptoms	Treat with the following CD4 values: Age 1 to <3 y with CD4 <1,000 or <25% (AII) Age 3 to <5 y with CD4 <750 <25% (AII) Age ≥5 y with CD4 <350 (AI) with CD4 350–500 (BII)	Preferred regimens comprise either zidovudine plus lamivudine (at any age) OR abacavir plus lamivudine (>3 mo) OR tenofovir plus emtricitabene aka Truvada (adolescents/Tanner stage 4 or 5) PLUS either lopinavir/ritonavir (any age >2 wk) OR efavirenz (≥3 y) OR atazanavir/ritonavir (≥6 y).
– HIV-infected children ≥1 y who are asymptomatic or have mild symptoms	Consider treatment with the following CD4 values: Age 1 to <3 y with CD4 ≥1,000 or ≥25% (BIII) Age 3 to <5 y with CD4 ≥750 or ≥25% (BIII) Age ≥5 y with CD4 >500 (BIII)	Expert opinion has migrated toward treatment consideration even in mild clinical situations. Treatment deferral and monitoring of clinical course, CD4 count, and plasma HIV RNA on a 3- to 4-mo basis is an option.
– Any child ≥1 y	Treat when viral load ≥100,000 copies/mL (AII).	Most experts now recommend treatment in settings of high viral load.
– Antiretroviral-experienced child	Consult with HIV specialist.	Consider treatment history and drug resistance testing and assess adherence.
– HIV exposures, nonoccupational	Therapy recommendations for exposures available on the CDC Web site given on page 117, based on assessment of risk of HIV exposure.	Prophylaxis remains unproven; consider individually regarding risk, time from exposure, and likelihood of adherence; prophylactic regimens administered for 4 wk.
– Negligible exposure risk (urine, nasal secretions, saliva, sweat, or tears—no visible blood in secretions) OR >72 h since exposure	Prophylaxis not recommended (BII)	
– Significant exposure risk (blood, semen, vaginal, or rectal secretions from a known HIV-infected individual) AND <72 h since exposure	Prophylaxis recommended (BIII): combivir (zidovudine/lamivudine) or Truvada (tenofovir/emtricitabine) PLUS efavirenz or Kaletra (lopinavir/ritonavir). Since the last DHHS/CDC guidelines in 2005, raltegravir or darunavir/ritonavir in place of either efavirenz or lopinavir/ritonavir has gained some favor among experts	Preferred prophylactic regimens – Based on treatment regimens for infected individuals – 28-day regimen In the event of poor adherence or toxicity, some experts consider 2 NRTI regimens, such as combivir (zidovudine/lamivudine) or Truvada (tenofovir/emtricitabine) (BIII).
– HIV exposure, occupational	See guidelines on CDC Web site given on page 117.	

Influenza virus

Frequent changes in recommendations have occurred recently regarding influenza due to antiviral resistance that can vary from season to season; therefore, the reader should access the AAP Web site (www.aap.org) and the CDC Web site (www.cdc.gov/flu/professionals/antivirals/antiviral-agents-flu.htm) for the most current, accurate information.

Influenza A and B

– Treatment	**Oseltamivir** Preterm, <38 wk postmenstrual age: 1.0 mg/kg/dose PO bid Preterm, 38–40 wk postmenstrual age: 1.5 mg/kg/dose PO bid Preterm, >40 wk postmenstrual age: 3.0 mg/kg/dose PO bid[53] Term, birth–8 mo: 3.0 mg/kg/dose PO bid 9–11 mo: 3.5 mg/kg/dose PO bid 12–23 mo: 3.5 mg/kg/dose PO bid[r] 2–12 y: ≤15 kg: 30 mg, bid; 16–23 kg: 45 mg, bid; 24–40 kg: 60 mg, bid; >40 kg: 75 mg, bid ≥13 y: 75 mg, bid, OR Zanamivir ≥7 y: 10 mg by inhalation, bid for 5 days	Oseltamivir currently is drug of choice for treatment of influenza infections. Preliminary data in premature infants (median gestational age 27.5 wk, median weight 1,680 g, median age 2.5 wk) suggest 1 mg/kg/dose q12h. The adamantanes, amantadine and rimantadine, currently are not effective for treatment due to near-universal resistance of influenza A.
– Chemoprophylaxis	**Oseltamivir** 3 mo–12 y: Same as treatment for patients 3 mo–12 y, except dose given qd for 2–12-y (given bid to 0–23 mo) ≥13 y: 75 mg, qd **Zanamivir** ≥5 y: 10 mg by inhalation, qd for as long as 28 days (community outbreaks) or 10 days (household setting)	Oseltamivir currently is drug of choice for chemoprophylaxis of influenza infection. The adamantanes, amantadine and rimantadine, currently are not effective for chemoprophylaxis due to near-universal resistance of influenza A.
Measles[55]	No prospective data on antiviral therapy. Ribavirin is active against measles virus in vitro. Vitamin A is beneficial to children who may be deficient (qd dosing for 2 days): for children ≥1 y: 200,000 IU; for infants 6–12 mo: 100,000 IU; for infants <6 mo: 50,000 IU (BII).	IG prophylaxis for exposed, susceptible children: 0.25 mL/kg IM; and for immunocompromised children: 0.5 mL/kg (max 15 mL) IM

Infection	Therapy (evidence grade)	Comments
Respiratory syncytial virus (RSV)[56]		
– Therapy (severe disease in compromised host)	Ribavirin (6-g vial to make 20 mg/mL solution in sterile water), aerosolized over 18–20 h daily for 3–5 days (BII)	Aerosol ribavirin provides a small benefit and should only be used for life-threatening infection with RSV. Airway reactivity with inhalation precludes routine use.
– Palivizumab (Synagis) prophylaxis for high-risk infants (AII) (for definition of high risk, see Comments)	Palivizumab (Synagis, a monoclonal antibody) 15 mg/kg IM monthly. For all high-risk groups except premature infants with GA between 32 and 35 wk, a maximum of 5 doses should be provided during the RSV season, with the first dose given on November 1, and the last dose on March 1 (currently defined as the RSV season for most of the United States). For infants with GA between 32 and <35 wk, a maximum of 3 doses should be provided during the RSV season. No infants should routinely receive a dose of palivizumab after the March 1 dose.	Palivizumab will not treat an active infection. In Florida, the RSV season lasts 5 mo but starts earlier than in the rest of the United States.[27] 1. Infants <24 mo with chronic lung disease who are receiving or have received medical therapy (oxygen, bronchodilator, diuretic, or corticosteroid therapy) within 6 mo before start of the RSV season (since May 1). 2. Infants <24 mo with hemodynamically significant congenital heart disease (congestive heart failure requiring therapy, moderate–severe pulmonary hypertension, cyanotic heart disease). 3. Infants with congenital abnormalities of the airway or a neuromuscular disorder, who will be <12 mo on November 1. 4. Extremely premature infants: GA <28 wk, and CA <12 mo on November 1. 5. Very premature infants: GA 29 to <32 wk (31 wk, 6 days), and CA <6 mo on November 1. 6. Premature infants: GA between 32 wk (32 wk, 0 days) to <35 wk (34 wk, 6 days), and CA <3 mo on November 1, AND 1 of 2 additional risk factors should be present to receive palivizumab: child care attendance; or a sibling <5 y.

Varicella-zoster virus[57]

– Infection in a normal host	Acyclovir 80 mg/kg/day (max 3.2 g/day) PO div qid for 5 days (AI)	The sooner antiviral therapy can be started, the greater the impact.
– Severe primary chickenpox, disseminated infection (cutaneous, pneumonia, encephalitis, hepatitis); immunocompromised host with primary chickenpox or disseminated zoster	Acyclovir 30 mg/kg/day IV as 1–2 h infusion div q8h; for 10 days (acyclovir doses of 45–60 mg/kg/day in 3 divided doses IV should be used for disseminated or central nervous system infection). Dosing can also be provided as: 1,500 mg/m²/day IV div q8h. Duration in immunocompromised children: 7–14 days, based on clinical response (AI).	Valacyclovir, famciclovir, foscarnet also active

10. Preferred Therapy for Specific Parasitic Pathogens

NOTES
- For some parasitic diseases, therapy may be available only from the Centers for Disease Control and Prevention (CDC), as noted. Consultation is available from the CDC for parasitic disease diagnostic services (www.cdc.gov/parasites/health_professionals.html), parasitic disease testing, and experimental therapy Monday through Friday, 8:00 am to 4:30 pm EST, at 404/718-4745 (emergency, after-hours hotline 770/488-7100); for malaria Monday through Friday, 9:00 am to 5:00 pm EST, 770/488-7788 or toll-free 855/856-4713 (emergency, after-hours hotline 770/488-7100). Antiparasitic drugs available from the CDC can be viewed and requested at www.cdc.gov/ncidod/srp/drugs/formulary.html.

- The US Food and Drug Administration provides a number of useful resources.
  - New Pediatric Labeling Information Database (www.fda.gov/NewPedLabeling)
  - Safety Reporting on products presented to the Pediatric Advisory Committee (www.fda.gov/PedDrugSafety)
  - Pediatric Studies Characteristics (www.fda.gov/PedStudies)

- **Abbreviations:** AFB, acid-fast bacteria; bid, twice daily; BP, blood pressure; CDC, Centers for Disease Control and Prevention; CNS, central nervous system; CSF, cerebrospinal fluid; CrCl, creatinine clearance; DEC, diethylcarbamazine; div, divided; ECG, electrocardiogram; FDA, US Food and Drug Administration; G6PD, glucose-6-phosphate dehydrogenase; GI, gastrointestinal; HAART, highly active antiretroviral therapy; HIV, human immunodeficiency virus; IM, intramuscular; IV, intravenous; PO, orally; qd, once daily; qid, 4 times daily; qod, every other day; tab, tablet; tid, 3 times daily; TMP/SMX, trimethroprim/sulfamethoxazole; UV, ultraviolet.

Disease/Organism	Treatment	Comments
AMEBIASIS[1–4]		
ENTERITIS/LIVER ABSCESS		
Entamoeba histolytica		
– Asymptomatic carrier	Paromomycin 30 mg/kg/day PO tid for 7 days; OR iodoquinol 30–40 mg/kg/day (max 2 g) PO tid for 20 days; OR diloxanide furoate (not commercially available in the US) 20 mg/kg/day PO div tid for 10 days (CII)	Follow-up stool examination to ensure eradication of carriage; screen/treat positive close contacts.
– Mild to moderate colitis	Metronidazole 30–40 mg/kg/day PO div tid for 10 days; OR tinidazole 50 mg/kg/day PO (max 2 g) qd for 3 days FOLLOWED by paromomycin or iodoquinol as above to eliminate cysts (BII)	Avoid antimotility drugs, steroids. Take tinidazole with food to decrease GI side effects; if unable to take tablets, pharmacists can crush tablets and mix with syrup. Nitazoxanide (see *Giardia*) may also be effective.
– Severe colitis, liver abscess	Metronidazole 35–40 mg/kg/day IV q8h, switch to PO when tolerated, for 10 days; OR tinidazole (age ≥3 y) 50 mg/kg/day PO (max 2 g) qd for 5 days FOLLOWED by paromomycin or iodoquinol as above to eliminate cysts (BII)	Serologic assays >95% positive in extraintestinal amebiasis. Percutaneous or surgical drainage may be indicated for large liver abscesses or inadequate response to medical therapy. Chloroquine plus metronidazole or tinidazole followed by luminal agent considered alternative for liver abscess.
MENINGOENCEPHALITIS[5–10]		
Naegleria, Acanthamoeba, Balamuthia, Hartmanella spp	Amphotericin B 1.5 mg/kg/day IV in 2 doses for 3 days then 1 mg/kg/day for 6 days plus 1.5 mg/day intrathecally for 2 days, then 1 mg/day qod for 8 days; consider alternative 1–1.5 mg/kg/day qd for 3–4 wk or longer, PLUS azithromycin for *Naegleria*; for *Naegleria*, also consider rifampicin 10 mg/kg/day IV and/or fluconazole 10 mg/kg/d IV; miltefosine (from CDC as IND in association with FDA) may be of benefit to treat free-living amoeba infections (especially *Acanthamoeba* and *Balamuthia*); miltefosine dose for <45 kg, 100 mg daily (ie, one 50-mg cap PO bid), for ≥45 kg: 150 mg daily (ie, one 50-mg cap PO tid). Give miltefosine with food to decrease gastrointestinal side effects.	Treatment outcomes usually unsuccessful; early therapy (even before diagnostic confirmation if indicated) may improve survival. *Acanthamoeba* may be susceptible in vitro to ketoconazole, flucytosine, and pentamidine; voriconazole and miltefosine active against *Acanthamoeba* (alone or in combination with pentamidine). *Balamuthia* may be susceptible in vitro to pentamidine, azithromycin/clarithromycin, fluconazole, sulfadiazine, and flucytosine (CIII). Surgical resection of CNS lesions may be beneficial. Miltefosine may be of benefit. Keratitis should be evaluated by an ophthalmologist.

Ancylostoma caninum	See EOSINOPHILIC COLITIS.	
Ancylostoma duodenale	See HOOKWORM.	
ANGIOSTRONGYLIASIS[1,12,13]		
Angiostrongylus cantonensis	Albendazole 20 mg/kg/day PO div bid for 9 days (CIII)	Most patients recover without antiparasitic therapy; treatment may provoke severe neurologic symptoms but may shorten duration of headache. Corticosteroids, analgesics, and repeat lumbar puncture may be of benefit.
Angiostrongylus costaricensis	Thiabendazole 50–75 mg/kg/day (max 3 g) PO div tid for 3 days (CIII)	No well-proven treatment for either *Angiostrongylus* spp
ASCARIASIS (*Ascaris lumbricoides*)[14,15]	Albendazole 400 mg PO once (BII); OR ivermectin 150–200 µg/kg PO once (CII)	Follow-up stool ova and parasite examination after therapy not essential. Take albendazole with food. Nitazoxanide also effective against intestinal helminths. Albendazole has theoretical risk of causing seizures in patients coinfected with cysticercosis.
BABESIOSIS (*Babesia* spp)[16–18]	Clindamycin 30 mg/kg/day PO div tid, PLUS quinine 25 mg/kg/day PO div tid for 7 days (BII); OR atovaquone 40 mg/kg/day div bid, PLUS azithromycin 12 mg/kg/day for 7 days (CII)	Clindamycin (IV) and quinine preferred for severe disease; prolonged therapy, daily monitoring of hematocrit and percentage of parasitized RBCs, and exchange blood transfusion may be of benefit for severe disease.
Balantidium coli[19]	Tetracycline (patient >7 y) 40 mg/kg/day PO div qid for 10 days (max 2 g/day) (BII); OR metronidazole 35–50 mg/kg/day PO div tid for 5 days; OR iodoquinol 40 mg/kg/day (max 2 g/day) PO div tid for 20 days (CII)	Repeated stool examination may be needed for diagnosis; prompt stool examination may increase detection of rapidly degenerating trophozoites.
Baylisascaris procyonis (raccoon roundworm)[20,21]	For CNS infection: albendazole 25–40 mg/kg/day PO div q12h AND high-dose corticosteroid therapy (CIII)	Therapy generally unsuccessful to prevent fatal outcome or severe neurologic sequelae once CNS disease present. Steroids may be of value in decreasing inflammation with therapy of CNS or ocular infection. Retinal worms may be killed by direct photocoagulation. Consider prophylactic albendazole (25–50 mg/kg PO daily for 10–20 days) for children who may have ingested soil contaminated with raccoon feces.

Preferred Therapy for Specific Parasitic Pathogens

10

Disease/Organism	Treatment	Comments
Blastocystis hominis[22,23]	Metronidazole 30 mg/kg/day PO div tid for 10 days; OR iodoquinol 40 mg/kg/day (max 2 g) PO div tid for 20 days; OR nitazoxanide (as for Cryptosporidium) (CII)	Normal hosts may not need therapy; reexamination of stool for other parasites (eg, Giardia) may be of value. Metronidazole resistance may occur.
CHAGAS DISEASE (Trypanosoma cruzi)[24,25]	See TRYPANOSOMIASIS.	
Clonorchis sinensis	See FLUKES.	
CRYPTOSPORIDIOSIS (Cryptosporidium parvum)[26–30]	Nitazoxanide, age 12–47 mo, 5 mL (100 mg) bid for 3 days; age 4–11 y, 10 mL (200 mg) bid for 3 days (BII); OR paromomycin 30 mg/kg/day div bid–qid (CII); OR azithromycin 10 mg/kg/day for 5 days (CII); repeated treatment courses may be needed.	Disease may be self-limited in immunocompetent hosts. In HIV-infected patients not receiving HAART, medical therapy may have limited efficacy.
CUTANEOUS LARVA MIGRANS or CREEPING ERUPTION[31,32] (dog and cat hookworm) Ancylostoma caninum, Ancylostoma braziliense, Uncinaria stenocephala	Albendazole 15 mg/kg/day PO qd for 3 days (BII); OR ivermectin 200 µg/kg PO once (BII)	
Cyclospora spp[33,34] (cyanobacterium-like agent)	TMP/SMX (10 mg TMP/kg/day) PO div bid for 5–10 days (BIII); OR ciprofloxacin 30 mg/kg/day div bid for 7 days	HIV-infected patients may require higher doses/longer therapy.
CYSTICERCOSIS[35–37] (Cysticercus cellulosae)	Albendazole 15 mg/kg/day PO bid (max 800 mg/day) for 8–30 days (CII); OR praziquantel 50–100 mg/kg/day PO div for 15–30 days (phenytoin decreases praziquantel concentration) (CII)	For CNS disease with multiple lesions, give steroids and anticonvulsants before first dose; for CNS disease with few lesions, steroid pretreatment not required.[30,31] Contraindicated for eye or spinal cord lesions (surgery as indicated). Treatment controversial, especially for single lesion disease.
DIENTAMEBIASIS[38,39] (Dientamoeba fragilis)	Paromomycin 25 mg/kg/day PO div tid for 7 days; OR iodoquinol 40 mg/kg/day (max 2 g) PO div tid for 20 days; OR metronidazole 30 mg/kg/day PO div tid for 10 days (BII)	Asymptomatic colonization more common in adults than children
Diphyllobothrium latum	See TAPEWORMS.	

ECHINOCOCCOSIS		
Echinococcus granulosus, Echinococcus multilocularis[40,41]	Albendazole 15 mg/kg/day PO div bid (max 800 mg/day) for 1–6 mo alone (CIII), or combined with praziquantel 50–75 mg/kg daily (BII) for 5–14 days ± once weekly dose for additional 3–6 mo	Surgical excision may be the only reliable therapy; ultrasound-guided percutaneous aspiration-injection-reaspiration (PAIR) plus albendazole may be effective for hepatic hydatid cysts.
Entamoeba histolytica	See AMEBIASIS.	
Enterobius vermicularis	See PINWORMS.	
Fasciola hepatica	See FLUKES.	
EOSINOPHILIC COLITIS (*Ancylostoma caninum*)[42]	Albendazole 15 mg/kg/day PO div bid (max 400 mg/day) (BII)	Endoscopic removal may be considered if medical treatment not successful.
EOSINOPHILIC MENINGITIS	See ANGIOSTRONGYLIASIS.	
FILARIASIS[43]		Ivermectin may be effective for killing *Wuchereria, Brugia,* and *Loa loa* microfilariae; in heavy infections or when coinfection with *O volvulus* possible, consider ivermectin initially to reduce microfilaremia before giving DEC (decreased risk of encephalopathy or severe allergic or febrile reaction).
– River blindness (*Onchocerca volvulus*)	Ivermectin 150 µg/kg PO once (AII); repeat q6–12 mo until asymptomatic and no chronic, ongoing exposure	Antihistamines or corticosteroids are of benefit for allergic reactions.
– *Wuchereria bancrofti, Brugia malayi, Mansonella streptocerca*	*W bancrofti, B malayi, M streptocerca*: DEC (from CDC) 1 mg/kg PO after food on day 1; then 3 mg/kg/day div tid on day 2; then 3–6 mg/kg/day div tid on day 3; then 6 mg/kg/day div tid on days 4–14 (AII)	
Mansonella ozzardi	Ivermectin 150 µg/kg PO once may be effective	DEC not reported to be effective.
Mansonella perstans	Albendazole 400 mg PO bid for 10 days	
Loa loa	DEC (from CDC) as above, then 9 mg/kg/day div tid on days 14–21 (AII)	
Tropical pulmonary eosinophilia (TPE)[44]	DEC (from CDC) 6 mg/kg/day PO tid for 14 days; antihistamines/corticosteroids for allergic reactions (CII)	

10

Preferred Therapy for Specific Parasitic Pathogens

10

Disease/Organism	Treatment	Comments
FLUKES		
Chinese liver fluke[45] *(Clonorchis sinensis)* and others *(Fasciolopsis, Heterophyes, Metagonimus, Metorchis, Nanophyetus, Opisthorchis)*	Praziquantel 75 mg/kg PO tid for 2 days (BII); OR albendazole 10 mg/kg/day PO qd for 7 days (CIII)	Take praziquantel with liquids and food.
Lung fluke[46,47] *(Paragonimus westermani* and other *Paragonimus* lung flukes)*	Praziquantel 75 mg/kg PO tid for 2 days (BII)	Triclabendazole (see below) (5 mg/kg qd for 3 days or 10 mg/kg bid for 1 day) may also be effective; triclabendazole should be taken with food to facilitate absorption.
Sheep liver fluke[48] *(Fasciola hepatica)*	Triclabendazole (from CDC) 10 mg/kg PO once (BIII); OR nitazoxanide PO (take with food), age 12–47 mo, 100 mg/dose bid for 7 days; age 4–11 y, 200 mg/dose bid for 7 days; age ≥12 y, 1 tab (500 mg)/dose bid for 7 days (CII)	Triclabendazole is not approved by the FDA or available in the United States; physicians may seek individual use IND through FDA.
GIARDIASIS *(Giardia lamblia)*[49-51]	Metronidazole 30–40 mg/kg/day PO tid for 7–10 days (BII); OR nitazoxanide PO (take with food), age 12–47 mo, 100 mg/dose bid for 7 days; age 4–11 y, 200 mg/dose bid for 7 days; age ≥12 y, 1 tab (500 mg)/dose bid for 7 days (BII); OR tinidazole 50 mg/kg/day (max 2 g) for 1 day (BII)	If therapy inadequate, another course of the same agent usually curative. Alternatives: furazolidone 6 mg/kg/day in 4 doses for 7–10 days; OR paromomycin 30 mg/kg/day div tid for 5–10 days; OR albendazole 10 mg/kg/day PO for 5 days (CII). Prolonged courses may be needed for immunocompromising conditions (eg, hypogammaglobulinemia). Treatment of asymptomatic carriers not usually recommended.
HOOKWORM[52]		
Necator americanus, Ancylostoma duodenale	Albendazole 10 mg/kg (max 400 mg) once (repeat dose may be necessary) (BII); OR pyrantel pamoate 11 mg/kg (max 1 g/day) (BII) PO qd for 3 days	Perform repeat stool examination 2 weeks after treatment, re-treat if positive.

Hymenolepis nana	See TAPEWORMS.
ISOSPORIASIS (*Isospora belli*)[19], now also known as cystoisosporiasis	TMP/SMX (10 mg TMP/kg/day) PO div qid for 10 days; then 5 mg TMP/kg/day PO div bid for 3 wk; pyrimethamine may be effective (CII). HIV-infected children may need longer courses of therapy (consider long-term maintenance therapy for multiple relapses).	Infection often self-limited in immunocompetent hosts. Repeated stool examinations and special techniques (eg, modified AFB staining or UV microscopy) may be needed to detect low oocyst numbers.
LEISHMANIASIS,[53-58] including kala azar		
Leishmania spp	Visceral: liposomal amphotericin B, 3 mg/kg/day on days 1–5, day 14, and day 21 (BIII); OR sodium stibogluconate (from CDC) 20 mg/kg/day IM, IV for 20–28 days (or longer) (BIII); OR miltefosine 2.5 mg/kg/day PO (max 150 mg/day) for 28 days (BIII); OR amphotericin B 1 mg/kg/day IV daily for 15–20 days or every second day for 4–8 wk (BIII); OR paromomycin sulfate 15 mg/kg/day IM for 21 days (BII) Cutaneous: sodium stibogluconate 20 mg/kg/day IM, IV for 20 days (BIII); OR miltefosine (as above) (BIII); OR pentamidine isethionate 2–4 mg/kg/day IM daily or every second day for 14 days (BII) Mucosal: sodium stibogluconate 20 mg/kg/day IM, IV for 28 days; OR amphotericin B 0.5–1 mg/kg/day IV daily for 15–20 days or every second day for 4–8 wk; OR miltefosine (as above)	Consult with tropical medicine specialist if unfamiliar with leishmaniasis. Patients infected in south Asia (especially India, Nepal) should receive non-antimonial regimens because of high rates of resistance. Azoles (eg, fluconazole, ketoconazole) may be effective for cutaneous disease but should be avoided in treating mucosal or visceral disease. Topical paromomycin (15%) applied twice daily for 10–20 days may be considered for cutaneous leishmaniasis in areas where the potential for mucosal disease is rare.

Preferred Therapy for Specific Parasitic Pathogens

10

Disease/Organism	Treatment	Comments
LICE		
Pediculus capitis or humanus, Phthirus pubis[59,60]	Follow manufacturer's instructions for topical use: permethrin 1% (BII); OR pyrethrins (BII); OR malathion 0.5% (BII); OR lindane; OR benzyl alcohol lotion 5% (BII); OR ivermectin lotion 0.5% (BII); OR spinosad 0.9% topical suspension (BII); for topical therapies repeat in 1 wk; OR ivermectin 200 µg/kg PO once	Launder bedding and clothing; for eyelash infestation, use petrolatum; for head lice, remove nits with comb designed for that purpose. Use benzyl alcohol lotion and ivermectin lotion for children aged ≥6 mo and spinosad for children aged ≥4 y. Benzyl alcohol can be irritating to skin. Consult health care provider before re-treatment with ivermectin lotion; re-treatment with spinosad topical suspension usually not needed (unless live lice seen 1 wk after first treatment). Administration of 3 doses of ivermectin (1 dose/wk separately by weekly intervals) may be needed to eradicate infection.
MALARIA[61–66]		
Plasmodium falciparum, Plasmodium vivax, Plasmodium ovale, Plasmodium malariae	CDC Physician's Malaria Hotline 770/488-7788 (or, after hours, 7100); online information at www.cdc.gov/malaria. Consult tropical medicine specialist if unfamiliar with malaria.	No antimalarial drug provides absolute protection against malaria; fever after return from an endemic area should prompt an immediate evaluation. Emphasize personal protective measures (insecticides, bed nets, clothing, avoidance of dusk-dawn mosquito exposures).

Prophylaxis	
For areas with chloroquine-resistant *P falciparum* or *P vivax*	Atovaquone-proguanil (A-P): 11–20 kg, 1 pediatric tab (62.5 mg atovaquone/25 mg proguanil); 21–30 kg, 2 pediatric tabs; 31–40 kg, 3 pediatric tabs; >40 kg, 1 adult tab (250 mg atovaquone/100 mg proguanil) PO daily starting 1–2 days before travel and continuing 7 days after last exposure; for children <10 kg, data on A-P are limited (BIII); OR mefloquine: for children <5 kg, 5 mg/kg; 5–9 kg, ⅛ tab; 10–19 kg, ¼ tab; 20–30 kg, ½ tab; 31–45 kg, ¾ tab; >45 kg (adult dose) 1 tab PO once weekly starting 1 wk before arrival in area and continuing for 4 wk after leaving area (BII); OR doxycycline (patients >7 y): 2 mg/kg (max 100 mg) PO daily starting 1–2 days before arrival in area and continuing for 4 wk after leaving area (BIII); OR primaquine (check for G6PD deficiency before administering): 0.5 mg/kg base daily starting 1–2 days before travel and continuing for 2 days after last exposure (BII)	Avoid mefloquine for persons with a history of seizures or psychosis, active depression, or cardiac conduction abnormalities. Avoid atovaquone-proguanil in severe renal impairment (CrCl <30). *P falciparum* resistance to mefloquine exists along the borders between Thailand and Myanmar and Thailand and Cambodia, Myanmar and China, and Myanmar and Laos; isolated resistance has been reported in southern Vietnam. Take doxycycline with adequate fluids to avoid esophageal irritation and food to avoid GI side effects; use sunscreen and avoid excessive sun exposure.
For areas without chloroquine-resistant *P falciparum* or *P vivax*	Chloroquine phosphate 5 mg base/kg (max 300 mg base) PO once weekly, beginning 1 wk before arrival in area and continuing for 4 wk after leaving area (available in suspension outside the United States and Canada) (AII) For heavy or prolonged (months) exposure to mosquitoes: treat with primaquine (check for G6PD deficiency before administering) 0.3–0.6 mg base/kg PO qd with final 2 wk of chloroquine for prevention of relapse with *P ovale* or *P vivax*	
Treatment of disease		Consider exchange blood transfusion for >10% parasitemia, altered mental status, pulmonary edema, or renal failure.

Preferred Therapy for Specific Parasitic Pathogens

Disease/Organism	Treatment	Comments
– Chloroquine-resistant *P falciparum* or *P vivax*	Oral therapy: atovaquone-proguanil: for children <5 kg, data limited; 5–8 kg, 2 pediatric tabs (62.5 mg atovaquone/25 mg proguanil) PO qd for 3 days; 9–10 kg, 3 pediatric tabs qd for 3 days; 11–20 kg, 1 adult tab (250 mg atovaquone/100 mg proguanil) qd for 3 days; 21–30 kg, 2 adult tabs qd for 3 days; 31–40 kg, 3 adult tabs qd for 3 days; >40 kg, 4 adult tabs qd for 3 days OR quinine 25 mg/kg/day (max 2 g/day) PO div tid for 3–7 days AND doxycycline (patients >7 y) 2 mg/kg/day for 7 days, or pyrimethamine-sulfadoxine: <1 y, ¼ tab; 1–3 y, ½ tab; 4–8 y, 1 tab; 9–14 y, 2 tab; >14 y, 3 tabs as a single dose on last day of quinine; or clindamycin 30 mg/kg/day div tid (max 900 mg tid) for 5 days OR artemether/lumefantrine 6 doses over 3 days at 0, 8, 24, 36, 48, and 60 h; <15 kg, 1 tab/dose; 15–25 kg, 2 tabs/dose; 25–35 kg, 3 tabs/dose; >35 kg, 4 tabs/dose (not available in US) (BII) *Parenteral therapy* (check with CDC): quinidine 10 mg/kg (max 600 mg) IV (1 h infusion in normal saline) followed by continuous infusion of 0.02 mg/kg/min until oral therapy can be given (after 48-h therapy, decrease dose by ⅓ to ½); (BII) alternative: artesunate 2.4 mg/kg/dose IV for 3 days at 0, 12, 24, 48, and 72 h (from CDC) (BI) For prevention of relapse with *P vivax, P ovale*: primaquine (check for G6PD deficiency before administering) 0.3–0.6 mg base/kg/day PO for 14 days	Mild disease may be treated with oral antimalarial drugs; severe disease (impaired level of consciousness, convulsion, hypotension, or parasitemia >5%) should be treated parenterally. Avoid mefloquine for treatment of malaria if possible given higher dose and increased incidence of adverse events. Do not use primaquine during pregnancy; for relapses of primaquine-resistant *P vivax* or *P ovale*, consider retreating with primaquine 30 mg (base) for 28 days. Continuously monitor ECG, BP, and glucose in patients receiving quinidine. Use artesunate for quinidine intolerance, lack of quinidine availability, or treatment failure; www.cdc.gov/malaria/resources/pdf/treatmenttable.pdf; artemisinins should be used in combination with other drugs to avoid resistance.
– Chloroquine-susceptible *P falciparum*, chloroquine-susceptible *P vivax, P ovale, P malariae*	Oral therapy: chloroquine 10 mg/kg base (max 600 mg base) PO then 5 mg/kg 6 h, 24 h, and 48 h after initial dose Parenteral therapy: quinidine, as above See above for prevention of relapse due to *P vivax* and *P ovale*.	

Paragonimus westermani	See FLUKES.
PINWORMS (*Enterobius vermicularis*)[67]	Albendazole 10 mg/kg (max 400 mg) PO once (BII); OR pyrantel pamoate 11 mg/kg (max 1 g) PO once (BII); repeat treatment in 2 wk	Treatment of entire household (and if this fails, consider close child care/school contacts) often recommended; re-treatment of contacts after 2 wk may be needed to prevent reinfection.
PNEUMOCYSTIS	See Chapter 8, Preferred Therapy for Specific Fungal Pathogens, *Pneumocystis*.	
SCABIES (*Sarcoptes scabei*)[68,69]	Permethrin 5% cream applied to entire body (including scalp in infants), left on for 8–14 h then bathe (BII); OR lindane lotion applied to body below neck, leave on overnight, bathe in am (BII); OR ivermectin 200 µg/kg PO once (BII)	Launder bedding and clothing. Reserve lindane for patients who do not respond to other therapy. Treatment may need to be repeated in 10–14 days.
SCHISTOSOMIASIS (*Schistosoma haematobium,* *Schistosoma japonicum,* *Schistosoma mansoni,* *Schistosoma mekongi,* *Schistosoma intercalatum*)[70–73]	Praziquantel 40 (for *S haematobium* and *S mansoni*) or 60 (for *S japonicum* and *S mekongi*) mg/kg/day PO div bid (if 40 mg/day) or tid (if 60 mg/day) for 1 day (AII); OR oxamniquine (not commercially available in the US) 15 mg/kg PO once (West Africa, Brazil), or 40–60 mg/kg/day for 2–3 days (most of Africa) for praziquantel-resistant *S mansoni* infections (BII)	Take praziquantel with food and liquids.
STRONGYLOIDIASIS (*Strongyloides stercoralis*)[74–76]	Ivermectin 200 µg/kg PO qd for 1–2 days (BII); OR thiabendazole 50 mg/kg/day (max 3 g/day) PO div bid for 2 days (≥5 days for disseminated disease) (BII)	Albendazole is less effective but may be adequate if longer courses used; thiabendazole has been discontinued in the United States.
TAPEWORMS		
– *Cysticercus cellulosae*	See CYSTICERCOSIS.	
– *Echinococcus granulosus*	See ECHINOCOCCOSIS.	
– *Taenia saginata, T solium,* *Hymenolepis nana,* *Diphyllobothrium latum,* *Dipylidium caninum*	Praziquantel 5–10 mg/kg PO once (25 mg/kg once for *H nana*) (BII); OR niclosamide tab 50 mg/kg PO once, chewed thoroughly (all but *H nana*)	

10

Preferred Therapy for Specific Parasitic Pathogens

Disease/Organism	Treatment	Comments
TOXOPLASMOSIS (*Toxoplasma gondii*)[77-79]	Pyrimethamine 2 mg/kg/day PO div bid for 3 days (max 100 mg) then 1 mg/kg/day (max 25 mg) PO qd AND sulfadiazine 120 mg/kg/day PO div qid (max 6 g/day); with supplemental folinic acid and leucovorin 10–25 mg with each dose of pyrimethamine (AI). For treatment in pregnancy, spiramycin 50–100 mg/kg/day PO div qid (available as investigational therapy through the FDA at 301/827-2335) (CII). See Chapter 5 for congenital infection.	Treatment continued for 2 wk after resolution of illness; concurrent corticosteroids given for ocular or CNS infection. Prolonged therapy if HIV positive. Take pyrimethamine with food to decrease GI adverse effects; sulfadiazine should be taken on an empty stomach with adequate liquids. Atovaquone plus pyrimethamine may be effective for patients intolerant of sulfa-containing drugs.
TRAVELER'S DIARRHEA[80-82]	Azithromycin 10 mg/kg qd for 3–5 days (BIII); OR rifaximin 200 mg PO tid for 3 days (ages ≥12 y) (BIII); OR ciprofloxacin (BIII); OR cefixime (CII)	Azithromycin preferable to ciprofloxacin for travelers to SE Asia given high prevalence of quinolone-resistant *Campylobacter*. Rifaximin may not be as efficacious for *Shigella* and other enterics in patients with bloody diarrhea and invasive infection.
TRICHINELLOSIS (*Trichinella spiralis*)[83]	Albendazole 20 mg/kg/day (max 400 mg/dose) PO div bid for 8–14 days (BII)	Therapy ineffective for larvae already in muscles. Anti-inflammatory drugs, steroids for CNS or cardiac involvement or severe symptoms.
TRICHOMONIASIS (*Trichomonas vaginalis*)[84]	Metronidazole 40 mg/kg (max 2 g) PO for 1 dose, or metronidazole 500 mg PO bid for 7 days (AII); OR tinidazole 50 mg/kg (max 2 g) PO for 1 dose (BII)	Treat sex partners simultaneously. Metronidazole resistance occurs and may be treated with higher-dose metronidazole or tinidazole.
Trichuris trichiura	See WHIPWORM (TRICHURIASIS).	
TRYPANOSOMIASIS		
– **Chagas disease**[85] (*Trypanosoma cruzi*)	Nifurtimox PO (from CDC): children 1–10 y, 15–20 mg/kg/day div qid for 90–120 days; 11–16 y, 12.5–15 mg/kg/day div qid for 90–120 days; ≥17 y; 8–10 mg/kg/day div tid-qid for 90–120 days (BIII); OR benznidazole PO (not commercially available in the US): children <12 y, 10 mg/kg/day div bid for 30–90 days; ≥12 y; 5–7 mg/kg/day div bid for 30–90 days (BIII)	Therapy recommended for acute and congenital infection, reactivated infection, and chronic infection in children aged <18 y. Take benznidazole with meals to avoid GI adverse effects. Interferon-γ in addition to nifurtimox may shorten acute disease duration.

– Sleeping sickness[86-89] Trypanosoma brucei gambiense (West African) T brucei rhodesiense (East African) Acute (hemolymphatic) stage	*Tb gambiense*: pentamidine isethionate 4 mg/kg/day (max 300 mg) IM for 7 days (BII); *Tb rhodesiense*: suramin (from CDC) 20 mg/kg (max 1.5 g) IV on days 1, 3, 7, 14, and 21 (BIII)	Consult with tropical medicine specialist if unfamiliar with trypanosomiasis. Examination of the buffy coat of peripheral blood may be helpful. *Tb gambiense* may be found in lymph node aspirates.
Late (CNS) stage	*Tb gambiense*: eflornithine (not available commercially in the US) 400 mg/kg/day IV div q6h for 14 days (BIII); OR melarsoprol (from CDC) 2.2 mg/day (max 180 mg) IV for 10 days (BIII); *Tb rhodesiense*: melarsoprol, 2–3.6 mg/kg/day IV for 3 days; repeat again after 7 days, 3.6 mg/kg/day IV for 3 days; repeat again after 7 days; (max 180 mg); corticosteroids given with melarsoprol to decrease risk of CNS toxicity	CSF examination needed for management (double- centrifuge technique recommended); perform repeat CSF examinations every 6 mo for 2 y to detect relapse. Addition of nifurtimox (approved for *T cruzi* infection, available for late-stage *Tb gambiense* infection from WHO) may shorten required duration of therapy and may be more effective vs standard melarsoprol regimens.
VISCERAL LARVA MIGRANS (TOXOCARIASIS)		
Toxocara canis; Toxocara cati	Albendazole 15 mg/kg/day PO bid for 3–5 days (BII), OR DEC (from CDC) 6 mg/kg/day PO div tid for 7–10 days	Some experts advocate longer therapy (eg, 20 days). Corticosteroids if severe or ocular involvement.
WHIPWORM (TRICHURIASIS)		
Trichuris trichiura[90]	Albendazole 400 mg PO for 3 days; OR ivermectin 200 µg/kg/day PO daily for 3 days (BII)	Stool reexamination after treatment usually not necessary.
Wuchereria bancrofti	See FILARIASIS.	

11. Alphabetic Listing of Antimicrobials

NOTES

- Higher dosages in a dose range are generally indicated for illnesses that are more serious.

- For most antimicrobials, a maximum dosage is provided, based on US Food and Drug Administration (FDA)-reviewed and approved clinical data. However, data may be published on higher dosages than originally approved by the FDA, particularly for generic drugs. Whenever possible, these dosages are also provided.

- For additional information on dosing in obesity, see Chapter 12. No single accurate adjustment for dosing can be made for all drug classes and tissue sites. Most published data result from single patient reports or a study of a small group. As a rough guide, to achieve serum concentrations that are achieved in patients of normal body weight,

Aminoglycosides	Start with standard mg/kg dose based on ideal body weight (IBW), then use a 40% correction factor for additional kg of weight above IBW.
Vancomycin	Dose based on body surface area.
Beta-lactams	Start with standard mg/kg dose based on IBW, then use a 30% correction factor for additional kg of weight above IBW. Because of the wide safety margin of beta-lactams, a simpler acceptable strategy is to dose based on mg/kg of total body weight, not to exceed the adult maximum dose.
Fluoroquinolones	Increase dose based on a 45% correction factor for additional kg of weight above standard mg/kg dosing for IBW.

In situations in which aggressive therapy is indicated, the benefits of using a high or adult-sized dose in an obese child may outweigh the unknown risks at that higher dosage.

- Drugs with FDA-approved pediatric dosage, or dosages based on multiple randomized clinical trials, are given a Level of Evidence I. For dosages for which data are collected from adults, from noncomparative trials, or from small comparative trials, the Level of Evidence is II. For dosages that are based on expert or consensus opinion, or case reports, the Level of Evidence given is III.

- All commercially available dosage forms for children and adults are listed. If no oral liquid form is available, round the child's dose to the nearest value using a combination of commercially available solid dosage form strengths OR consult pediatric pharmacist for recommendations on mixing with food (eg, crushing tablets, emptying capsule contents) or the availability of a valid extemporaneously compounded liquid formulation if the child is unable to take solid dosage forms.

- **Abbreviations:** AOM, acute otitis media; bid, twice daily; BSA, body surface area; CA-MRSA, community-associated methicillin-resistant *Staphylococcus aureus;* cap, capsule or caplet; CABP, community-acquired bacterial pneumonia; CNS, central nervous system; CMV, cytomegalovirus; CrCl, creatinine clearance; DRV, darunavir; EC, enteric coated; ER, extended release; FDA, US Food and Drug Administration; hs, at bedtime; HSV, herpes simplex virus; IBW, ideal body weight; IM, intramuscular; IR, instant release; IV, intravenous; ivpb, intravenous piggyback (premixed bag); MAC, *Mycobacterium avium* complex; oint, ointment; ophth, ophthalmic; PCP, *Pneumocystis* pneumonia; PIP, piperacillin; PK, pharmacokinetic; PMA, post menstrual age; PO, oral; pwd, powder; soln, solution; qd, once daily; qhs, every bedtime; qid, 4 times daily; RTV, ritonavir; SPAG-2, small particle aerosol generator model-2; SQ, subcutaneous; susp, suspension; tab, tablet; TB, tuberculosis; TBW, total body weight; tid, 3 times daily; SMX, sulfamethoxazole; TMP, trimethoprim; top, topical; UTI, urinary tract infection; vag, vaginal; VZV, varicella-zoster virus.

A. SYSTEMIC ANTIMICROBIALS WITH DOSAGE FORMS AND USUAL DOSAGES

Generic and Trade Names	Dosage Form	Route	Dose (evidence grade)	Interval
Abacavir, Ziagen	100-mg/5-mL soln 300-mg tab	PO	16 mg/kg/day (adults 600 mg/day) (I) Not approved for ages <3 mo	q12–24h
Epzicom	Combination tab with 600 mg abacavir + 300 mg lamivudine	PO	Adolescents ≥16 y/Adults 1 tab	q24h
Trizivir	Combination tab with 300 mg abacavir, 300 mg zidovudine, 150 mg lamivudine	PO	Adolescents ≥40 kg/Adults 1 tab	q12h
Acyclovir*, Zovirax	500-, 1,000-mg vial	IV	15–60 mg/kg/day (I) (See Chapter 9.) Use IBW in obese children ≥12 y	q8h
	200-mg/5-mL susp, 200-mg cap; 400-, 800-mg tab	PO	900 mg/m²/day (I) (See Chapter 5.) 60–80 mg/kg/day (max 3.2 g/day) (I)	q8h q6–8h
Sitavig	50-mg tab	Buccal	Adults 50 mg, for herpes labialis	one time
Albendazole, Albenza	200-mg tab	PO	15 mg/kg/day (max 800 mg/day) (I)	q12h
Amantadine*, Symmetrel	100-mg cap, tab 100-mg cap, 50-mg/5-mL soln	PO	5–9 mg/kg/day (max 150 mg/day <9 y) 200 mg/day if ≥9 y (I)	q12h
Amikacin*, Amikin	500-mg/2 mL, 1,000-mg/4-mL vials	IV, IM	15–22.5 mg/kg/day (See Chapter 1 regarding q24h dosing.) (I)	q8–24h
Amoxicillin*, Amoxil	125-, 200-, 250-, 400-mg/5-mL susp 125-, 250-mg chew tab 250, 500-mg cap 500-, 875-mg tab	PO	40–100 mg/kg/day if <40 kg (II) Max 150 mg/kg/day divided q8h for penicillin-resistant S pneumoniae otitis media (III) >40 kg and adults 750–1,750 mg/day (I)	q8–12h
Amoxicillin extended release*, Moxatag	775-mg tab	PO	≥12 y and adults 775 mg/day	q24h

*Available in a generic formulation.

11

Alphabetic Listing of Antimicrobials

Alphabetic Listing of Antimicrobials

A. SYSTEMIC ANTIMICROBIALS WITH DOSAGE FORMS AND USUAL ≠DOSAGES (cont)

Generic and Trade Names	Dosage Form	Route	Dose (evidence grade)	Interval
Amoxicillin/clavulanate*, Augmentin	**16:1** Formulation (Augmentin XR): **1000**/62.5-mg tab	PO	**16:1** Formulation: ≥40 kg and adults (I) 4,000 mg amoxicillin component/day	q12h
	14:1 Formulation (Augmentin ES-600): **600**/42.9-mg/5-mL susp	PO	**14:1** Formulation: 90 mg amoxicillin component/kg/day if <40 kg (I). Not for use in children ≥40 kg or adults	q12h
	7:1 Formulation: **875**/125-mg tab **200**/28.5-, 400/57-mg chew tab; **200**/28.5-, 400/57-mg/5-mL susp	PO	**7:1** Formulation: 25–45 mg amoxicillin component/kg/day (adult max 1,750 mg/day) (I)	q12h
	4:1 Formulation: **500**/125-mg tab **125**/31.25-, **250**/62.5-mg chew tab; **125**/31.25-, **250**/62.5-mg/5-mL susp	PO	**4:1** Formulation: 20–40 mg amoxicillin component/kg/day (adults 1,500 mg/day) (I)	q8h
Amphotericin B deoxycholate (AmB-D)*, Fungizone	50-mg vial	IV	0.7–1 mg/kg (II) Adults 1–1.5 mg/kg (I)	q24h
Amphotericin B cholesteryl sulfate, Amphotec	50-, 100-mg vial	IV	3–4 mg/kg pediatric and adult dose (I)	q24h
Amphotericin B, lipid complex (ABLC), Abelcet	100-mg/20-mL vial	IV	5 mg/kg pediatric and adult dose (I)	q24h
Amphotericin B, liposomal (AmB-LP), AmBisome	50-mg vial	IV	3–5 mg/kg pediatric and adult dose (I)	q24h
Ampicillin/ampicillin trihydrate*	250-, 500-mg cap 125-, 250-mg/5-mL susp	PO	50–100 mg/kg/day if <20 kg (I) ≥20 kg and adults 1–2 g/day (I)	q6h
Ampicillin sodium*	0.125-, 0.25-, 0.5-, 1-, 2-, 10-g vial	IV, IM	50–200 mg/kg/day (I) 300–400 mg/kg/day endocarditis/meningitis (III) Adults 2–12 g/day (I)	q6h q4–6h

Ampicillin and sulbactam*, Unasyn	1/0.5-, 2/1-, 10/5-g vial	IV/IM	200 mg/kg/day (amp) if <40 kg (I) ≥40 kg and adults 4–8 g ampicillin/day (I)	q6h
Anidulafungin, Eraxis	50-, 100-mg vial	IV	1.5–3 mg/kg loading dose followed by 0.75–1.5 mg/kg (II) Adult loading dose 100–200 mg followed by 50-100 mg (I)	q24h
Atazanavir, Reyataz	100-, 150-, 200-, 300-mg cap	PO	≥6 y (I): 15 to <20 kg: 150 mg + RTV 80 mg 20 to <40 kg: 200 mg + RTV 100 mg ≥40 kg: 300 mg + RTV 100 mg OR 400 mg if w/o RTV	q24h
Atovaquone, Mepron	750-mg/5-mL susp	PO	30 mg/kg/day if 1–3 mo or >24 mo (I) 45 mg/kg/day if 4–24 mo (I) Adolescents/adults 1,500 mg/day (I)	q12h q24h for prophylaxis
Atovaquone and proguanil, Malarone	62.5/25-mg pediatric tab 250/100-mg adult tab	PO	Prophylaxis for malaria: 11–20 kg: 1 ped tab, 21–30 kg: 2 ped tabs, 31–40 kg: 3 ped tabs, >40 kg: 1 adult tab (I) Treatment: 5–8 kg: 2 ped tabs, 9–10 kg: 3 ped tabs, 11–20 kg: 1 adult tab, 21–30 kg: 2 adult tabs, 31–40 kg: 3 adult tabs, >40 kg: 4 adult tabs (I)	q24h
Azithromycin*, Zithromax, Zmax	250-, 500-, 600-mg tab 100-, 200-mg/5-mL susp 27-mg/mL extended release susp (Zmax)	PO	Otitis: 10 mg/kg/day for 1 day, then 5 mg/kg for 4 days; or 10 mg/kg/day for 3 days; or 30 mg/kg once (I). Pharyngitis: 12 mg/kg/day for 5 days (I). Sinusitis: 10 mg/kg/day for 3 days (I). CABP: 10 mg/kg for 1 day, then 5 mg/kg/day for 4 days or 60 mg/kg once of ER (Zmax) susp (I). Adult single or total course dose: 1.5–2 g (I). MAC/PCP prophylaxis: 5 mg/kg/day (I). See Chapter 6 for other specific disease dosing recommendations.	q24h
	500-mg vial	IV	10 mg/kg (II)	q24h
Aztreonam, Azactam	500-mg, 1-, 2-g vial*, 1-, 2-g ivpb	IV, IM	90–120 mg/kg/day (adults 3–6 g/d) (I)	q6–8h
Aztreonam inhalation, Cayston	75-mg vial	Inhaled	≥7 y: 75 mg/dose via Altera nebulizer (I)	q8h

11 Alphabetic Listing of Antimicrobials

*Available in a generic formulation.

Alphabetic Listing of Antimicrobials

11

A. SYSTEMIC ANTIMICROBIALS WITH DOSAGE FORMS AND USUAL DOSAGES (cont)

Generic and Trade Names	Dosage Form	Route	Dose (evidence grade)	Interval
Capreomycin, Capastat	1-g vial	IV, IM	15–30 mg/kg (III) Adults 1 g, max 20 mg/kg (I)	q24h
Caspofungin, Cancidas	50-, 70-mg vial	IV	70 mg/m² once, then 50 mg/m² maximum dose 70 mg (I)	q24h
Cefaclor*, Ceclor	125-, 187-, 250-, 375-mg/5-mL susp 250-, 500-mg cap 375-, 500-mg ER tab	PO	20–40 mg/kg/day, max 1 g/day (I)	q12h
Cefadroxil*, Duricef	250-, 500-mg/5-mL susp 500-mg cap, 1-g tab	PO	30 mg/kg/day (adults 1–2 g/day) (I)	q12–24h
Cefazolin*, Ancef	0.5-, 1-, 10-, 20-g vial, 1-, 2-g ivpb	IV, IM	25–100 mg/kg/day (adults 3–6 g/day) (I) For serious infections, up to 150 mg/kg/day (III)	q6–8h
Cefdinir*, Omnicef	125-, 250-mg/5-mL susp, 300-mg cap	PO	14 mg/kg/day, max 600 mg/day (I)	q24h
Cefditoren, Spectracef	200-, 400-mg tab	PO	≥12 y and adults, 400–800 mg/day (I)	q12h
Cefepime*, Maxipime	1-, 2-g vial 1-, 2-g ivpb	IV, IM	100 mg/kg/day (adults 2–4 g/day) (I)	q12h
			150 mg/kg/day empiric therapy of fever with neutropenia (adults 6 g/day) (I)	q8h
Cefixime, Suprax	100-, 200-, 500-mg/5-mL susp 100-, 150-, 200-mg chew tab 400-mg tab, cap	PO	8 mg/kg/day if <50 kg (adults 400 mg/day) (I) For convalescent oral therapy of serious infections, up to 20 mg/kg/day (III)	q12–24h
Cefotaxime*, Claforan	0.5-, 1-, 2-, 10-g vial	IV, IM	50–180 mg/kg/day (adults 3–8 g/day) (I)	q6–8h
			200–225 mg/kg/day for meningitis (adults 12 g/day) (I)	q6h
Cefotetan*, Cefotan	1-, 2-, 10-g vial 1-, 2-g ivpb	IV, IM	60–100 mg/kg/day (II)	q12h
			Adults 2–4 g/day (I)	q12h

Drug	Formulations	Route	Dosage	Interval
Cefoxitin,* Mefoxin	1-, 2-, 10-g vial, 1-, 2-g ivpb	IV, IM	80–160 mg/kg/day, max 12 g/day (I)	q6h
Cefpodoxime,* Vantin	50-, 100-mg/5-mL susp 100-, 200-mg tab	PO	10 mg/kg/day, max 400 mg/day (I)	q12h
Cefprozil,* Cefzil	125-, 250-mg/5-mL susp 250-, 500-mg tab	PO	15–30 mg/kg/day (adults 0.5–1 g/d) (I)	q12h
Ceftaroline, Teflaro (Doses are investigational in children.)	400-, 600-mg vial	IV	<6 months (II): 24 mg/kg/day for skin or CABP 30 mg/kg/day for complicated CABP ≥6 months (II): 36 mg/kg/day for skin or CABP, max 1,200 mg/day 45 mg/kg/day for complicated CABP, max 1,800 mg/day	q8h
Ceftazidime,* Ceptaz, Fortaz	0.5-, 1-, 2-, 6-g vial 1-, 2-g ivpb	IV, IM	90–150 mg/kg/day (adults 3–6 g/d) (I)	q8h
			200–300 mg/kg/day for serious Pseudomonas infection (III)	q8h
Ceftibuten, Cedax	90-mg/5-mL susp 400-mg cap	PO	9 mg/kg/day (adults 400 mg/day) (I)	q24h
Ceftriaxone,* Rocephin	0.25-, 0.5-, 1-, 2-, 10-g vial 1-, 2-g ivpb	IV, IM	50–75 mg/kg/day, max 2 g/day (I) 100 mg/kg/day for meningitis, max 4 g/day (I) 50 mg/kg, max 1 g, q24h for 1–3 doses IM for AOM (II)	q12–24h
Cefuroxime axetil,* Ceftin	125-, 250-mg/5-mL susp 250-, 500-mg tab	PO	20–30 mg/kg/day (adults 0.5–1 g/d) (I) For bone and joint infections, up to 100 mg/kg/day (III)	q12h
Cefuroxime sodium,* Zinacef	0.75-, 1.5-g vial, ivpb	IV, IM	100–150 mg/kg/day (adults 1.5–3 g/day) (I)	q8h
Cephalexin,* Keflex	125-, 250-mg/5-mL susp 250-, 500-mg caps and tabs	PO	25–50 mg/kg/day, max 1 g/day (I)	q12h
			75–100 mg/kg/day for bone and joint, or severe infections (II) Adults 2–4 g/day (I)	q6–8h

*Available in a generic formulation.

11 Alphabetic Listing of Antimicrobials

Alphabetic Listing of Antimicrobials

11

A. SYSTEMIC ANTIMICROBIALS WITH DOSAGE FORMS AND USUAL DOSAGES (cont)

Generic and Trade Names	Dosage Form	Route	Dose (evidence grade)	Interval
Chloramphenicol sodium succinate*, Chloromycetin	1-g vial	IV	50–75 mg/kg/day 75–100 mg/kg/day for meningitis (I) Adults max 100 mg/kg/day	q6h
Chloroquine phosphate*, Aralen	250-, 500-mg (150-, 300-mg base) tabs	PO	See Chapter 10.	
Cidofovir*, Vistide	375-mg/5-mL vial	IV	5 mg/kg (III), see also Chapter 9.	weekly
Ciprofloxacin*, Cipro	250-, 500-mg/5-mL susp 100-, 250-, 500-, 750-mg tab	PO	20–40 mg/kg/day, max 1.5 g/day (I)	q12h
	200-, 400-mg vial, ivpb	IV	20–30 mg/kg/day, max 1.2 g/day (I)	q12h
Ciprofloxacin extended release*, Cipro XR	500-, 1,000-mg ER tab	PO	Adults 500–1,000 mg (I)	q24h
Clarithromycin*, Biaxin	125-, 250-mg/5-mL susp 250-, 500-mg tab	PO	15 mg/kg/day, max 1 g/day (I)	q12h
Clarithromycin extended release*, Biaxin XL*	500-, 1,000-mg ER tab	PO	Adults 1,000 mg (I)	q24h
Clindamycin*, Cleocin	75 mg/5-mL soln 75-, 150-, 300-mg cap	PO	10–25 mg/kg/day (adults 1.2–1.8 g/day) (I) 30–40 mg/kg/day for CA-MRSA, intra-abdominal infection, or AOM (III)	q8h
	0.3-, 0.6-, 0.9-g vial, ivpb	IV, IM	20–40 mg/kg/day (adults 1.8–2.7 g/day) (I)	q8h
Clotrimazole*, Mycelex	10-mg lozenge	PO	≥3 y and adults, dissolve lozenge in mouth (I)	5 times daily
Colistimethate*, Coly-Mycin M	150-mg (colistin base) vial	IV, IM	2.5–5 mg/kg/day based on IBW (I) up to 5–7 mg/kg/day (III)	q8h
Cycloserine, Seromycin	250-mg cap	PO	10–20 mg/kg/day (III) Adults max 1 g/day (I)	q12h

Dapsone*	25-, 100-mg tab	PO	2 mg/kg, max 100 mg (I)	q24h
			4 mg/kg, max 200 mg (I)	Once weekly
Daptomycin, Cubicin (Doses are investigational in children.)	500-mg vial	IV	2–5 y: 10 mg/kg (III) ≥6–11 y: 7 mg/kg (II) ≥12 y and adults: 4–6 mg/kg TBW (I)	q24h
Darunavir, Prezista	500-mg/5-mL susp 75-, 150-, 400-, 600-, 800-mg tab	PO	≥3 y and ≥10 kg (I): ARV naive and experienced as well as with or without one or more DRV-associated resistance mutations (dose, twice daily with food): 10 to <11 kg: DRV 200 mg (2.0 mL) + RTV 32 mg (0.4 mL) 11 to <12 kg: DRV 220 mg (2.2 mL) + RTV 32 mg (0.4 mLb) 12 to <13 kg: DRV 240 mg (2.4 mL) + RTV 40 mg (0.5 mLb) 13 to <14 kg: DRV 260 mg (2.6 mL) + RTV 40 mg (0.5 mLb) 14 to <15 kg: DRV 280 mg (2.8 mL) + RTV 48 mg (0.6 mLb) 15 to <30 kg: DRV 375 mg (combination of tablets or 3.8 mLc) + RTV 48 mg (0.6 mLb) 30 to <40 kg: DRV 450 mg (combination of tablets or 4.6 mLc) + RTV 100 mg (tablet or 1.25 mLb) ≥40 kg: DRV 600 mg (tablet or 6 mL) + RTV 100 mg (tablet or 1.25 mL)	q24h q12h if ≥30 kg and using suspension
Delavirdine, Rescriptor	100-, 200-mg tab	PO	≥16 y: 1,200 mg/day (I)	q8h
Demeclocycline*, Declomycin	150-, 300-mg tab	PO	≥8 y: 7–13 mg/kg/day, max 600 mg/day (I)	q6h
Dicloxacillin*, Dynapen	125-, 250-, 500-mg cap	PO	12–25 mg/kg/day (adults 0.5–1 g/day) (I) For bone and joint infections, up to 100 mg/kg/day (III)	q6h

*Available in a generic formulation.

11 Alphabetic Listing of Antimicrobials

Alphabetic Listing of Antimicrobials

11

A. SYSTEMIC ANTIMICROBIALS WITH DOSAGE FORMS AND USUAL DOSAGES (cont)

Generic and Trade Names	Dosage Form	Route	Dose (evidence grade)	Interval
Didanosine (ddI)*, Videx	50-mg/5-mL oral soln	PO	2 wk–2 mo: 100 mg/m²/day (II) ≥3–8 mo: 200 mg/m²/day (I) >8 mo: 240 (180–300) mg/m²/day (I) Max 400 mg/day (I)	q12h
Videx-EC	125-, 200-, 250-, 400-mg cap	PO	20 to <25 kg: 200 mg, 25 to <60 kg: 250 mg, ≥60 kg: 400 mg (I)	q24h
Diiodohydroxyquin (see Iodoquinol)				
Doxycycline*	50-, 75-, 100-mg cap, tab 50-mg/5-mL susp	PO	≥8 y, ≤45 kg: 2–4 mg/kg/day (adults 100–200 mg/day) (I)	q12h
	100-mg vial	IV		
Efavirenz, Sustiva	50-, 200-mg cap, 600-mg tab See also Emtricitabine for combination forms	PO	≥3 mo (I) (Note: generally not recommended for use in children <3 y): 3.5 to <5 kg: 100 mg 5 to <7.5 kg: 150 mg 7.5 to <15 kg: 200 mg 15 to <20 kg: 250 mg 20 to <25 kg: 300 mg 25 to <32.5 kg: 350 mg 32.5 to <40 kg: 400 mg ≥40 kg and adults: 600 mg (I)	q24h
Emtricitabine, Emtriva	50-mg/5-mL soln 200-mg cap	PO	0–3 mo: 3 mg/kg (I) ≥3 mo: 6 mg/kg, max 240-mg soln (I) >33 kg and adults: 200-mg cap (I)	q24h
Truvada	Combination tab with 200 mg emtricitabine + 300 mg tenofovir	PO	≥12 y (if ≥35 kg) and adults: 1 tab (I)	q24h

Drug	Formulation	Route	Dose	Interval
Atripla	Combination tab with 200 mg emtricitabine, 300 mg tenofovir, 600 mg efavirenz	PO	≥12 y (if ≥40 kg) and adults: 1 tab (I)	q24h
Complera	Combination tab with 200 mg emtricitabine, 300 mg tenofovir, 25 mg rilpivirine	PO	Adults 1 tab (I)	q24h
Stribild	Combination tab with 200 mg emtricitabine, 300 mg tenofovir, 150 mg elvitegravir, 150 mg cobicistat	PO	Adults 1 tab (I)	q24h
Enfuvirtide, Fuzeon	108-mg vial (90 mg/mL)	SQ	≥6 y: 4 mg/kg/day, max 180 mg/day (I)	q12h
Ertapenem, Invanz	1-g vial	IV, IM	30 mg/kg/day, max 1 g/day (I) ≥13 y and adults: 1 g/day (I)	q12h q24h
Erythromycin* base	250-, 500-mg tab, film coated	PO	50 mg/kg/day (adults 1–4 g/day) (I)	q6–8h
coated pellets*, ERYC	250-mg cap, EC			
coated particles, PCE	333-, 500-mg tabs of EC particles			
delayed release*, Ery-Tab	250-, 333-, 500-mg tab, EC			
Erythromycin ethylsuccinate*, EES, EryPed	200-, 400-mg/5-mL susp	PO	50 mg/kg/day (adults 1–4 g/day) (I)	q6–8h
Erythromycin lactobionate*, Erythrocin	0.5-, 1-g vial	IV	20 mg/kg/day (adults 1–4 g/day) (I)	q6h
Erythromycin stearate*	250-mg tab, film coated	PO	50 mg/kg/day (adults 1–4 g/day) (I)	q6–8h
Ethambutol*, Myambutol	100-, 400-mg tab	PO	15–25 mg/kg, max 2.5 g (I)	q24h

*Available in a generic formulation.

11 Alphabetic Listing of Antimicrobials

Alphabetic Listing of Antimicrobials

A. SYSTEMIC ANTIMICROBIALS WITH DOSAGE FORMS AND USUAL DOSAGES (cont)

Generic and Trade Names	Dosage Form	Route	Dose (evidence grade)	Interval
Ethionamide, Trecator	250-mg tab	PO	15–20 mg/kg/day, max 1 g/day (III)	q12h
Etravirine, Intelence	25-, 100-, 200-mg tab	PO	≥6 y (if ≥16 kg) (I): 16 to <20 kg: 200 mg/day 20 to <25 kg: 250 mg/day 25 to <30 kg: 300 mg ≥30 kg and adults: 400 mg/day (I)	q12h
Famciclovir*, Famvir	125-, 250-, 500-mg tab	PO	Adults 0.5–1.5 g/day (I)	q8–12h
Fluconazole*, Diflucan	50-, 100-, 150-, 200-mg tab 50-, 200-mg/5-mL susp	PO	3–12 mg/kg/day, max 600 mg/day (I). Max 800–1,000 mg/day may be used for some CNS fungal infections. See Chapter 8.	q24h
	100-, 200-, 400-mg vial, ivpb	IV		
Flucytosine*, Ancobon	250-, 500-mg cap	PO	50–150 mg/kg/day (III)	q6h
Fosamprenavir, Lexiva	250-mg/5-mL susp 700-mg tab	PO	≥6 mo (I): <11 kg: 90 mg/kg/d + RTV 14 mg/kg/d 11 to <15 kg: 60 mg/kg/d + RTV 6 mg/kg/d 15 to <20 kg: 46 mg/kg/d + RTV 6 mg/kg/d ≥20 kg: 36 mg/kg/day + RTV 6 mg/kg/d Max 1,400 mg/day + RTV 200 mg/d	q12h
Foscarnet*, Foscavir	6-, 12-g vial	IV	CMV/VZV: 180 mg/kg/day (I)	q8h
			CMV suppression: 90–120 mg/kg (I)	q24h
			HSV: 120 mg/kg/day (I)	q8–12h
Ganciclovir*, Cytovene	500-mg vial	IV	CMV treatment: 10–15 mg/kg/day (I)	q12h
			CMV suppression: 5 mg/kg (I)	q24h
			VZV: 10 mg/kg/day (III)	q12h

11

Gemifloxacin, Factive	320-mg tab	PO	Adults 320 mg (I)	q24h
Gentamicin*	20-mg/2-mL pediatric vial 80-mg/2-mL, 800-mg/20-mL adult vial, numerous ivpb	IV, IM	3–7.5 mg/kg/day (cystic fibrosis 7–10); see Chapter 1 regarding q24h dosing.	q8–24h
Griseofulvin microsized*, Grifulvin V	125-mg/5-mL susp 500-mg tab	PO	20–25 mg/kg (II) Adults 0.5–1 g (I)	q24h
Griseofulvin ultramicrosized*, Gris-PEG	125-, 250-mg tab	PO	10–15 mg/kg (II) Adults 0.375–0.75 g (I)	q24h
Imipenem/cilastatin, Primaxin	250/250-, 500/500-mg vial for IV 500/500-mg vial for IM	IV, IM	60–100 mg/kg/day (I) IM form not approved for <12 y	q6h
Iodoquinol*, Yodoxin	210-, 650-mg tab	PO	30–40 mg/kg/day, max 1.95 g/day (I)	q8h
Isoniazid*, Nydrazid	50-mg/5-mL syrup; 100-, 300-mg tab 1,000-mg vial	PO IV, IM	10–15 mg/kg/day, max 300 mg/day (I)	q12–24h
			With directly observed biweekly therapy, dosage is 20–30 mg/kg, max 900 mg/dose (I).	twice weekly
Itraconazole, Sporanox	50-mg/5-mL soln 100-mg cap*, 200-mg tab	PO	10 mg/kg/day (III), max 200 mg/day	q12h
			5 mg/kg/day for chronic mucocutaneous *Candida* (III)	q24h
Ivermectin, Stromectol	3-mg tab	PO	150–200 µg/kg (I)	1 dose
Ketoconazole*, Nizoral	200-mg tab	PO	≥2 y: 3.3–6.6 mg/kg/day (II)	q24h
Lamivudine, Epivir	50-mg/5-mL soln 150-, 300-mg tab*	PO	Neonates (<4 wk): 4 mg/kg/day Infants/children: 8 mg/kg/day max 300 mg/day (I) ≥50 kg: 150 mg/dose q12h or 300 mg once daily (I)	q12h
Epivir HBV	100-mg tab, 25-mg/5-mL soln	PO	3 mg/kg (max 100 mg)	q24h
Combivir*	Combination tab: 150 mg lamivudine + 300 mg zidovudine		≥30 kg and adults 1 tab/dose	q12h

*Available in a generic formulation.

11 **Alphabetic Listing of Antimicrobials**

Alphabetic Listing of Antimicrobials

11

A. SYSTEMIC ANTIMICROBIALS WITH DOSAGE FORMS AND USUAL DOSAGES (cont)

Generic and Trade Names	Dosage Form	Route	Dose (evidence grade)	Interval
Epzicom	Combination tab with 300 mg lamivudine + 600 mg abacavir		>50 kg and adults 1 tab	q24h
Trizivir	Combination tab with 150 mg lamivudine, 300 mg zidovudine, 300 mg abacavir		>40 kg and adults 1 tab/dose	q12h
Levofloxacin*, Levaquin	125-mg/5-mL soln 250-, 500-, 750-mg tab, 500-, 750-mg vial 250-, 500-, 750-mg ivpb	PO, IV	16 mg/kg/day div q12h up to 50 kg body weight, then 500 mg qd for post-exposure anthrax prophylaxis (I) For respiratory infections: <5 y: 20 mg/kg/day (II) ≥5 y: 10 mg/kg/day (II)	q12h q12h q24h
Linezolid, Zyvox	100-mg/5-mL susp 600-mg tab 200-, 600-mg ivpb	PO, IV	<5 y: 30 mg/kg/day (I) 5–11 y for uncomplicated skin infection: 20 mg/kg/day 5–11 y for complicated skin infection: 30 mg/kg/day ≥12 y, adults: 1,200 mg/day (I)	q8h q12h q8h q12h
Lopinavir/ritonavir, Kaletra	400 mg lopinavir/100 mg ritonavir per 5-mL oral soln 100/25-mg pediatric tab 200/50-mg adult tab	PO	≥14 d–1 y: 600/150 mg/m²/day (I) >1 y and ARV naïve: 460/115 mg/m²/day >1 y ARV experienced: same as ≤1 y Adult dose 800/200 mg/day	q12h
Maraviroc (Selzentry)	150-, 300-mg tab	PO	Adolescents ≥16 y/adults: 300–1,200 mg/day based on drug interactions (I)	q12h
Mefloquine*, Lariam	250-mg tab	PO	See Chapter 10 for detailed weight-based recommendations for malaria.	
Meropenem*, Merrem	0.5-, 1-g vial	IV	60 mg/kg/day, max 3 g/day (I) 120 mg/kg/day meningitis, max 6 g/day (I)	q8h q8h
Methenamine hippurate*, Hiprex	1-g tab	PO	6–12 y: 1–2 g/day (I) >12 y: 2 g/day (I)	q12h

Metronidazole*, Flagyl	250-, 500-mg tab, 375-mg cap	PO	30–50 mg/kg/day (adults 750–2,250 mg/day) (I)	q8h
	500-mg vial, ivpb	IV	22.5–40 mg/kg/day (II) Adults 1,500 mg/day (I)	q8h
Micafungin, Mycamine	50-, 100-mg vial	IV	2–4 mg/kg, max 150 mg (I)	q24h
Miconazole, Oravig	50-mg buccal tab	PO	≥16 y and adults: 50-mg buccal tab (I)	q24h
Minocycline, Minocin	50-, 75-, 100-mg cap*, tab* 100-mg vial	PO, IV	≥8 y: 4 mg/kg/day (adults 200 mg/d) (I)	q12h
Moxifloxacin, Avelox	400-mg tab, 400-mg ivpb	PO, IV	Adults 400 mg/day (I)	q24h
Nafcillin*, Nallpen	1-, 2-, 10-g vial, 1-, 2-g ivpb	IV, IM	150–200 mg/kg/day (II) Adults 3–6 g/day q4h (I)	q6h
Nelfinavir, Viracept	250-, 625-mg tab	PO	≥2 y: 90–110 mg/kg/day max 2.5 g/d (I)	q12h
Neomycin sulfate*	500-mg tab	PO	50–100 mg/kg/day (II)	q6–8h
Nevirapine, Viramune, Viramune XR	50-mg/5-mL susp*, 200-mg tab* 100-, 400-mg ER tab	PO	See Chapter 5 for neonatal dosing. <8 y: 400 mg/m²/day (I). ≥8 y: 240–300 mg/m²/day max 400 mg/day (I). Initiate above regimens with half daily dose q24h for 14 days (I).	q12h
			ER tab ≥6 y (I): BSA 0.58–0.83 m² 200 mg BSA 0.84–1.16 m² 300 mg BSA >1.16 m² 400 mg	q24h Begin after 14-day initiation with IR forms
Nitazoxanide, Alinia	500-mg tab; 100-mg/5-mL susp	PO	1–3 y: 200 mg/day 4–11 y: 400 mg/day ≥12 y: 1 g/day (I)	q12h
Nitrofurantoin*, Furadantin	25-mg/5-mL susp	PO	5–7 mg/kg/day (I)	q6h
			1–2 mg/kg for UTI prophylaxis (I)	q24h

*Available in a generic formulation.

11 Alphabetic Listing of Antimicrobials

Alphabetic Listing of Antimicrobials

11

A. SYSTEMIC ANTIMICROBIALS WITH DOSAGE FORMS AND USUAL DOSAGES (cont)

Generic and Trade Names	Dosage Form	Route	Dose (evidence grade)	Interval
Nitrofurantoin, macrocrystalline*, Macrodantin	25-, 50-, 100-mg cap	PO	Same as susp	
Nitrofurantoin monohydrate and macrocrystalline*, Macrobid	100-mg cap	PO	>12 y: 200 mg/day (I)	q12h
Norfloxacin, Noroxin	400-mg tab	PO	Adults 800 mg/day (I)	q12h
Nystatin*, Mycostatin	500,000-unit/5-mL susp	PO	Infants 2 mL/dose, children 4–6 mL/dose, to coat oral mucosa	q6h
Oseltamivir, Tamiflu	30-mg/5-mL susp 30-, 45-, 75-mg cap	PO	Preterm, <38 wk PMA (II): 1 mg/kg/dose PO bid Preterm, 38–40 wk PMA (II): 1.5 mg/kg/dose PO bid Preterm, >40 wk PMA (II), and Term, birth–8 mo (I): 3 mg/kg/dose PO bid 9–23 mo (II): 3.5 mg/kg/dose PO bid ≥24 mo (I): ≤15 kg: 60 mg/day >15–23 kg: 90 mg/day >23–40 kg: 120 mg/day >40 kg: 150 mg/day	q12h
			Prophylaxis: give ½ above dosages	q24h
Oxacillin*, Bactocill	1-, 2-, 10-g vial, 1-, 2-g ivpb	IV, IM	100 mg/kg/day (adults 4–12 g/day) (I) 150–200 mg/kg/day for meningitis (III)	q4–6h
Palivizumab, Synagis	50-, 100-mg vial	IM	15 mg/kg (I)	monthly
Paromomycin*, Humatin	250-mg cap	PO	25–35 mg/kg/day (adult max 4 g/day) (I)	q8h

Drug	Formulation	Route	Dose	Frequency
Penicillin G benzathine*, Bicillin L-A	600,000 units/mL in 1-, 2-, 4-mL prefilled syringes	IM	50,000 units/kg for newborns and infants, children <60 lb: 300,000–600,000 units, children ≥60 lb: 900,000 units (I) (First FDA-approved in 1952 for dosing by pounds body weight)	1 dose for treatment
Penicillin G benzathine/procaine*, Bicillin C-R	1,200,000 units per 2 mL prefilled syringe as 600,000 units benzathine + 600,000 units procaine per mL	IM	<30 lb: 600,000 units 30–60 lb: 900,000–1,200,000 units >60 lb: 2,400,000 units (I)	1 dose usually (may need repeat injections q 2–3 days)
Penicillin G procaine*	600,000 units/mL in 1-, 2-mL prefilled syringes	IM	50,000 units/kg/day, max 1,200,000 units per dose (I)	q12–24h
Penicillin G K*, Pfizerpen	5-, 20-million unit vial 1-, 2-, 3-million unit ivpb	IV, IM	100,000–250,000 units/kg/day (I)	q4–6h
Penicillin G sodium*	5-million unit vial			
Penicillin V K*	125-, 250-mg/5-mL soln 250-, 500-mg tab	PO	25–50 mg/kg/day (I)	q6h
Pentamidine*, Pentam	300-mg vial	IV, IM	4 mg/kg/day (I)	q24h
Nebupent	300-mg vial	Inhaled	300 mg q month for prophylaxis (I)	q24h
Piperacillin/tazobactam*, Zosyn	2/0.25-, 3/0.375-, 4/0.5-g vial ivpb 36/4.5-g vial	IV	≤40 kg: 240–300 mg PIP/kg/day (adults 12–16 g PIP/day q6h) (I)	q8h
Posaconazole, Noxafil	200-mg/5-mL susp	PO	≥13 y and adults (I): 100 mg q12h for 2 doses then 100 mg/day for oropharyngeal candidiasis (OPC) 600 mg/day for prophylaxis of invasive infection 800 mg/day for refractory OPC	q24h q8h q12h
Praziquantel, Biltricide	600-mg triscored tab	PO	20–25 mg/kg (I)	q4–6h for 3 doses
Primaquine phosphate*	15-mg base tab	PO	0.3 mg (base)/kg for PCP, max 30 mg/day (with clindamycin) (III) See also Chapter 10.	q24h

*Available in a generic formulation.

11 **Alphabetic Listing of Antimicrobials**

Alphabetic Listing of Antimicrobials

11

A. SYSTEMIC ANTIMICROBIALS WITH DOSAGE FORMS AND USUAL DOSAGES (cont)

Generic and Trade Names	Dosage Form	Route	Dose (evidence grade)	Interval
Pyrantel*, Pin-X	250-mg chew tab 250-mg/5-mL susp	PO	11 mg/kg, max 1 g (I)	once
Pyrazinamide*	500-mg tab	PO	15–30 mg/kg/day, max 2 g/day (I)	q24h
			Directly observed biweekly therapy, 40–50 mg/kg (I)	twice weekly
Quinupristin/ dalfopristin, Synercid	150/350-mg vial (500 mg total)	IV	22.5 mg/kg/day (II) Adults 15–22.5 mg/kg/day (I)	q8h q8–12h
Raltegravir, Isentress	25-, 100-mg chew tab 400-mg tab	PO	2 to <12 y (I): chew tabs 10 to <14 kg: 150 mg/day 14 to <20 kg: 200 mg/day 20 to <28 kg: 300 mg/day 28 to <40 kg: 400 mg/day ≥40 kg: 600 mg/day ≥12 y: 800 mg/day regular tab (I)	q12h
Ribavirin*, Rebetol	200-mg cap/tab 400-, 500-, 600-mg tab 200-mg/5-mL soln	PO	15 mg/kg/day (with interferon, see Chapter 9) (II)	q12h
Ribavirin, inhalation, Virazole	6-g vial	Inhaled	1 vial by SPAG-2, see Chapter 9	
Rifabutin, Mycobutin	150-mg cap	PO	5 mg/kg for MAC prophylaxis (II) 10–20 mg/kg for MAC or TB treatment (I) Max 300 mg/day	q24h
Rifampin*, Rifadin	150-, 300-mg cap, 600-mg vial	PO, IV	10–20 mg/kg, max 600 mg for TB (I)	q24h
			With directly observed biweekly therapy, dosage is still 10–20 mg/kg/dose (max 600 mg)	twice weekly
			20 mg/kg/day for 2 days for meningococcus prophylaxis, adult dose 1,200 mg/day (I)	q12h

Drug	Formulation	Route	Dose	Interval
Rifampin/isoniazid/pyrazinamide, Rifater	120/50/300-mg tab	PO	Refer to individual agents.	
Rifapentine, Priftin	150-mg tab	PO	≥12 y and adults: 600 mg/dose (I)	twice weekly
Rifaximin, Xifaxan	200-, 550-mg tab	PO	≥12 y and adults: 600 mg/day (I)	q8h
Rilpivirine, Edurant	25-mg tab. See also Emtricitabine.	PO	Adults 25 mg (I)	q24h
Rimantadine*, Flumadine	100-mg tab	PO	≥1 y: 5 mg/kg/day, max 150 mg/day (III) ≥10 y and adults: 200 mg/day (I)	q12h
Ritonavir, Norvir	100-mg cap, tab 400-mg/5-mL soln	PO	Pharmacokinetic enhancer of other HIV protease inhibitors. Dose varies.	q12–24h
Saquinavir, Invirase	200-mg hard gel cap 500-mg tab	PO	≥2 y: 100 mg/kg/day + RTV 5–6 mg/kg/day (II) Adolescent/adults: 2,000 mg/day + RTV 200 mg/day (I)	q12h
Stavudine*, Zerit	5-mg/5-mL soln 15-, 20-, 30-, 40-mg cap	PO	Birth–13 days: 1 mg/kg/day (I) ≥14 days <30 kg: 2 mg/kg/day (I) ≥30 kg and adults: 60 mg/day (I)	q12h
Streptomycin*	1-g vial	IM, IV	20–30 mg/kg/day, max 1 g/day (I)	q12h
Sulfadiazine*	500-mg tab	PO	120–150 mg/kg/day, max 4–6 g/day (I)	q6h
			Rheumatic fever secondary prophylaxis 500 mg once daily if ≤27 kg 1,000 mg once daily if >27 kg (II)	q24h
			See also Chapter 10.	
Telbivudine, Tyzeka	600-mg tab	PO	≥16 y and adults: 600 mg/day (I)	q24h
Telithromycin, Ketek	300-, 400-mg tab	PO	Adults 800 mg/day (I)	q24h
Tenofovir, Viread	40 mg/scoop powder 150-, 200-, 250-, 300-mg tab See also Emtricitabine for combination forms.	PO	≥2 y: 8 mg/kg ≥12 y and ≥35 kg and adults: 300 mg (I)	q24h

*Available in a generic formulation.

11 Alphabetic Listing of Antimicrobials

11

A. SYSTEMIC ANTIMICROBIALS WITH DOSAGE FORMS AND USUAL DOSAGES (cont)

Generic and Trade Names	Dosage Form	Route	Dose (evidence grade)	Interval
Terbinafine, Lamisil	125-, 187.5-mg oral granules 250-mg tab*	PO	>4 y <25 kg: 125 mg/day, 25–35 kg: 187.5 mg/day, >35 kg: 250 mg/day (I)	q24h
Tetracycline*	250-, 500-mg cap, tab	PO	≥8 y: 25–50 mg/kg/day (I)	q6h
Ticarcillin/clavulanate, Timentin	3/0.1-g vial, ivpb, 30/1-g vial	IV	200–300 mg ticarcillin/kg/day (adults 12–18 g/day) (I)	q4–6h
Tinidazole*, Tindamax	250-, 500-mg tab	PO	50 mg/kg, max 2 g (I) See also Chapter 10.	q24h
Tipranavir, Aptivus	500-mg/5-mL soln, 250-mg cap	PO	≥2 y: 28 mg/kg/day + RTV 12 mg/kg/day max 1,000 mg/day + RTV 400 mg/d (I)	q12h
Tobramycin*, Nebcin	20-mg/2-mL pediatric vial 80-mg/2-mL, 1.2-g vial	IV, IM	3–7.5 mg/kg/day (cystic fibrosis 7–10); see Chapter 1 regarding q24h dosing.	q8–24h
Tobraycin inhalation, Tobi*	300-mg ampule	Inhaled	≥6 y: 600 mg/day (I)	q12h
Tobi Podhaler	28-mg capsules for inhalation	Inhaled	≥6 y: 224 mg/day via Podhaler device (I)	q12h
Trimethoprim/ sulfamethoxazole*, Bactrim, Septra	80-mg TMP/400-mg SMX tab (single strength) 160-mg TMP/800-mg SMX tab (double strength) 40-mg TMP/200-mg SMX per 5-mL susp 16-mg TMP/80-mg SMX per mL inj soln in 5-, 10-, 30-mL vials	PO, IV	8–10 mg TMP/kg/day (I)	q12h
			2 mg TMP/kg/day for UTI prophylaxis (I)	q24h
			15–20 mg TMP/kg/day for PCP treatment (I)	q6–8h
			150 mg TMP/m²/day, OR 5 mg TMP/kg/day for PCP prophylaxis (I)	q12h 3 x week OR q24h

Valacyclovir*, Valtrex	500-mg, 1-g tab	PO	VZV: ≥3 mo: 60 mg/kg/day (I,II) HSV: ≥3 mo: 40 mg/kg/day (II) Max single dose 1 g (I)	q8h q12h
Valganciclovir, Valcyte	250-mg/5-mL soln 450-mg tab	PO	CMV treatment: 32 mg/kg/day (II). CMV prophylaxis: 7 x BSA x CrCl (using the modified Schwartz formula for CrCl). Max 900 mg (I). See also Chapters 9 and 14.	q12h q24h
			Adults 900–1,800 mg/day (I)	q12–24h
Vancomycin*, Vancocin	125-, 250-mg cap	PO	40 mg/kg/day (I), max 500 mg/day (III)	q6h
	0.5-, 0.75-, 1-, 5-, 10-g vial* 0.5-, 0.75-, 1-g ivpb	IV	30–40 mg/kg/day (adjusted based on therapeutic drug monitoring) (I) For life-threatening invasive MRSA infection, 60–70 mg/kg/day adjusted to achieve AUC >400 mg•h/L (III)	q6–8h
Voriconazole, Vfend	200-mg vial	IV	2–12 y: 18 mg/kg/day loading dose x 1 day, then 16 mg/kg/day (II) >12 y: 12 mg/kg/day loading dose x 1 day, then 8 mg/kg/day (max 600 mg/day) (I)	q12h
	200-mg/5-mL susp 50-, 200-mg tab	PO	18 mg/kg/day (II) Adults 400–600 mg/day (I)	
Zanamivir, Relenza	5-mg blister cap for inhalation	Inhaled	Prophylaxis: ≥5 y: 10 mg (I)	q24h
			Treatment: ≥7 y: 10 mg (I)	q12h
Zidovudine*, Retrovir	50-mg/5-mL syrup 100-mg cap, 300-mg tab 200-mg/20-mL vial See also Lamivudine for combination forms.	PO	See Chapter 5 for neonatal dosing. 4 to <9 kg: 24 mg/kg/day, 9 to <30 kg: 18 mg/kg/day, ≥30 kg and adults: 600 mg/day (I). 480 mg/m²/day (max 600 mg/day) (I).	q12h
		IV	480 mg/m²/day (max 600 mg/day) (II) 20 mg/m²/hour continuous infusion (II)	q6h

*Available in a generic formulation.

11 Alphabetic Listing of Antimicrobials

Alphabetic Listing of Antimicrobials

11

B. TOPICAL ANTIMICROBIALS (SKIN, EYE, EAR)

Generic and Trade Names	Dosage Form	Route	Dose	Interval
Acyclovir, Zovirax	5% cream	Top	≥12 y: apply to oral lesion	5 times a day
	5% oint[a]		Apply to genital lesion	6 times a day
Azithromycin, AzaSite	1% ophth soln	Ophth	1 gtt	bid for 2 days then daily for 5 days
Bacitracin	ophth oint	Ophth	Apply to affected eye	q3–4h
	oint[b,c]	Top	Apply to affected area	bid–qid
Benzyl alcohol, Ulesfia	5% lotion	Top	Apply to scalp and hair	once; repeat application in 7 days
Besifloxacin, Besivance	0.6% ophth susp	Ophth	≥1 y: 1 gtt to affected eye	tid
Butenafine, Mentax	1% cream	Top	≥12 y: apply to affected area	qd
Butoconazole[a], Gynazole-1	2% cream	Vag	Insert intravaginally	qd for 1 day
Femstat-3				qd for 3 days
Ciclopiroxb, Loprox, Penlac	0.77% cream, gel, lotion	Top	≥10 y: apply to affected area	bid
	1% shampoo[a]		≥16 y: apply to scalp	twice weekly
	8% nail lacquer		≥12 y: apply to infected nail	qd
Ciprofloxacin, Ciloxan	0.3% ophth soln[b]	Ophth	≥12 y: apply to affected eye	q2h for 2 days then q4h for 5 days
	0.3% ophth oint[a]			q8h for 2 days then q12h for 5 days
Ciprofloxacin, Cetraxal Cipro HC (plus hydrocortisone) Otic	0.2% otic soln	Otic	≥1 y: apply 3 drops to affected ear	bid for 7 days
Ciprofloxacin + dexamethasone, Ciprodex	0.3% otic soln	Otic	≥6 mo: apply 4 drops to affected ear	bid for 7 days

Drug	Formulation	Route	Dosage	Frequency
Clindamycin, Clindesse	2% cream	Vag	1 applicatorful intravaginally	one time
Cleocin[b]	100-mg supp		1 supp intravaginally	qhs for 3 days
	2% cream		1 applicatorful intravaginally	qhs for 3–7 days
Cleocin-T[b]	1% soln, gel, lotion	Top	Apply to affected area	qd–bid
Evoclin	1% foam			qd
Clindamycin + benzoyl peroxide, Benzaclin	1% gel	Top	≥12 y: apply to affected area	bid
Acanya	1.2% gel		Apply small amount to face	q24h
Clindamycin + tretinoin, Ziana, Veltin	1.2% gel	Top	Apply small amount to face	hs
Clotrimazole[b,c] Lotrimin	1% cream, lotion, soln	Top	Apply to affected area	bid
Gyne-Lotrimin-7	1% cream, 100-mg supp	Vag	Adolescents intravaginally	qhs for 7–14 days
Gyne-Lotrimin-3	2% cream, 200-mg supp			qhs for 3 days
Clotrimazole + betamethasone, Lotrisone[b]	1% cream, lotion	Top	≥12 y: apply to affected area	bid
Coly-Mycin S, Colistin + neomycin + hydrocortisone	otic susp	Otic	Apply 3–4 drops to affected ear canal; may use with wick.	q6–8h

11 Alphabetic Listing of Antimicrobials

11

B. TOPICAL ANTIMICROBIALS (SKIN, EYE, EAR) (cont)

Generic and Trade Names	Dosage Form	Route	Dose	Interval
Cortisporin, Bacitracin + neomycin + polymyxin b + hydrocortisone	oint[a]	Ophth	Apply to affected eye	q4h
		Top	Apply to affected area	bid–qid
Cortisporin, Neomycin + polymyxin b + hydrocortisone	ophth soln[a]	Ophth	1–2 drops to affected eye	q4h
	otic soln, susp	Otic	3 drops to affected ear	bid–qid
	cream[a]	Top	Apply to affected area	
Dapsone, Aczone	5% gel	Top	Apply to affected area	bid
Econazole[b], Spectazole	1% cream	Top	Apply to affected area	qd–bid
Erythromycin	0.5% ophth oint[b]	Ophth	Apply to affected eye	q4h
Eryderm, Erygel	2% soln[b], gel[a,b]	Top	Apply to affected area	bid
Ery Pads	2% pledgets[b]			
Akne-mycin	2% oint			
Erythromycin + benzoyl peroxide, Benzamycin[b]	3% gel	Top	≥12 y: apply to affected area	qd–bid
Gatifloxacin, Zymaxid	0.5% ophth soln	Ophth	Apply to affected eye	q2h for 1 day then q6h
Gentamicin[b], Garamycin	0.1% cream, oint	Top	Apply to affected area	tid–qid
	0.3% ophth soln, oint	Ophth[a]	Apply to affected eye	q1–4h (sol) q4–8h (oint)

Gentamicin + prednisolone, Pred-G[a]	0.3% ophth soln, oint	Ophth	Apply to affected eye	q1–4h (sol) qd–tid (oint)
Ivermectin, Sklice	0.5% lotion	Top	≥6 mo: thoroughly coat hair and scalp, rinse after 10 minutes	once
Ketoconazole				
Nizoral	2% shampoo[a,b]	Top	Apply to affected area	qd
	2% cream[b]	Top	≥12 y: apply to affected area	qd–bid
Nizoral A-D[c]	1% shampoo	Top	≥12 y: apply to affected area	bid
Extina, Xolegel	2% foam[b], gel	Top	≥12 y: apply to affected area	bid
Levofloxacin		Ophth	Apply to affected eye	q1–4h
Iquix	1.5% ophth soln			
Quixin	0.5% ophth soln			
Mafenide, Sulfamylon	8.5% cream	Top	Apply to burn	qd–bid
	5-g pwd for reconstitution		To keep burn dressing wet	q4–8h as needed
Malathion, Ovide	0.5% soln	Top	≥6 y: apply to hair and scalp	once
Maxitrol[a,b], neomycin + polymyxin b + dexamethasone	susp, oint	Ophth	Apply to affected eye	q4h (oint) q1–4h (susp)
Metronidazole[a]				
MetroGel-Vaginal[b]	0.75% vag gel	Vag	1 applicatorful intravaginally	qd–bid
MetroCream-gel,	0.75% cream[b], gel[b], lotion[b]	Top		bid
– lotion				
Noritate, MetroGel	1% cream, gel			qd

Alphabetic Listing of Antimicrobials

11

B. TOPICAL ANTIMICROBIALS (SKIN, EYE, EAR) (cont)

Generic and Trade Names	Dosage Form	Route	Dose	Interval
Miconazole				
Micatin[b,c] and others	2% cream, pwd, oint, spray, lotion, gel	Top	Apply to affected area	qd–bid
Fungoid[c]	2% tincture			bid
Vusion	0.25% oint	Top	≥1 mo: to diaper dermatitis	Each diaper change for 7 days
Monistat-1	1.2-g vag supp	Vag	Adolescents: intravaginally	once
Monistat-3[b,c]	4% cream, 200-mg supp			qhs for 3 days
Monistat-7[b,c]	2% cream, 100-mg supp			qhs for 7 days
Moxifloxacin, Vigamox	0.5% ophth soln	Ophth	Apply to affected eye	tid
Mupirocin, Bactroban	2% oint[b], cream, nasal oint	Top	Apply to infected skin or nasal mucosa	tid
Naftifine, Naftin[a]	2% cream, gel	Top	Apply to affected area	qd
Natamycin, Natacyn[a]	5% ophth soln	Ophth	Apply to affected eye	q1–4h
Neosporin[b]				
bacitracin + neomycin	ophth oint[a]	Ophth	Apply to affected eye	q4h
+ polymyxin B	top oint[c]	Top	Apply to affected area	bid–qid
gramicidin + neomycin + polymyxin B	ophth soln[a]	Ophth	Apply to affected eye	q4h
Nystatin[b], Mycostatin	100,000 units/g cream, oint, pwd	Top	Apply to affected area	bid–qid

Nystatin + triamcinolone 0.1% Mycolog II[b]	100,000 units/g cream, oint	Top	Apply to affected area	bid
Ofloxacin[b], Floxin Otic	0.3% otic soln	Otic	5–10 drops to affected ear	qd–bid
Ocuflox	0.3% ophth soln	Ophth	Apply to affected eye	q1–6h
Oxiconazole, Oxistat	1% cream, lotion	Top	Apply to affected area	qd–bid
Penciclovir, Denavir	1% top cream	Top	Apply to affected area	q2h while awake for 4 days
Permethrin, Nix[b,c]	1% cream	Top	Apply to hair/scalp	once for 10 min
Elimite[b]	5% cream	Top	Apply to all skin surfaces	once for 8–14 h
Polysporin[b]	ophth oint[a]	Ophth	Apply to affected eye	qd–tid
polymyxin B + bacitracin	oint[c], pwd[c]	Top	Apply to affected area	
Polytrim[b] trimethoprim + polymyxin B	ophth soln	Ophth	Apply to affected eye	q3–4h
Pyrethrins[b], Rid	0.3% lotion, gel, shampoo	Top	Apply to affected area	once for 10 min
Retapamulin, Altabax	1% oint	Top	Apply thin layer to affected area	bid for 5 days
Selenium sulfide[b], Selsun	2.5% suspension/lotion	Top	Lather into scalp or affected area	twice weekly then every 1–2 weeks
Selsun Blue[b,c]	1% shampoo	Top		qd
Sertaconazole, Ertaczo	2% cream	Top	≥12 y: apply to affected area	bid
Silver Sulfadiazine[a,b], Silvadene	1% cream	Top	Apply to affected area	qd–bid
Spinosad[b], Natroba	0.9% susp	Top	Apply to scalp and hair	once; may repeat in 7 days
Sulconazole[a], Exelderm	1% soln, cream	Top	Apply to affected area	qd–bid

11

Alphabetic Listing of Antimicrobials

Alphabetic Listing of Antimicrobials

11

B. TOPICAL ANTIMICROBIALS (SKIN, EYE, EAR) (cont)

Generic and Trade Names	Dosage Form	Route	Dose	Interval
Sulfacetamide sodium[b]	10%, 15%, 30% soln	Ophth	Apply to affected eye	q1–3h qid
Sodium-Sulamyd	10% ophth oint			
Klaron	10% top lotion	Top	≥12 y: apply to affected area	bid–qid
Sulfacetamide sodium	10% ophth oint	Ophth	Apply to affected eye	tid–qid
+ prednisolone, Blephamide[b]	10% opth soln			
Sulfacetamide sodium + fluorometholone, FML-S	10% opth soln	Ophth	Apply to affected eye	qid
Terbinafine, Lamisil-AT[c]	1% cream[b], spray, gel, soln	Top	Apply to affected area One applicator full	qd–bid, hs for 7 days
Terconazole[a,b], Terazol-7	0.4% cream	Vag	One applicator full or 1 supp	hs for 3 days
Terazol-3	0.8% cream, 80 mg supp	Vag		
Tobramycin[b], Tobrex	0.3% ophth soln, oint	Ophth	Apply to affected eye	q1–4h (sol) q4–8h (oint)
Tobramycin + dexamethasone, Tobradex	0.3% ophth soln[b], oint	Ophth	Apply to affected eye	q2–6h (sol) q6–8h (oint)
Trifluridine[b], Viroptic	1% ophth soln	Ophth	1 drop (max 9 drops/day)	q2h
Tolnaftate[b], Tinactin	1% cream, soln, pwd, spray	Top	Apply to affected area	bid

[a]Not approved for children.
[b]Generic available.
[c]Over the counter

12. Antibiotic Therapy for Obese Children

The dose of antimicrobial for an obese child that is required to achieve the same tissue site exposure to pathogens as children of average body weight is most often not available. When antimicrobials are first investigated for US Food and Drug Administration approval, obese children are excluded from pharmacokinetic and drug exposure analysis. During the treatment studies required for drug approval, obese children are also excluded, so unless specific studies are performed on this population, no dosing or exposure data exist.

In general, different classes of drugs distribute in a predictable way into different tissue compartments, so a reasonable guess for the proper dose, by class of antibiotic, is possible. For drugs that do not distribute into adipose tissue, dosing should be based on lean body weight. For those that do distribute into adipose tissue, increasing the dose, based on body weight, is logical, although high-dosage regimens may represent an increased risk of toxicity or poor tolerance. For other classes of drugs, distribution into adipose tissue may be intermediate, and the dose should be somewhere in between that calculated for lean body weight and total body weight.

Listed below are the major classes of antimicrobials and guidance on how to calculate the most appropriate dose. The level of evidence to support these recommendations is Level II–III (based on adult studies). Whenever a dose is used that is greater than one prospectively investigated for efficacy and safety, the clinician must monitor the child closely for unanticipated adverse events. Data are not available on all agents.

Drug Class	Dosing Recommendations		
	By Ideal Body Weight	Intermediate Dosing	By Total Body Weight[a]
ANTIBACTERIALS			
Beta-lactams		IBW + 0.3 (TBW-IBW)	
Penicillins		X	
Cephalosporins		X	
Carbapenems		X	
Macrolides			
Erythromycins	X		
Azithromycin	X (for gastrointestinal infections)		X
Clarithromycin	X		
Lincosamides			
Clindamycin			X

Drug Class	Dosing Recommendations		
	By Ideal Body Weight	Intermediate Dosing	By Total Body Weight[a]
ANTIBACTERIALS (cont)			
Glycopeptides			
Vancomycin		1,500–2,000 mg/m²/day	
Aminoglycosides		IBW + 0.4 (TBW-IBW)	
Gentamicin		X	
Tobramycin		X	
Amikacin		X	
Fluoroquinolones		IBW + 0.45 (TBW-IBW)	
Ciprofloxacin		X	
Levofloxacin		X	
Rifamycins			
Rifampin	X		
Miscellaneous			
TMP/SMX			X
Metronidazole	X		
Linezolid	X		
Daptomycin			X
ANTIFUNGALS			
Amphotericin B (conventional and lipid formulations)			X
Echinocandins			
Caspofungin			X
Micafungin		X	
Azoles			
Fluconazole			X
Voriconazole	X		
Flucytosine	X		

Drug Class	Dosing Recommendations		
	By Ideal Body Weight	Intermediate Dosing	By Total Body Weight[a]
ANTIVIRALS (non-HIV)			
Nucleoside analogues (acyclovir, ganciclovir)	X		
ANTIMYCOBACTERIALS			
Isoniazid	X		
Rifampin	X		
Pyrazinamide	X		
Ethambutol	X		
Streptomycin	X		

Abbreviations: HIV, human immunodeficiency virus; IBW, ideal body weight; TBW, total body weight.
[a]Actual measured body weight.

Bibliography

Camaione L, Elliott K, Mitchell-Van Steele A, Lomaestro B, Pai MP. Vancomycin dosing in children and young adults: back to the drawing board. *Pharmacotherapy.* 2013;33(12):1278–1287

Heble DE Jr, McPherson C, Nelson MP, Hunstad DA. Vancomycin trough concentrations in overweight or obese pediatric patients. *Pharmacotherapy.* 2013;33(12):1273–1277

Janson B, Thursky K. Dosing of antibiotics in obesity. *Curr Opin Infect Dis.* 2012;25(6):634–649

Reynolds DC, Waite LH, Alexander DP, DeRyke CA. Performance of a vancomycin dosage regimen developed for obese patients. *Am J Health Syst Pharm.* 2012;69:944–950

Antibiotic Therapy for Obese Children

12

13. Antibiotic Therapy for Patients With Renal Failure

For anti-infective drugs recently approved by the US Food and Drug Administration (FDA), information on drug exposure in patients with varying degrees of renal failure is placed in the package label and posted on the National Library of Medicine/National Institutes of Health Web site as a collaborative project with the FDA (http://dailymed.nlm.nih.gov/dailymed/about.cfm). Information on older agents is often lacking, and information on children in particular may never have been collected prospectively. A complete list of antibiotics and dosing recommendations in renal failure, and for children on dialysis, is beyond the scope of this chapter. An exhaustive, annually updated reference that includes information on dosing adjustments in renal failure, *AHFS Drug Information 2014,* is available in print, online, and mobile formats from the American Society of Health-System Pharmacists, Inc. (www.ahfsdruginformation.com).

Many commonly used antimicrobials are excreted primarily by the kidneys; therefore, when significant renal impairment is present, either downward adjustments in dosages must be made or the intervals between doses must be lengthened. Drugs that are excreted by the kidney and have a narrow therapeutic index, with toxicity documented at serum concentrations not too much greater than therapeutic concentrations, must be monitored closely. The aminoglycosides and vancomycin are prime examples of these antibiotics. For those antibiotics excreted by the kidney but with little toxicity at high serum concentrations, such as the beta-lactam antibiotics, only moderate changes in dosages need to be made. Drugs such as metronidazole that are metabolized by the liver and those excreted significantly by the liver, such as azithromycin, nafcillin, and ceftriaxone, do not usually require adjustments in dosing in renal failure.

In some circumstances, dosing drugs in children with decreased renal function is best achieved by therapeutic drug monitoring of serum antibiotic concentrations. Many computer programs are available that integrate information on the serum creatinine (or creatinine clearance [CrCl]) and population pharmacokinetics which allows for estimation of the best mg/kg dosage, administered at a specified interval to attain therapeutic but nontoxic peak and trough serum concentrations (or time-above-minimum inhibitory concentration [MIC], or area under the curve [AUC], depending on the antibiotic) to achieve the most appropriate antibiotic exposure profile for cure. Many hospital-based pharmacists can assist with this determination. The following calculation, from the 2009 Schwartz equation and now based on the new enzymatic methods for determining serum creatinine concentrations,[1,2] is used for estimating CrCl (and, therefore, antibiotic clearance) in infants and children (1–18 years of age) with stable renal function:

CrCl (mL/min/1.73 m^2 BSA) = (0.413 x height [cm])/serum creatinine (mg/dL)
BSA = body surface area
(In the previous Schwarz equations, different adjustment constants were used based on age and sex.)

In the absence of a software program, one can administer the customary initial loading mg/kg dose, and until antibiotic assay results are available, make an estimate of the appropriate dosage based on rates of excretion roughly related to the estimated degree of renal failure, with this information frequently available on the antibiotic's package label, available online as noted above. Alterations in dosage and/or interval are subsequently made, based on measured antibiotic values, to achieve serum concentrations and, therefore, exposure of antibiotic at the site of infection, similar to those in patients with normal renal function.

14. Antimicrobial Prophylaxis/Prevention of Symptomatic Infection

This chapter provides a summary of recommendations for prophylaxis of infections, defined as providing therapy prior to the onset of clinical signs or symptoms of infection. Prophylaxis can be considered in several clinical scenarios.

A. Postexposure Prophylaxis

Given for a short, specified period after exposure to specific pathogens/organisms, where the risks of acquiring the infection are felt to justify antimicrobial treatment to eradicate the pathogen or prevent symptomatic infection in situations in which the child (either healthy or with increased susceptibility to infection) is likely to have been inoculated (eg, asymptomatic child closely exposed to meningococcus; a neonate born to a mother with active genital herpes simplex virus).

B. Long-term Symptomatic Disease Prophylaxis

Given to a particular, defined population of children who are of relatively high risk of acquiring a severe infection (eg, a child post-splenectomy; a child with documented rheumatic heart disease to prevent subsequent streptococcal infection), with prophylaxis provided during the period of risk, potentially months or years.

C. Preemptive Treatment/Latent Infection Treatment ("Prophylaxis of Symptomatic Infection")

Where a child has a documented but asymptomatic infection, and targeted antimicrobials are given to prevent the development of symptomatic disease (eg, latent tuberculosis infection or therapy of a stem cell transplant patient with documented cytomegalovirus viremia but no symptoms of infection or rejection). Treatment period is usually defined, but certain circumstances, such as reactivation of a herpesvirus, may require re-treatment.

D. Surgical/Procedure Prophylaxis

A child receives a surgical/invasive catheter procedure, planned or unplanned, where the risk of infection postoperatively or post-procedure may justify prophylaxis to prevent an infection from occurring (eg, prophylaxis to prevent infection following spinal rod placement). Treatment is usually short-term, beginning just prior to the procedure and ending at the conclusion of the procedure, or within 24 to 48 hours.

E. Travel-Related Exposure Prophylaxis

Not discussed in this chapter; please refer to information on specific disease entities (eg, traveler's diarrhea, Chapter 6) or pathogens (eg, malaria, Chapter 10). Updated, current information for travelers about prophylaxis and current worldwide infection risks can be found on the Centers for Disease Control and Prevention Web site at www.cdc.gov/travel (accessed November 14, 2013).

Note

- **Abbreviations:** ACOG, American College of Obstetricians and Gynecologists; amox/clav, amoxicillin/clavulanate; bid, twice daily; CDC, Centers for Disease Control and Prevention; CMV, cytomegalovirus; div, divided; GI, gastrointestinal; HSV, herpes simplex virus; IGRA, interferon-gamma release assay; IM, intramuscular; INH, isoniazid; IV, intravenous; MRSA, methicillin-resistant *Staphylococcus aureus;* MRSE, methicillin-resistant *S epidermidis;* PO, orally; PPD, purified protein derivative; qd, once daily; qid, 4 times daily; TB, tuberculosis; tid, 3 times daily; TIG, tetanus immune globulin; TMP/SMX, trimethoprim/sulfamethoxazole; UTI, urinary tract infection.

A. POSTEXPOSURE PROPHYLAXIS

Prophylaxis Category	Therapy (evidence grade)	Comments
Bacterial		
Bites, animal and human[1–4] (*Pasteurella multocida* [animal], *Eikenella corrodens* [human], *Staphylococcus* spp and *Streptococcus* spp)	Amox/clav 45 mg/kg/day PO div tid (amox/clav 7:1, see Chapter 1, Aminopenicillins) for 5–10 days (AII) OR ampicillin and clindamycin (BII)	Consider rabies prophylaxis for animal bites (AI); consider tetanus prophylaxis. Human bites have a very high rate of infection (do not close open wounds routinely). *S aureus* coverage is only fair with amox/clav and provides no coverage for MRSA. For penicillin allergy, consider ciprofloxacin (for *Pasteurella*) plus clindamycin (BIII).

Endocarditis Prophylaxis[5]: Given that (1) endocarditis is rarely caused by dental/GI procedures and (2) prophylaxis for procedures prevents an exceedingly small number of cases, the risks of antibiotics most often outweigh benefits. However, some "highest risk" conditions are currently recommended for prophylaxis: (1) prosthetic heart valve (or prosthetic material used to repair a valve); (2) previous endocarditis; (3) cyanotic congenital heart disease that is unrepaired (or palliatively repaired with shunts and conduits); (4) congenital heart disease that is repaired but with defects at the site of repair adjacent to prosthetic material; (5) completely repaired congenital heart disease using prosthetic material, for the first 6 months after repair; or (6) cardiac transplant patients with valvulopathy. Routine prophylaxis no longer is required for children with native valve abnormalities. Follow-up data suggest that following these new guidelines, no increase in endocarditis has been detected.[6]

– In highest risk patients: dental procedures that involve manipulation of the gingival or periodontal region of teeth	Amoxicillin 50 mg/kg PO 1 h before procedure OR ampicillin or ceftriaxone or cefazolin, all at 50 mg/kg IM/IV 30–60 min before procedure	If penicillin allergy: clindamycin 20 mg/kg PO (60 min before) or IV (30 min before); OR azithromycin 15 mg/kg or clarithromycin 15 mg/kg, 1 h before
– Genitourinary and gastrointestinal procedures	None	No longer recommended

14

Antimicrobial Prophylaxis/Prevention of Symptomatic Infection

A. POSTEXPOSURE PROPHYLAXIS (cont)

Prophylaxis Category	Therapy (evidence grade)	Comments

Bacterial (cont)

Tetanus
(*Clostridium tetani*)[10,11]

	Need for tetanus vaccine or TIG			
	Clean wound		Contaminated wound	
Number of past tetanus vaccine doses	Need for tetanus vaccine	Need for TIG 250 U IM	Need for tetanus vaccine	Need for TIG 250 U IM
<3 doses	Yes	No	Yes	Yes
≥3 doses	No (if <10 y) Yes (if ≥10 y)	No	No (if <5 y) Yes (if ≥5 y)	No

For deep, contaminated wounds, wound debridement is essential. For wounds that cannot be fully debrided, consider metronidazole 30 mg/kg/day PO div q8h until wound healing is underway and anaerobic conditions no longer exist, as short as 3–5 days (BIII).

Tuberculosis
(*Mycobacterium tuberculosis*)
Exposed infant <4 y, or immunocompromised patient (high risk of dissemination)[12,13]

Exposed infant <4 y, or immunocompromised patient (high risk of dissemination): INH 10–15 mg/kg PO daily for 2–3 mo after last exposure AND with repeat skin test or IGRA test negative (AIII)

If PPD or IGRA remains negative at 2–3 mo and child remains well, consider stopping empiric therapy. However, tests at 2–3 mo may not be reliable in immunocompromised patients.
This regimen is to PREVENT infection in a compromised host after exposure, rather than to treat latent asymptomatic infection.

Viral		
Herpes Simplex Virus		
During pregnancy	For women with recurrent genital herpes: acyclovir 400 mg PO bid; valacyclovir 500 mg PO qd OR 1 g PO qd from 36 wk gestation until delivery (CII)	ACOG recommends maternal antiviral prophylaxis beginning at 36 weeks' gestation in women with active recurrent genital herpes. Development of neonatal HSV disease after maternal suppression has been documented.[14]
Neonatal	300 mg/m^2/dose PO tid for 6 mo following cessation of IV acyclovir treatment of acute disease (AI)	Follow absolute neutrophil counts at 2 and 4 wk, then monthly during prophylactic/suppressive therapy
Keratitis (ocular)	300 mg/m^2/dose PO tid for at least 12 mo following cessation of treatment of acute disease (AII)	Based on data from adults. Watch for severe recurrence at conclusion of suppression.
Influenza virus (A or B)[15]	Oseltamivir (AI) 3 mo through ≤8 mo: 3.0 mg/kg/dose once daily for 10 days 9–23 months 3.5 mg/kg/dose PO bid once daily for 10 days[16] Based on body weight for children ≥24 mo ≤15 kg: 30 mg once daily for 10 days >15–23 kg: 45 mg once daily for 10 days >23–40 kg: 60 mg once daily for 10 days >40 kg: 75 mg once daily for 10 days Zanamivir (AI) Children ≥5 y: 10 mg (two 5-mg inhalations) qd for as long as 28 days (community outbreaks) or 10 days (household settings)	Amantadine and rimantadine are not recommended for prophylaxis. Not recommended for infants 0 to ≤3 mo unless situation judged critical because of limited data on use in this age group.
Rabies virus[17]	Rabies immune globulin, 20 IU/kg, infiltrate around wound, with remaining volume injected IM (AII). Rabies immunization should be provided postexposure (AII).	For dog, cat, or ferret bite, immediate RIG and immunization for symptomatic animal; otherwise, can wait 10 days for observation of animal, if possible, prior to RIG or vaccine. Bites of squirrels, hamsters, guinea pigs, gerbils, chipmunks, rats, mice and other rodents, rabbits, hares, and pikas almost never require antirabies prophylaxis.

14

Antimicrobial Prophylaxis/Prevention of Symptomatic Infection

14

A. POSTEXPOSURE PROPHYLAXIS (cont)

Prophylaxis Category	Therapy (evidence grade)	Comments
Fungal		
– *Pneumocystis jiroveci* (previously *Pneumocystis carinii*)[18,19]	TMP/SMX as 5 mg TMP/kg/day PO, divided in 2 doses, q12h, either daily or 3 times/wk (AI); OR TMP/SMX 5 mg TMP/kg/day PO as a single dose, once daily, given 3 times/wk (AI); OR dapsone 2 mg/kg (max 100 mg) PO once daily, or 4 mg/kg (max 200 mg) once weekly, until no longer immunocompromised, based on oncology or transplant treatment regimen	Prophylaxis in specific immunocompromised hosts

B. LONG-TERM SYMPTOMATIC DISEASE PROPHYLAXIS

Prophylaxis Category	Therapy (evidence grade)	Comments
Bacterial otitis media[20,21]	Amoxicillin or other antibiotics can be used in one-half the therapeutic dose qd or bid to prevent infections if the benefits outweigh the risks of development of resistant organisms for that child, and the risk of antibiotic side effects.	To prevent recurrent infections, also consider the risks and benefits of placing tympanostomy tubes to improve middle ear ventilation. Studies have demonstrated that amoxicillin, sulfisoxazole, and TMP/SMX are effective. However, antimicrobial prophylaxis may alter the nasopharyngeal flora and foster colonization with resistant organisms, compromising long-term efficacy of the prophylactic drug. Continuous PO-administered antimicrobial prophylaxis should be reserved for control of recurrent acute otitis media, only when defined as ≥3 distinct and well-documented episodes during a period of 6 mo or ≥4 episodes during a period of 12 mo. Although prophylactic administration of an antimicrobial agent limited to a period when a person is at high risk of otitis media has been suggested (eg, during acute viral respiratory tract infection), this method has not been evaluated critically.
Acute rheumatic fever	For >27.3 kg (>60 lb): 1.2 million U penicillin G benzathine, q4wk For <27.3 kg: 600,000 U penicillin G benzathine, q4wk OR penicillin V (phenoxymethyl) oral, 250 mg PO bid	Doses studied many years ago, with no new data; ARF an uncommon disease currently in the US. Alternatives to penicillin include sulfasoxazole or macrolides, including erythromycin, azithromycin, and clarithromycin.

| **Urinary tract infection, recurrent**[22-25] | TMP/SMX (2 mg/kg/dose of TMP) PO qd OR nitrofurantoin 1–2 mg/kg PO qd at bedtime; more rapid resistance may develop using beta-lactams (BII). | Only for those with grade III–V reflux or with recurrent febrile UTI: prophylaxis no longer recommended for patients with grade I–II (some also exclude grade III) reflux and no evidence of renal damage. Early treatment of new infections is recommended for these children. Resistance eventually develops to every antibiotic; follow resistance patterns for each patient. |

C. PREEMPTIVE TREATMENT/LATENT INFECTION TREATMENT ("PROPHYLAXIS OF SYMPTOMATIC INFECTION")

| **Tuberculosis**[12,13] *(latent tuberculosis infection [asymptomatic infection], defined by a positive skin test or IGRA, with no clinical or x-ray evidence of active disease)* | INH 10–15 mg/kg/day (max 300 mg) PO daily for 9 mo (12 mo for immunocompromised patients) (AII); treatment with INH at 20–30 mg twice weekly for 9 mo is also effective (AIII). | Single drug therapy if no clinical or radiographic evidence of active disease. For exposure to known INH-R but rifampin-S strains, use rifampin 6 mo (AIII). For exposure to multidrug-resistant strains, consult with TB specialist. |

14

D. SURGICAL/PROCEDURE PROPHYLAXIS[26-30]

The CDC and National Healthcare Safety Network use a classification of surgical procedure-related wound infections based on an estimation of the load of bacterial contamination: Class I, clean; Class II, clean-contaminated; Class III, contaminated; and Class IV, dirty/infected.[27,31] Other major factors creating risk for postoperative surgical site infection include the duration of surgery (a longer duration operation, defined as one that exceeded the 75th percentile for a given procedure) and the medical comorbidities of the patient, as determined by an American Society of Anesthesiologists score of III, IV, or V (presence of severe systemic disease that results in functional limitations, is life-threatening, or is expected to preclude survival from the operation). The virulence/pathogenicity of bacteria inoculated and the presence of foreign debris/devitalized tissue/surgical material in the wound are also considered risk factors for infection.

For all categories of surgical prophylaxis, dosing recommendations are derived from (1) choosing agents likely to be responsible for inoculation of the surgical site; (2) giving the agents shortly before starting the operation to achieve appropriate serum and tissue exposures at the time of incision through the end of the procedure; (3) providing additional doses during the procedure at times based on the standard dosing guideline for that agent; and (4) stopping the agents at the end of the procedure, but no longer than 24 to 48 hours after the procedure.[28-30,32]

Procedure/Operation	Recommended Agents	Preoperative Dose
Cardiovascular		
Cardiothoracic *S epidermidis, S aureus,* *Corynebacterium* spp	Cefazolin, OR	30 mg/kg
	Vancomycin, if MRSA likely	15 mg/kg
Vascular *S epidermidis, S aureus,* *Corynebacterium* spp, gram-negative enteric bacilli, particularly for procedures in the groin	Cefazolin, OR	30 mg/kg
	Vancomycin, if MRSA likely	15 mg/kg
Gastrointestinal		
Gastroduodenal Enteric gram-negative bacilli, respiratory tract gram-positive cocci	Cefazolin	30 mg/kg
Biliary Procedure, Open Enteric gram-negative bacilli, enterococci, *Clostridia*	Cefazolin	30 mg/kg

Appendectomy, non-perforated	Cefoxitin, OR	40 mg/kg
	Cefazolin and metronidazole	30 mg/kg cefazolin and 10 mg/kg metronidazole
Complicated appendicitis or other ruptured viscus	Cefoxitin, OR	40 mg/kg
Enteric gram-negative bacilli, enterococci, anaerobes. May require additional therapy for treatment of infection.	Cefazolin and metronidazole, OR	30 mg/kg cefazolin and 10 mg/kg metronidazole
	Meropenem, OR	20 mg/kg
	Imipenen, OR	20 mg/kg
	Ertapenem	30 mg/kg
Genitourinary		
Cystoscopy (only requires prophylaxis for children with suspected active UTI or those having foreign material placed) Enteric gram-negative bacilli, enterococci	Cefazolin, OR	30 mg/kg
	TMP/SMX (if low local resistance), OR Select a 3rd-generation cephalosporin (cefotaxime) or fluoroquinolone (ciprofloxacin) if the child is colonized with cefazolin-resistant, TMP/SMX-resistant strains.	4–5 mg/kg
Open or laparoscopic surgery Enteric gram-negative bacilli, enterococci	Cefazolin	30 mg/kg
Head and Neck Surgery		
Assuming incision through respiratory tract mucosa	Clindamycin, OR	10 mg/kg
Anaerobes, enteric gram-negative bacilli, S aureus	Cefazolin and metronidazole	30 mg/kg cefazolin and 10 mg/kg metronidazole
Neurosurgery		
Craniotomy, ventricular shunt placement S epidermidis, S aureus	Cefazolin, OR	30 mg/kg
	Vancomycin, if MRSA likely	15 mg/kg

14   Antimicrobial Prophylaxis/Prevention of Symptomatic Infection

Antimicrobial Prophylaxis/Prevention of Symptomatic Infection

14

D. SURGICAL/PROCEDURE PROPHYLAXIS[26-30] (cont)

Procedure/Operation	Recommended Agents	Preoperative Dose
Orthopedic		
Internal fixation of fractures, spinal rod placement, prosthetic joints	Cefazolin, OR	30 mg/kg
S epidermidis, S aureus	Vancomycin, if MRSA likely	15 mg/kg
Trauma		
Exceptionally varied; agents should focus on skin flora (*S epidermidis, S aureus*) as well as the flora inoculated into the wound, based on the trauma exposure, that may include enteric gram-negative bacilli, anaerobes (including *Clostridia* spp), fungi. Cultures at time of wound exploration are critical to focus therapy.	Cefazolin (for skin) OR	30 mg/kg
	Vancomycin (for skin), if MRSA likely, OR	15 mg/kg
	Meropenem OR imipenem (for anaerobes, including *Clostridia* spp, and non-fermenting gram-negative bacilli) OR	20 mg/kg for either
	Gentamicin and metronidazole (for anaerobes, including *Clostridia* spp, and non-fermenting gram-negative bacilli), OR	2.5 mg/kg gentamicin and 10 mg/kg metronidazole
	Piperacillin/tazobactam	100 mg/kg piperacillin component

15. Sequential Parenteral-Oral Antibiotic Therapy (Oral Step-down Therapy) for Serious Infections

Bacterial pneumonias, bone and joint infections,[1–3] deep-tissue abscesses, and appendicitis,[4,5] as well as cellulitis or pyelonephritis,[6] may require initial parenteral therapy to control the growth and spread of pathogens and minimize injury to tissues. However, intravenous (IV) therapy carries risks of catheter-related complications that are unpleasant for the child whether therapy is provided in the hospital or on an outpatient basis. For the beta-lactam class of antibiotics, absorption of orally administered antibiotics in standard dosages provides peak serum concentrations that are routinely only 5% to 20% of those achieved with IV or intramuscular administration. However, clindamycin and many newer antibiotics of the fluoroquinolone class (ciprofloxacin)[7] and oxazolidinone class (linezolid) have excellent absorption of their oral formulations and provide virtually the same tissue antibiotic exposure at a particular mg/kg dose, compared with the exposure when the antibiotic is given at that dose IV. Following initial parenteral therapy of serious infections, it may be possible to provide oral antibiotic therapy to achieve the tissue antibiotic exposure that is required for cure. One must also assume that the parent and child are compliant with the administration of each antibiotic dose, and that the parents will seek medical care if the clinical course does not continue to improve for their child.

High-dose oral beta-lactam antibiotic therapy of osteoarticular infections, associated with achieving a particular level of bactericidal activity in serum, has been associated with treatment success since 1978.[1] While most hospital laboratories no longer offer bactericidal assays, the need to achieve bactericidal activity with high-dose oral therapy, explained below, remains important. Comparable mg/kg dosages of parenteral and oral beta-lactam medications often result in comparable tissue concentrations 4 to 6 hours after a dose (although the high mg/kg doses given orally may not always be well tolerated). The momentary high serum concentrations that occur during IV administration of beta-lactam antibiotics may provide for better tissue penetration; however, killing of bacteria by beta-lactam antibiotics is not dependent on the height of the antibiotic concentration but on the time that the antibiotic is present at the site of infection at concentrations above the minimum inhibitory concentration of the antibiotic for that pathogen.

For abscesses in soft tissues, joints, and bones, most organisms are removed by surgical drainage and killed by the initial parenteral therapy. When the signs and symptoms of infection begin to resolve, usually within 3 to 5 days, continuing IV therapy may not be required as a normal host response begins to assist in clearing the infection. Following objective laboratory markers such as C-reactive protein (CRP) or procalcitonin (PCT) during the hospitalization may help the clinician better assess the response to therapy, particularly in the infant or child who is difficult to examine.[8]

Large dosage oral beta-lactam therapy (based on in vitro susceptibilities) provides the tissue antibiotic exposure required to eradicate the remaining pathogens at the infection site as the tissue perfusion improves. For beta-lactams, begin with a dosage 2 to 3 times the normal dosage (eg, 75–100 mg/kg/day of amoxicillin or 100 mg/kg/day of cephalexin). High-dose prolonged oral beta-lactam therapy may be associated with reversible neutropenia; checking for hematologic toxicity every few weeks during therapy should be considered.

For methicillin-resistant *Staphylococcus aureus* (MRSA) infections, prospective evaluations of clindamycin or trimethoprim/sulfamethoxazole have not been published yet, but data on clindamycin for osteomyelitis were published decades ago.[9] Dose-limiting diarrhea prevents increasing the clindamycin dose above 30 to 40 mg/kg/day, divided 3 times daily.

Monitor the child clinically for a continued response on oral therapy; follow CRP or PCT after the switch to oral therapy if there are concerns about continue response, to make sure that the antibiotic and dosage you selected are appropriate.

16. Adverse Reactions to Antimicrobial Agents

A good rule of clinical practice is to be suspicious of an adverse drug reaction when a patient's clinical course deviates from the expected. This section focuses on reactions that may require close observation or laboratory monitoring either because of their frequency or because of their severity. For more detailed listings of reactions, review the US Food and Drug Administration (FDA)-approved package labels available at the National Library of Medicine (NLM) site at http://dailymed.nlm.nih.gov (accessed November 14, 2013) with more recently approved agents actually having adverse events listed for both the new agent and the comparator agent from the phase 3 prospective clinical trials. This allows one to assign drug-attributable side effects for specific drugs such as oseltamivir, used for influenza, when both influenza and the antiviral may cause nausea. The NLM also provides an online drug information service (MedlinePlus) at www.nlm.nih.gov/medlineplus/druginformation.html.

Antibacterial Drugs

Aminoglycosides. Any of the aminoglycosides can cause serious nephrotoxicity and ototoxicity. Monitor all patients receiving aminoglycoside therapy for more than a few days for renal function with periodic determinations of blood urea nitrogen and creatinine to assess potential problems of drug accumulation with deteriorating renal function. Common practice has been to measure the peak serum concentration 0.5 to 1.0 hour after a dose to make sure one is in a safe and therapeutic range and to measure a trough serum concentration immediately preceding a dose to assess for drug accumulation and pending toxicity. Monitoring is especially important in patients with any degree of renal insufficiency. Elevated trough concentrations (>2 mg/mL for gentamicin and tobramycin, and >10 mg/mL for amikacin) suggest drug accumulation and should be a warning to decrease the dose, even if the peak is not yet elevated. Renal toxicity may be related to the total exposure of the kidney to the aminoglycoside over time. With once-daily administration regimens, peak values are 2 to 3 times greater, and trough values are usually very low. Nephrotoxicity seems to be less common in adults with once-daily (as opposed to 3 times daily) dosing regimens, but data are generally lacking in children.[1] In cystic fibrosis patients with pulmonary exaserbations, once-daily aminoglycosides appear less toxic and equally effective.[2]

The "loop" diuretics (furosemide and bumetanide) potentiate the ototoxicity of the aminoglycosides. Aminoglycosides potentiate botulinum toxin and are to be avoided in young infants with infant botulism.

The aminoglycosides are well tolerated via intramuscular and intravenous (IV) routes of administration. Minor side effects, such as allergies, rashes, and drug fever, are rare.

Beta-Lactam Antibiotics. The most feared reaction to penicillins, anaphylactic shock, is extremely rare, and no absolutely reliable means of predicting its occurrence exists. For most infections, alternative therapy to penicillin or beta-lactams exists. However, in certain situations, the benefits of penicillin or a beta-lactam may outweigh the risk of anaphylaxis, requiring that skin testing and desensitization be performed in a medically supervised environment. The commercially available skin testing material, benzylpenicilloyl polylysine (Pre-Pen, AllerQuest) was approved and marketed in September 2009. It contains the major determinants thought to be primarily responsible for urticarial reactions but does not contain the minor determinants that are more often associated with anaphylaxis. No commercially available minor determinant mixture is available. Some authorities use a dilute solution of freshly prepared benzyl penicillin G as the skin test material in place of a standardized mixture of minor determinants. Testing should be performed on children with a credible history of a possible reaction to a penicillin before these drugs are used in either oral or parenteral formulations. Anaphylaxis has been reported in adults receiving penicillin skin testing. Recent reviews provide more in-depth discussion,[3,4] with additional information on desensitization available at the Centers for Disease Control and Prevention Web site (www.cdc.gov/STD/treatment/2006/penicillin-allergy.htm#skintesting [accessed November 14, 2013]). Cross-reactions between classes of beta-lactam antibiotics (penicillins, cephalosporins, carbapenems, and monobactams) occur at a rate of less than 5% to 20%, with the rate of reaction to cephalosporins in patients without a serious reaction to penicillin of 0.1%.[5] No commercially available skin testing reagent has been developed for beta-lactam antibiotics other than penicillin.

Amoxicillin and other aminopenicillins are associated with minor adverse effects. Diarrhea, oral or diaper area candidiasis, morbilliform, and blotchy rashes are not uncommon. The kinds of non-urticarial rashes that may occur while a child is receiving amoxicillin are not known to predispose to anaphylaxis and may not actually be caused by amoxicillin itself; they do not represent a routine contraindication to subsequent use of amoxicillin or any other penicillins. Rarely, beta-lactams cause serious, life-threatening pseudomembranous enterocolitis due to suppression of normal bowel flora and overgrowth of toxin-producing strains of *Clostridium difficile*. Drug-related fever may occur; serum sickness is uncommon. Reversible neutropenia and thrombocytopenia may occur with any of the beta-lactams and seem to be related to dose and duration of therapy but do not appear to carry the same risk of bacterial superinfection that is present with neutropenia in oncology patients.

The cephalosporins have been a remarkably safe series of antibiotics. The third-generation cephalosporins cause profound alteration of normal flora on mucosal surfaces, and all have caused pseudomembranous colitis on rare occasions. Ceftriaxone commonly causes loose stools, but it is rarely severe enough to require stopping therapy. Ceftriaxone in high dosages may cause fine "sand" (a calcium complex of ceftriaxone) to develop in the gallbladder. In adults, and rarely in children, these deposits may cause biliary tract symptoms; these are not gallstones, and the deposits are reversible after stopping the drug. In neonates receiving calcium-containing hyperalimentation concurrent with IV ceftriaxone, precipitation of ceftriaxone-calcium in the bloodstream resulting in death has been reported,[6] leading to an FDA warning against the concurrent use of ceftriaxone and parenteral calcium in infants younger than 28 days (www.fda.gov/Drugs/DrugSafety/PostmarketDrugSafety InformationforPatientsandProviders/ucm109103.htm). As ceftriaxone may also displace bilirubin from albumin-binding sites and increase free bilirubin in serum, the antibiotic is not routinely used in neonatal infections until the normal physiologic jaundice is resolving after the first few weeks of life. Cefotaxime is the preferred IV third-generation cephalosporin for neonates.

Imipenem/cilastatin, meropenem, and ertapenem have rates of adverse effects on hematopoietic, hepatic, and renal systems that are similar to other beta-lactams. However, children treated with imipenem for bacterial meningitis were noted to have an increase in probable drug-related seizures not seen with meropenem therapy in controlled studies.[7] For children

2014 Nelson's Pediatric Antimicrobial Therapy — 185

requiring carbapenem therapy, meropenem is preferred for those with any underlying central nervous system inflammatory condition.

Fluoroquinolones (FQs). All quinolone antibiotics (nalidixic acid, ciprofloxacin, levofloxacin, gatifloxacin, and moxifloxacin) cause cartilage damage to weight-bearing joints in toxicity studies in various immature animals; however, no conclusive data indicate similar toxicity in young children. Studies to evaluate cartilage toxicity and failure to achieve predicted growth have not consistently found statistically significant differences between those children treated with FQs and controls, although in an FDA-requested, blinded, prospective study of complicated urinary tract infections, the number of muscular/joint/tendon events was greater in the ciprofloxacin-treated group than in the comparator (www.fda.gov/downloads/Drugs/ DevelopmentApproval Process/DevelopmentResources/UCM162536.pdf). This continues to be an area of active investigation by the pediatric infectious diseases community as well as the FDA. Fluoroquinolone toxicities in adults, which vary in incidence considerably between individual agents, include cardiac dysrhythmias, hepatotoxicity, and photodermatitis; other reported side effects include gastrointestinal symptoms, dizziness, headaches, tremors, confusion, seizures, and alterations of glucose metabolism producing both hyper- and hypoglycemia. The American Academy of Pediatrics published a clinical report on the use of fluoroquinolones, and based on the best available evidence, concluded that IV fluoroquinolones should be used when safer IV antibiotic alternatives were not available, and that PO fluoroquinolones should be used if no other safe and effective oral therapy existed, even if effective alternative IV therapy existed.[8]

Lincosamides. Clindamycin can cause nausea, vomiting, and diarrhea. Pseudomembranous colitis due to suppression of normal flora and overgrowth of *C difficile* is uncommon, especially in children, but potentially serious. Urticaria, glossitis, pruritus, and skin rashes occur occasionally. Serum sickness, anaphylaxis, and photosensitivity are rare, as are hematologic and hepatic abnormalities. Extensive use of clindamycin since 2000 for treatment of community-associated methicillin-resistant *Staphylococcus aureus* infections has not been accompanied by reports of increasing rates of *C difficile*–mediated colitis in children.

Macrolides. Erythromycin is one of the safest antimicrobial agents. However, it commonly produces nausea and epigastric distress. Azithromycin and clarithromycin cause fewer gastrointestinal side effects than erythromycin. Alteration of normal flora is generally not a problem, but oral or perianal candidiasis occasionally develops. Transient cholestatic hepatitis is a rare complication that occurs with approximately equal frequency among the various formulations of erythromycin. Intravenous erythromycin lactobionate causes phlebitis and should be administered slowly (1–2 hours); the gastrointestinal side effects seen with oral administration also accompany IV use. However, IV azithromycin is better tolerated than IV erythromycin and has been evaluated for pharmacokinetics in limited numbers of children.[9]

Erythromycin therapy has been associated with pyloric stenosis in newborns and young infants; due to this toxicity and with limited data on safety of azithromycin in the first months of life, azithromycin is now the preferred macrolide for treatment of pertusis in neonates and young infants.[10]

Oxazolidinones. Linezolid represents the first oxazolidinone antibiotic approved for all children, including neonates, by the FDA. Toxicity is primarily hematologic, with thrombocytopenia and neutropenia that is dependent on dosage and duration of therapy, occurring most often with treatment courses of 2 weeks or longer. Routine monitoring for bone

Adverse Reactions to Antimicrobial Agents

marrow toxicity every 1 to 2 weeks is recommended for children on long-term therapy. Peripheral neuropathy and optic neuritis may also occur with long-term therapy.[11]

Sulfonamides and Trimethoprim. The most common adverse reaction to sulfonamides is a hypersensitivity rash, which occurs much more commonly in children with HIV infection on therapy. The frequency and types of reactions to the trimpethoprim/sulfamethoxazole (TMP/SMX) combination are said to be the same as with sulfamethoxazole alone, but it is not clear whether the most significant reaction, Stevens-Johnson syndrome, is caused more often by the combination than by sulfamethoxazole alone. Neutropenia and anemia occur occasionally. Mild depression of platelet counts occurs in approximately one-half the patients treated with sulfas or TMP/SMX and seems to be dosage-related, but this rarely produces clinical bleeding problems. Sulfa drugs can precipitate hemolysis in patients with glucose-6-phosphate dehydrogenase deficiency. Drug fever and serum sickness are infrequent hypersensitivity reactions. Hepatitis with focal or diffuse necrosis is rare. A rare idiosyncratic reaction to sulfa drugs is acute aseptic meningitis.

Tetracyclines. Tetracyclines are used infrequently in pediatric patients because the major indications are uncommon diseases (rickettsial infections, brucellosis, Lyme disease), with the exception of acne. Tetracyclines are deposited in growing bones and teeth, with depression of linear bone growth, dental staining, and defects in enamelization in deciduous and permanent teeth. This effect is dose-related, and the risk extends up to 8 years of age. A single treatment course of tetracyclines has not been found to cause dental staining, leading to the recommendation for tetracyclines as the drugs of choice in children for a number of uncommon pathogens. Doxycycline is likely to produce less dental staining than tetracycline. A parenteral tetracycline approved for adults in 2005, tigecycline, produces the same "staining" of bones in experimental animals as seen with other tetracyclines.

Side effects include minor gastrointestinal disturbances, photosensitization, angioedema, glossitis, pruritus ani, and exfoliative dermatitis. Potential adverse drug reactions from tetracyclines involve virtually every organ system. Hepatic and pancreatic injuries have occurred with accidental overdosage and in patients with renal failure. (Pregnant women are particularly at risk for hepatic injury.)

Vancomycin. Vancomycin can cause phlebitis if the drug is injected rapidly or in concentrated form. Vancomycin has the potential for ototoxicity and nephrotoxicity, and serum concentrations should be monitored for children on more than a few days of therapy. Hepatic toxicity is rare. Neutropenia has been reported. If the drug is infused too rapidly, a transient rash of the upper body with itching may occur from histamine release (red man syndrome). It is not a contraindication to continued use and the rash is less likely to occur if the infusion rate is increased to 60 to 120 minutes and the children are pretreated with oral or IV antihistamines.

Antituberculous Drugs

Isoniazid (INH) is generally well tolerated and hypersensitivity reactions are rare. Peripheral neuritis (preventable or reversed by pyridoxine administration) and mental aberrations from euphoria to psychosis occur more often in adults than in children. Mild elevations of alanine transaminase in the first weeks of therapy, which disappear or remain stable with continued administration, are common. Rarely, hepatitis develops, but is reversible if INH is stopped; if INH is not stopped, liver failure may develop in these children. Monitoring of liver functions is not routinely required in children receiving INH single drug therapy for latent tuberculosis as long as the children can be followed closely and liver functions can be drawn if the child develops symptoms of hepatitis.

Rifampin can also cause hepatitis; it is more common in patients with preexisting liver disease or in those taking large dosages. The risk of hepatic damage increases when rifampin and INH are taken together in dosages of more than 15 mg/kg/day of each. Gastrointestinal, hematologic, and neurologic side effects of various types have been observed on occasion. Hypersensitivity reactions are rare.

Pyrazinamide also can cause hepatic damage, which again seems to be dosage-related. Ethambutol has the potential for optic neuritis, but this toxicity seems to be rare in children at currently prescribed dosages, and routine screening for color vision is no longer recommended.

Antifungal Drugs

Amphotericin B (deoxycholate) causes chills, fever, flushing, and headaches, the most common of the many adverse reactions. Some degree of decreased renal function occurs in virtually all patients given amphotericin B. Anemia is common and, rarely, hepatic toxicity and neutropenia occur. Patients should be monitored for hyponatremia and hypokalemia. However, much better tolerated (but more costly) lipid formulations of amphotericin B are now commonly used (see Chapter 2). For reasons of safety and tolerability, the lipid formulations should be used whenever possible.

Ketoconazole produces hepatic damage on rare occasions. The most common side effect is gastric distress; this can often be alleviated by dividing the daily dose. Gynecomastia is not rare in adult males. Itraconazole has a smaller incidence of adverse effects than ketoconazole.

Fluconazole is usually very well tolerated from both clinical and laboratory standpoints. Gastrointestinal symptoms, rash, and headache occur occasionally. Transient, asymptomatic elevations of hepatic enzymes have been reported but are rare.

Voriconazole, a new antifungal suspension, may interfere with metabolism of other drugs the child may be receiving due to hepatic P450 metabolism. However, a poorly understood visual field abnormality has been described, usually at the beginning of a course of therapy, and uniformly self-resolving, in which objects appear to glow. There is no pain and no known anatomic or biochemical correlate of this side effect; no lasting effects on vision have yet been reported. Hepatic toxicity has also been reported but is not so common as to preclude the use of voriconazole for serious fungal infections.

Caspofungin is very well tolerated, is now FDA approved for use in children down to 3 months of age, and has minimal side effects. Fever, rash, headache, and phlebitis at the site of infection have been reported in adults. Uncommon hepatic side effects have also been reported. Micafungin and anidulofungin seem to have the same benign side effect profile in adults as caspofungin. Flucytosine (5-FC) is seldom used due to the availability of safer, equally effective therapy. The major toxicity is bone marrow depression, which is dosage related, especially in patients treated concomitantly with amphotericin B. Renal function should be monitored.

Adverse Reactions to Antimicrobial Agents

16

Antiviral Drugs

After extensive clinical use, acyclovir has proved to be an extremely safe drug with only rare serious adverse effects. Renal dysfunction with IV acyclovir has occurred mainly with too rapid infusion of the drug. Neutropenia has been associated with administration of parenteral and oral acyclovir but is responsive to granulocyte colony-stimulating factor use and resolves spontaneously following halting of the drug. At very high doses, parenteral acyclovir can cause neurologic irritation, including seizures. Rash, headache, and gastrointestinal side effects are uncommon. There has been little controlled experience in children with famciclovir and valacyclovir.

Ganciclovir causes hematologic toxicity that is dependent on the dosage and duration of therapy. Gastrointestinal disturbances and neurologic damage are rarely encountered. Oral valganciclovir can have these same toxicities, but neutropenia is seen much less frequently following oral valganciclovir compared with intravenous ganciclovir.

Amantadine produces dizziness, drowsiness, and insomnia in many patients, but these effects are usually not severe. Rimantadine has fewer side effects. Visual disturbances, confusion, and psychosis are rare.

Oseltamivir is well tolerated except for nausea with or without vomiting, which may be more likely to occur with the first few doses but usually resolves within a few days while still on therapy. Neuropsychiatric events have been reported, primarily from Japan, in patients with influenza treated with oseltamivir (a rate of approximately 1:50,000), but also are seen in patients on all of the other influenza antivirals and in patients with influenza receiving no antiviral therapy. Based on an FDA assessment, it seems that these spontaneously reported side effects may be a function of influenza itself, oseltamivir itself, possibly a genetic predisposition to this clinical event, or a combination of all 3.

Foscarnet can cause renal dysfunction, anemia, and cardiac rhythm disturbances. Seizures and neuropathy are other serious but rare toxicities.

The many antiviral drugs for treatment for HIV infection have many adverse effects; consult the current FDA-approved package labels.

17. Drug Interactions

NOTES

- Antimicrobial drug-drug interactions that are known to be or have the potential to be clinically significant in children are listed in this chapter. Interactions involving probenecid, synergy-antagonism, and physical incompatibilities are not listed. Interactions involving antiretrovirals can be found at http://aidsinfo.nih.gov/contentfiles/lvguidelines/pediatricguidelines.pdf. Interactions involving QT interval prolongation can be found at www.crediblemeds.org. Citations at the end of this section provide more extensive details of all reported and theoretical interactions, including antimicrobial drug-disease interactions.

- **Abbreviations:** ACE, angiotensin-converting enzyme; ARB, angiotensin receptor blockers; CCB, calcium channel blockers; Conc, concentration; Decr, decreased; EIAED, enzyme-inducing antiepileptic drugs; FQ, fluoroquinolones; Incr, increased; MAO, monoamine oxidase; Poss, possible; NSAID, nonsteroidal anti-inflammatory drug; PPI, proton pump inhibitors; SRI, serotonin reuptake inhibitors; TMP/SMX, trimethoprim/sulfamethoxazole.

Anti-infective Agent	Interacting Drug(s)	Adverse Effect
Acyclovir/valacyclovir	Nephrotoxins[a]	Additive nephrotoxicity
	Phenytoin, valproic acid	Decr seizure control
Amantadine	Anticholinergics[b]	Additive anticholinergic toxicity
	Bupropion	Additive neurotoxicity
	Trimethoprim	Incr amantadine conc
Amikacin	(See Aminoglycosides[c].)	
Aminoglycosides[c] (parenteral)	Nephrotoxins[a]	Additive nephrotoxicity
	Neuromuscular blocking agents	Incr neuromuscular blockade
	Indomethacin, ibuprofen	Incr aminoglycoside conc
	Carbo-/cisplatin, ethacrynic acid	Additive ototoxicity
Amphotericin B	Nephrotoxins[a]	Additive nephrotoxicity
	Cisplatin, corticosteroids, diuretics	Additive hypokalemia
Atovaquone	Metoclopramide, rifamycins, tetracyline	Decr atovaquone conc
Carbapenems	Valproic acid	Decr conc of valproic acid

Drug Interactions

17

Anti-infective Agent	Interacting Drug(s)	Adverse Effect
Caspofungin	Cyclosporine	Incr caspofungin conc
	Tacrolimus, sirolimus	Decr tacrolimus/sirolimus conc
	Rifampin, EIAED[d]	Decr caspofungin conc
Cefdinir	Iron	Decr anti-infective oral absorption
Cefdinir, cefpodoxime, cefuroxime (oral), cefditoren	Antacids, H2 antagonists[e], PPI[f]	Decr anti-infective oral absorption
Ceftriaxone	Calcium intravenous	Precipitation, cardiopulmonary embolism
Cephalexin, ceftibuten	Zinc	Decr anti-infective oral absorption
Chloramphenicol[g]	Phenytoin, PPI[f], sulfonylureas	Incr conc of interacting drug
	EIAED[d], rifamycins	Decr chloramphenicol conc
Cidofovir	Nephrotoxins[a]	Additive nephrotoxicty
Ciprofloxacin	Caffeine, clozapine, diazepam, duloxetine, glyburide, methadone, olanzapine, sildenafil, theophylline, warfarin	Incr conc of interacting drug
	Phenytoin	Incr or decr conc of phenytoin
	Foscarnet	Additive seizure toxicity
	Antacids, bismuth, calcium, iron, sucralfate, zinc	Decr anti-infective oral absorption
Clarithromycin[g]	(See Erythromycin.)	
Clindamycin	Neuromuscular blocking agents	Incr neuromuscular blockade
Dapsone	Rifampin	Decr dapsone conc
	Trimethoprim	Incr dapsone and trimethoprim conc
Daptomycin	Statins	Additive myopathy
Doxycycline	Antacids, bismuth, calcium, iron, magnesium, sucralfate, zinc	Decr oral absorption
	EIAED[d], rifamycins	Decr doxycycline conc

Anti-infective Agent	Interacting Drug(s)	Adverse Effect
Erythromycin[g], clarithromycin, telithromycin	Theophylline	Incr conc of interacting drug
	Azole antifungals, diltiazem, verapamil	Incr anti-infective conc, additive cardiotoxicity
	Rifamycins	Decr anti-infective conc
Fluconazole[g]	Celecoxib, clopidogrel, cyclophosphamide, ibuprofen, naproxen, ifosfamide, phenytoin, PPI[f], sulfonylureas, warfarin	Incr conc of interacting drug-CYP 2C9 and 2C19 inhibition
	Losartan	Decr losartan activity
	Rifampin	Decr fluconazole conc
Foscarnet	Pentamidine	Hypocalcemia
	FQ	Additive seizure toxicity
	Nephrotoxins[a]	Additive nephrotoxicty
Ganciclovir/valganciclovir	Imipenem	Additive seizure toxicity
	Hemotoxins[h]	Additive hemotoxicity
Gentamicin	(See Aminoglycosides[c].)	
Griseofulvin	EIAED[d]	Decr griseofulvin conc
Imipenem	Cyclosporine, ganciclovir	Additive neurotoxicity
Isoniazid	Acetaminophen, carbamazepine	Hepatotoxicity
	Antacids	Decr conc of isoniazid
	Celecoxib, cyclophosphamide, ibuprofen, naproxen, ifosfamide, phenytoin, sulfonylureas, warfarin	Incr conc of interacting drug-CYP 2C9 inhibition
	Cycloserine	Dizziness, drowsiness
	Carbamazepine, valproate	Incr conc of interacting drug
	Atomoxetine, linezolid	Poss MAO inhibition toxicity
	Amphetamines, buspirone, mirtazipine, SRI[i], tramadol	Poss serotonin syndrome

Drug Interactions

17

Anti-infective Agent	Interacting Drug(s)	Adverse Effect
Itraconazole, ketoconazole[j]	Anthracyclines, aripiprazole, benzodiazepines[k], bosentan, buspirone, busulfan, CCB[l], carbamazepine, chlorpheniramine, corticosteroids, cyclophosphamide, cyclosporine, digoxin, docetaxel, ergotamine, etoposide, fentanyl, fexofenadine, fluoxetine, haloperidol, ifosfamide, irinotecan, loperamide, loratadine, methadone, phenytoin, pimozide, quetiapine, quinidine, rifabutin, sertraline, sildenafil, sirolimus, statins[m], tacrolimus, tiagabine, trazadone, vinca alkaloids, warfarin, zolpidem, zonisamide	Incr conc of interacting drug-CYP 3A4-7 inhibition
	Antacids, H2 antagonists[e], PPI[f]	Decr azole conc, itraconazole oral solution less affected
	Sucralfate	Decr ketoconazole conc
	EIAED[d] rifamycins	Decr azole conc
	Erythromycin, FQ, ziprasodone	Incr conc of interacting drugs with poss incr cardiotoxicity
	Methotrexate	Incr methotrexate conc
Levofloxacin	See Ciprofloxacin for drugs that decr oral absorption of FQ.	
Linezolid	Atomoxetine, isoniazid	Poss MAO inhibition toxicity
	Sympathomimetics	Poss hypertension
	Amphetamines, buspirone, mirtazipine, SRI[i], tramadol	Poss serotonin syndrome
	Rifampin	Decr linezolid conc
Metronidazole	Amiodarone, busulfan, carbamazepine, cyclosporine, 5-fluorouacil, lithium, phenytoin, tacrolimus, warfarin	Incr conc of interacting drug
	EIAED[d]	Decr metronidazole conc
Micafungin	Cyclosporine, sirolimus	Incr conc of interacting drug
Minocycline	Antacids, bismuth, calcium, iron, magnesium, sucralfate, zinc	Decr oral absorption
Nafcillin	Cyclosporine, CCB[l]	Decr conc of interacting drug
	Warfarin	Decr hypothrombinemic effect

Anti-infective Agent	Interacting Drug(s)	Adverse Effect
Norfloxacin	Cyclosporine	Incr cyclosporine conc
	See Ciprofloxacin for drugs that decr oral absorption of FQ.	
Oseltamivir	Methotrexate	Incr methotrexate conc
Penicillins	Methotrexate	Incr methotrexate conc
Posaconazole[g]	Phenytoin, H2 antagonists[e], PPI[f]	Decr conc of posaconazole
	Methotrexate	Incr methotrexate conc
Praziquantel	EIAED[d]	Decr conc of praziquantel
Quinupristin/dalfopristin[g]	(See Itraconazole.)	
Rifampin, Rifabutin	Numerous, including amiodarone, anticonvulsants, antidepressants, antipsychotics, barbiturates, benzodiazepines[k], beta-adrenergic blockers, buspirone, coxibs, calcium channel blockers[l], oral contraceptives, corticosteroids, digoxin, immuno-suppressants, NSAIDs, opioids, statins[m], sulfonylureas, warfarin, zolpidem	Decr conc of interacting drug; see also *Clinical Pharmacokinetics.* 2003;42(9):819–850.
Streptomycin	(See Aminoglycosides[c].)	
Telithromycin[g]	(See Erythromycin.)	
Terbinafine	Most SRI[i], tricyclic antidepressants	Incr conc of interacting drug
	Rifampin	Decr terbinafine conc
Tetracycline	Antacids, bismuth, calcium, iron, magnesium, sucralfate, zinc	Decr anti-infective oral absorption
	Atovaquone	Decr atovaquone conc
	Isotretinoin	Intracranial hypertension
TMP/SMX	Azathioprine, methotrexate	Additive hematological toxicity[h]
	Rifamycins	Decr TMP/SMX conc
	Amantadine, dapsone, phenytoin, sulfonylureas, warfarin	Incr conc of interacting drug
	ACE Inhibitors, ARB, spironolactone	Hyperkalemia
Tobramycin	(See Aminoglycosides[c].)	

Drug Interactions

17

Anti-infective Agent	Interacting Drug(s)	Adverse Effect
Vancomycin	Indomethacin, ibuprofen	Incr vancomycin conc
Voriconazole[g,j]	Methadone	Incr conc of interacting drug
	EIAED[d], rifamycins	Decr voriconazole conc

[a] Potentially nephrotoxic drugs include aminoglycosides, acyclovir, cidofovir, foscarnet,
  ACE inhibitors, cyclosporine, diuretics, NSAIDs, contrast agents, pentamidine, tacrolimus, tenofovir, vancomycin.
[b] Examples of anticholinergics: atropine, belladonna, benztropine, clidinium, dicyclomine, diphenhydramine,
  glycopyrrolate, homatropine, hyoscyamine, promethazine, propantheline, scopolamine.
[c] Gentamicin, tobramycin, amikacin, streptomycin.
[d] EIAED: carbamazepine, phenobarbital, phenytoin, and primidone.
[e] Famotidine, ranitidine.
[f] Pantoprazole, rabeprazole, omeprazole, lansoprazole, esomeprazole.
[g] Antibiotic is known to have or may potentially have the same interactions as itraconazole and ketoconazole due to
  similar inhibition of CYP3A4-7 drug metabolism.
[h] Notable hemotoxic drugs include antineoplastics, clozapine, dapsone, flucytosine, mycophenolate,
  pentamidine, primaquine, pyrimethamine, TMP/SMX, zidovudine.
[i] SRI: buproprion, citalopram, duloxetine, escitalopram, fluoxetine, fluvoxamine, nefazodone,
  paroxetine, sertraline, venlafaxine.
[j] Antibiotic is known to have or may potentially have the same interactions as fluconazole due to
  similar inhibition of CYP2C9 and CYP2C19 drug metabolism.
[k] CYP3A4 oxidized benzodiazepines: alprazolam, chlordiazepoxide, clonazepam, clorazepate,
  diazepam, midazolam, and triazolam.
[l] Amlodipine, bepridil, diltiazem, felodipine, isradipine, nicardipine, nifedipine, nimodipine, verapamil.
[m] Atorvastatin, lovastatin, simvastatin

Bibliography

Flockhart DA. P450 drug interaction table: abbreviated "clinically relevant" table.
  Indiana University Division of Clinical Pharmacology. http://medicine.iupui.edu/
  clinpharm/ddis/clinical-table. Accessed November 14, 2013

Hansten PD, Horn JR. *Drug Interactions Analysis and Management 2013.* St Louis, MO:
  Wolters Kluwer Health; 2013

Perucca E. Clinically relevant drug interactions with antiepileptic drugs. *Br J Clin Pharmacol.*
  2006;61(3):246–255 PMID: 16487217

Piscitelli SC, Rodvold KA, Pai MP, eds. *Drug Interactions in Infectious Diseases.* 3rd ed.
  New York, NY: Springer Science and Business Media; 2011

Ruggiero A, Arena R, Battista A, Rizzo D, Attinà G, Riccardi R. Azole interactions with
  multidrug therapy in pediatric oncology. *Eur J Clin Pharmacol.* 2013;69(1):1–10 PMID:
  22660443

Simkó J, Csilek A, Karászi J, Lorincz I. Proarrhythmic potential of antimicrobial agents.
  Infection. 2008;36(3):194–206 PMID: 18454341

Drug Interactions

7

Appendix

Nomogram for Determining Body Surface Area

Based on the nomogram shown below, a straight line joining the patient's height and weight will intersect the center column at the calculated body surface area (BSA). For children of normal height and weight, the child's weight in pounds is used, then the examiner reads across to the corresponding BSA in meters. Alternatively, Mosteller's formula can be used.

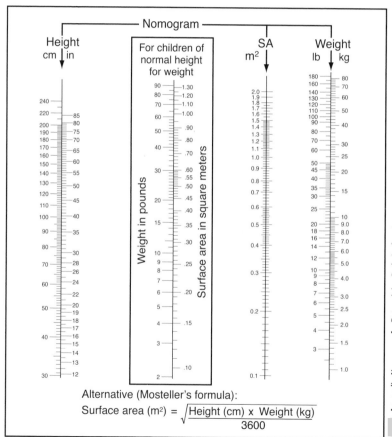

Nomogram and equation to determine body surface area. (From: Tschudy MM, Arcara KM, eds. *The Harriet Lane Handbook*. 19th ed. St Louis, MO: Mosby; 2012. |Data from Briars GL, Bailey BJ. Surface area estimation: pocket calculator v nomogram. *Arch Dis Child*. 1994;70[3]:246–247. Reprinted with permission from Elsevier.)

References

Chapter 2

1. Cornely OA, Maertens J, Bresnik M, et al. Liposomal amphotericin B as initial therapy for invasive mold infection: a randomized trial comparing a high-loading dose regimen with standard dosing (AmBiLoad trial). *Clin Infect Dis*. 2007;44(10):1289–1297 PMID: 17443465
2. Piper L, Smith PB, Hornik CP, et al. Fluconazole loading dose pharmacokinetics and safety in infants. *Pediatr Infect Dis J*. 2011;30(5):375–378 PMID: 21085048
3. Chen SC, Slavin MA, Sorrell TC. Echinocandin antifungal drugs in fungal infections: a comparison. *Drugs*. 2011;71(1):11–41 PMID: 21175238
4. Smith PB, Walsh TJ, Hope W, et al. Pharmacokinetics of an elevated dosage of micafungin in premature neonates. *Pediatr Infect Dis J*. 2009;28(5):412–415 PMID: 19319022
5. Kawada M, Fukuoka N, Kondo M, et al. Pharmacokinetics of prophylactic micafungin in very-low-birth-weight infants. *Pediatr Infect Dis J*. 2009;28(9):840–842 PMID: 19636279
6. Benjamin DK Jr, Smith PB, Arrieta A, et al. Safety and pharmacokinetics of repeat-dose micafungin in young infants. *Clin Pharmacol Ther*. 2010;87(1):93–99 PMID: 19890251
7. Cohen-Wolkowiez M, Benjamin DK Jr, Piper L, et al. Safety and pharmacokinetics of multiple-dose anidulafungin in infants and neonates. *Clin Pharmacol Ther*. 2011;89(5):702–707 PMID: 21412233

Chapter 4

1. Liu C, Bayer A, Cosgrove SE, et al. Clinical practice guidelines by the Infectious Diseases Society of America for the treatment of methicillin-resistant *Staphylococcus aureus* infections in adults and children. *Clin Infect Dis*. 2011;52(3):e18–e55 PMID: 21208910
2. Le J, Bradley JS, Murray W, et al. Improved vancomycin dosing in children using area under the curve exposure. *Pediatr Infect Dis J*. 2013;32(4):e155–e163 PMID: 23340565
3. Huang JT, Abrams M, Tlougar B, Rademaker A, Paller AS. Treatment of *Staphylococcus aureus* colonization in atopic dermatitis decreases disease severity. *Pediatrics*. 2009;123(5):e808–e814 PMID: 19403473

Chapter 5

1. Fox E, Balis FM. Drug therapy in neonates and pediatric patients. In: Atkinson AJ, Abernethy DR, Daniels C, Dedrick RL, Markey SP, eds. *Principles of Clinical Pharmacology*. Burlington, VT: Academic Press, Elsevier; 2007:359–373
2. Wagner CL, Wagstaff P, Cox TH, Annibale DJ. Early discharge with home antibiotic therapy in the treatment of neonatal infection. *J Perinatol*. 2000;20(6):346–350 PMID: 11002871
3. Ceftriaxone information. US Food and Drug Administration Web Site. http://www.fda.gov/Drugs/DrugSafety/DrugSafetyNewsletter/ucm189806.htm. Accessed November 14, 2013
4. Martin E, Fanconi S, Kalin P, et al. Ceftriaxone—bilirubin-albumin interactions in the neonate: an in vivo study. *Eur J Pediatr*. 1993;152(6):530–534 PMID: 8335024
5. Rours IG, Hammerschlag MR, Ott A, et al. Chlamydia trachomatis as a cause of neonatal conjunctivitis in Dutch infants. *Pediatrics*. 2008;121(2):e321–e326 PMID: 18245405
6. American Academy of Pediatrics. Chlamydial infections. In: Pickering LK, Baker CJ, Kimberlin DW, Long SS, eds. *Red Book: 2012 Report of the Committee on Infectious Diseases*. 29th ed. Elk Grove Village, IL: American Academy of Pediatrics; 2012:272–281
7. Hammerschlag MR, Gelling M, Roblin PM, et al. Treatment of neonatal chlamydial conjunctivitis with azithromycin. *Pediatr Infect Dis J*. 1998;17(11):1049–1050 PMID: 9849993
8. Zar HJ. Neonatal chlamydial infections: prevention and treatment. *Paediatr Drugs*. 2005;7(2):103–110 PMID: 15871630
9. Honein MA, Paulozzi LJ, Himelright IM, et al. Infantile hypertrophic pyloric stenosis after pertussis prophylaxis with erythromcyin: a case review and cohort study. *Lancet*. 1999;354(9196):2101–2105 PMID: 10609814
10. Laga M, Naamara W, Brunham RC, et al. Single-dose therapy of gonococcal ophthalmia neonatorum with ceftriaxone. *N Engl J Med*. 1986;315(22):1382–1385 PMID: 3095641

Chapter 5 (cont)

11. Workowski KA, Berman S. Sexually transmitted diseases treatment guidelines, 2010. *MMWR Recomm Rep.* 2010;59(RR-12):1–110 PMID: 21160459

12. Newman LM, Moran JS, Workowski KA. Update on the management of gonorrhea in adults in the United States. *Clin Infect Dis.* 2007;44(suppl 3):S84–S101 PMID: 17342672

13. MacDonald N, Mailman T, Desai S. Gonococcal infections in newborns and in adolescents. *Adv Exp Med Biol.* 2008;609:108–130 PMID: 18193661

14. American Academy of Pediatrics. Gonococcal infections. In: Pickering LK, Baker CJ, Kimberlin DW, Long SS, eds. *Red Book: 2012 Report of the Committee on Infectious Diseases.* 29th ed. Elk Grove Village, IL: American Academy of Pediatrics; 2012:336–344

15. Cimolai N. Ocular methicillin-resistant *Staphylococcus aureus* infections in a newborn intensive care cohort. *Am J Ophthalmol.* 2006;142(1):183–184 PMID: 16815280

16. Marangon FB, Miller D, Muallem MS, et al. Ciprofloxacin and levofloxacin resistance among methicillin-sensitive *Staphylococcus aureus* isolates from keratitis and conjunctivitis. *Am J Ophthalmol.* 2004;137(3):453–458 PMID: 15013867

17. American Academy of Pediatrics. Staphylococcal infections. In: Pickering LK, Baker CJ, Kimberlin DW, Long SS eds. *Red Book: 2012 Report of the Committee on Infectious Diseases.* 29th ed. Elk Grove Village, IL: American Academy of Pediatrics; 2012:653–668

18. Brito DV, Oliveira EJ, Matos C, et al. An outbreak of conjunctivitis caused by multiresistant *Pseudomonas aeruginosa* in a Brazilian newborn intensive care unit. *Braz J Infect Dis.* 2003;7(4):234–235 PMID: 14533982

19. Chen CJ, Starr CE. Epidemiology of gram-negative conjunctivitis in neonatal intensive care unit patients. *Am J Ophthalmol.* 2008;145(6):966–970 PMID: 18378213

20. Shah SS, Gloor P, Gallagher PG. Bacteremia, meningitis, and brain abscesses in a hospitalized infant: complications of *Pseudomonas aeruginosa* conjunctivitis. *J Perinatol.* 1999;19(6 pt 1):462–465 PMID: 10685281

21. Kimberlin DW, Lin CY, Sanchez PJ, et al. Effect of ganciclovir therapy on hearing in symptomatic congenital cytomegalovirus disease involving the central nervous system: a randomized, controlled trial. *J Pediatr.* 2003;143(1):16–25 PMID: 12915819

22. Kimberlin DW, Acosta EP, Sanchez PJ, et al. Pharmacokinetic and pharmacodynamic assessment of oral valganciclovir in the treatment of symptomatic congenital cytomegalovirus disease. *J Infect Dis.* 2008;197(6):836–845 PMID: 18279073

23. American Academy of Pediatrics. Cytomegalovirus infection. In: Pickering LK, Baker CJ, Kimberlin DW, Long SS, eds. *Red Book: 2012 Report of the Committee on Infectious Diseases.* 29th ed. Elk Grove Village, IL: American Academy of Pediatrics; 2012:300–305

24. Kimberlin DW, Jester PM, Sanchez PJ, et al, for the NIAID Collaborative Antiviral Study Group (CASG). Six months versus six weeks of oral valganciclovir for infants with symptomatic congenital cytomegalovirus (CMV) disease with and without central nervous system (CNS) involvement: results of a Phase III, randomized, double-blind, placebo-controlled, multinational study. IDWeek 2013 (annual meeting of the Pediatric Infectious Diseases Society, the Infectious Diseases Society of America, the HIV Medical Association, and the Society for Healthcare Epidemiology of America), San Francisco, CA, October 5, 2013; Late-Breaker Abstract #43178

25. American Academy of Pediatrics. Candidiasis. In: Pickering LK, Baker CJ, Kimberlin DW, Long SS, eds. *Red Book: 2012 Report of the Committee on Infectious Diseases.* 29th ed. Elk Grove Village, IL: American Academy of Pediatrics; 2012:265–269

26. Hundalani S, Pammi M. Invasive fungal infections in newborns and current management strategies. *Expert Rev Anti Infect Ther.* 2013;11(7):709–721 PMID: 23829639

27. Saez-Llorens X, Macias M, Maiya P, et al. Pharmacokinetics and safety of caspofungin in neonates and infants less than 3 months of age. *Antimicrob Agents Chemother.* 2009;53(3):869–875 PMID: 19075070

28. Wade KC, Benjamin DK Jr, Kaufman DA, et al. Fluconazole dosing for the prevention or treatment of invasive candidiasis in young infants. *Pediatr Infect Dis J.* 2009;28(8):717–723 PMID: 19593252

29. Smith PB, Walsh TJ, Hope W, et al. Pharmacokinetics of an elevated dosage of micafungin in premature neonates. *Pediatr Infect Dis J.* 2009;28(5):412–415 PMID: 19319022

30. Wurthwein G, Groll AH, Hempel G, et al. Population pharmacokinetics of amphotericin B lipid complex in neonates. *Antimicrob Agents Chemother.* 2005;49(12):5092–5098 PMID: 16304177

31. Heresi GP, Gerstmann DR, Reed MD, et al. The pharmacokinetics and safety of micafungin, a novel echinocandin, in premature infants. *Pediatr Infect Dis J.* 2006;25(12):1110–1115 PMID: 17133155

32. Kawaguchi C, Arai I, Yasuhara H, et al. Efficacy of micafungin in treating four premature infants with candidiasis. *Pediatr Int.* 2009;51(2):220–224 PMID: 19405920

33. Hsieh E, Smith PB, Jacqz-Aigrain E, et al. Neonatal fungal infections: when to treat? *Early Hum Dev.* 2012;88(Suppl 2):S6–S10 PMID: 22633516

34. Piper L, Smith PB, Hornik CP, et al. Fluconazole loading dose pharmacokinetics and safety in infants. *Pediatr Infect Dis J.* 2011;30(5):375–378 PMID: 21085048

35. Santos RP, Sanchez PJ, Mejias A, et al. Successful medical treatment of cutaneous aspergillosis in a premature infant using liposomal amphotericin b, voriconazole and micafungin. *Pediatr Infect Dis J.* 2007;26(4):364–366 PMID: 17414408

36. Frankenbusch K, Eifinger F, Kribs A, et al. Severe primary cutaneous aspergillosis refractory to amphotericin B and the successful treatment with systemic voriconazole in two premature infants with extremely low birth weight. *J Perinatol.* 2006;26(8):511–514 PMID: 16871222

37. Thomas L, Baggen L, Chisholm J, et al. Diagnosis and treatment of aspergillosis in children. *Expert Rev Anti Infect Ther.* 2009;7(4):461–472 PMID: 19400765

38. Shah D, Sinn JK. Antibiotic regimens for the empirical treatment of newborn infants with necrotising enterocolitis. *Cochrane Database Syst Rev.* 2012;8:CD007448 PMID: 22895960

39. Brook I. Microbiology and management of neonatal necrotizing enterocolitis. *Am J Perinatol.* 2008;25(2):111–118 PMID: 18236362

40. Alfaleh K, Bassler D. Probiotics for prevention of necrotizing enterocolitis in preterm infants. *Cochrane Database Syst Rev.* 2008;(1):CD005496 PMID: 18254081

41. Lin PW, Stoll BJ. Necrotising enterocolitis. *Lancet.* 2006;368(9543):1271–1283 PMID: 17027734

42. Cohen-Wolkowiez M, Poindexter B, Bidegain M, et al; Meropenem Study Team. Safety and effectiveness of meropenem in infants with suspected or complicated intra-abdominal infections. *Clin Infect Dis.* 2012;55(11):1495–1502 PMID: 22955450

43. Smith PB, Cohen-Wolkowiez M, Castro LM, et al; Meropenem Study Team. Population pharmacokinetics of meropenem in plasma and cerebrospinal fluid of infants with suspected or complicated intra-abdominal infections. *Pediatr Infect Dis J.* 2011;30(10):844–849 PMID: 21829139

44. American Academy of Pediatrics. *Salmonella* infections. In: Pickering LK, Baker CJ, Kimberlin DW, Long SS, eds. *Red Book: 2012 Report of the Committee on Infectious Diseases.* 29th ed. Elk Grove Village, IL: American Academy of Pediatrics; 2012:635–640

45. Pinninti SG, Kimberlin DW. Neonatal herpes simplex virus infections. *Pediatr Clin North Am.* 2013;60(2):351–365 PMID: 23481105

46. American Academy of Pediatrics. Herpes simplex. In: Pickering LK, Baker CJ, Kimberlin DW, Long SS, eds. *Red Book: 2012 Report of the Committee on Infectious Diseases.* 29th ed. Elk Grove Village, IL: American Academy of Pediatrics; 2012:398–408

47. Jones CA, Walker KS, Badawi N. Antiviral agents for treatment of herpes simplex virus infection in neonates. *Cochrane Database Syst Rev.* 2009;(3):CD004206 PMID: 19588350

48. Kimberlin DW, Whitley RJ, Wan W, et al for the NIAID Collaborative Antiviral Study Group. Oral acyclovir suppression and neurodevelopment after neonatal herpes. *N Engl J Med.* 2011;365(14):1284–1292 PMID: 21991950

49. Panel on Antiretroviral Therapy and Medical Management of HIV-Infected Children. Guidelines for the Use of Antiretroviral Agents in Pediatric HIV Infection. November 5, 2012. http://aidsinfo.nih.gov/ContentFiles/PediatricGuidelines.pdf. Accessed November 14, 2013

50. Panel on Treatment of HIV-Infected Pregnant Women and Prevention of Perinatal Transmission. Recommendations for Use of Antiretroviral Drugs in Pregnant HIV-1-Infected Women for Maternal Health and Interventions to Reduce Perinatal HIV Transmission in the United States. July 31, 2012. http://aidsinfo.nih.gov/guidelines. Accessed November 14, 2013

References

Chapter 5 (cont)

51. Nielsen-Saines K, Watts DH, Veloso VG, et al. Three postpartum antiretroviral regimens to prevent intrapartum HIV infection. *N Engl J Med.* 2012;366(25):2368–2379 PMID: 22716975

52. American Academy of Academy Committee on Infectious Diseases. Recommendations for prevention and control of influenza in children, 2013–2014. *Pediatrics.* 2013;132(4):e1089–e1104 PMID: 23999962

53. Acosta EP, Jester P, Gal P, et al. Oseltamivir dosing for influenza infection in premature neonates. *J Infect Dis.* 2010;202(4):563–566 PMID: 20594104

54. Kimberlin DW, Acosta EP, Prichard MN, et al, for the NIAID Collaborative Antiviral Study Group. Oseltamivir pharmacokinetics, dosing, and resistance among children aged <2 years with influenza. *J Infect Dis.* 2013;207(5):709–720 PMID: 23230059

55. Fraser N, Davies BW, Cusack J. Neonatal omphalitis: a review of its serious complications. *Acta Paediatr.* 2006;95(5):519–522 PMID: 16825129

56. Ulloa-Gutierrez R, Rodriguez-Calzada H, Quesada L, et al. Is it acute omphalitis or necrotizing fasciitis? Report of three fatal cases. *Pediatr Emerg Care.* 2005;21(9):600–602 PMID: 16160666

57. Sawardekar KP. Changing spectrum of neonatal omphalitis. *Pediatr Infect Dis J.* 2004;23(1):22–26 PMID: 14743041

58. Bingol-Kologlu M, Yildiz RV, Alper B, et al. Necrotizing fasciitis in children: diagnostic and therapeutic aspects. *J Pediatr Surg.* 2007;42(11):1892–1897 PMID: 18022442

59. Brook I. Cutaneous and subcutaneous infections in newborns due to anaerobic bacteria. *J Perinat Med.* 2002;30(3):197–208 PMID: 12122901

60. Kaplan SL. Challenges in the evaluation and management of bone and joint infections and the role of new antibiotics for gram positive infections. *Adv Exp Med Biol.* 2009;634:111–120 PMID: 19280853

61. Korakaki E, Aligizakis A, Manoura A, et al. Methicillin-resistant *Staphylococcus aureus* osteomyelitis and septic arthritis in neonates: diagnosis and management. *Jpn J Infect Dis.* 2007;60(2-3):129–131 PMID: 17515648

62. Dessi A, Crisafulli M, Accossu S, et al. Osteo-articular infections in newborns: diagnosis and treatment. *J Chemother.* 2008;20(5):542–550 PMID: 19028615

63. Berkun Y, Nir-Paz R, Ami AB, et al. Acute otitis media in the first two months of life: characteristics and diagnostic difficulties. *Arch Dis Child.* 2008;93(8):690–694 PMID: 18337275

64. Greenberg D, Hoffman S, Leibovitz E, et al. Acute otitis media in children: association with day care centers—antibacterial resistance, treatment, and prevention. *Paediatr Drugs.* 2008;10(2):75–83 PMID: 18345717

65. Spiegel R, Miron D, Sakran W, et al. Acute neonatal suppurative parotitis: case reports and review. *Pediatr Infect Dis J.* 2004;23(1):76–78 PMID: 14743054

66. Engle WD, Jackson GL, Sendelbach D, et al. Neonatal pneumonia: comparison of 4 vs 7 days of antibiotic therapy in term and near-term infants. *J Perinatol.* 2000;20(7):421–426 PMID: 11076325

67. Brook I. Anaerobic infections in children. *Microbes Infect.* 2002;4(12):1271–1280 PMID: 12467770

68. Darville T. *Chlamydia trachomatis* infections in neonates and young children. *Semin Pediatr Infect Dis.* 2005;16(4):235–244 PMID: 16210104

69. Waites KB, Schelonka RL, Xiao L, Grigsby PL, Novy MJ. Congenital and opportunistic infections: Ureaplasma species and Mycoplasma hominis. *Semin Fetal Neonatal Med.* 2009;14(4):190–199 PMID: 19109084

70. Morrison W. Infantile hypertrophic pyloric stenosis in infants treated with azithromycin. *Pediatr Infect Dis J.* 2007;26(2):186–188 PMID: 17259889

71. American Academy of Pediatrics. Pertussis. In: Pickering LK, Baker CJ, Kimberlin DW, Long SS, eds. *Red Book: 2012 Report of the Committee on Infectious Diseases.* 29th ed. Elk Grove Village, IL: American Academy of Pediatrics; 2012:553–566

72. Foca MD. *Pseudomonas aeruginosa* infections in the neonatal intensive care unit. *Semin Perinatol.* 2002;26(5):332–339 PMID: 12452505

73. American Academy of Pediatrics. Respiratory syncytial virus. In: Pickering LK, Baker CJ, Kimberlin DW, Long SS, eds. *Red Book: 2012 Report of the Committee on Infectious Diseases.* 29th ed. Elk Grove Village, IL: American Academy of Pediatrics; 2012:609–618

74. American Academy of Pediatrics Committee on Infectious Diseases. From the modified recommendations for use of palivizumab for prevention of respiratory syncytial virus infections. *Pediatrics.* 2009;124(6):1694–1701 PMID: 19736258

75. Vergnano S, Menson E, Smith Z, et al. Characteristics of invasive Staphylococcus aureus in United Kingdom neonatal units. *Pediatr Infect Dis J.* 2011;30(10):850–854 PMID: 21654546

76. Yee-Guardino S, Kumar D, Abughali N, et al. Recognition and treatment of neonatal community-associated MRSA pneumonia and bacteremia. *Pediatr Pulmonol.* 2008;43(2):203–205 PMID: 18085688

77. Lyseng-Williamson KA, Goa KL. Linezolid: in infants and children with severe gram-positive infections. *Paediatr Drugs.* 2003;5(6):419–431 PMID: 12765493

78. American Academy of Pediatrics. Group B streptococcal infections. In: Pickering LK, Baker CJ, Kimberlin DW, Long SS, eds. *Red Book: 2012 Report of the Committee on Infectious Diseases.* 29th ed. Elk Grove Village, IL: American Academy of Pediatrics; 2012:680–685

79. Schrag S, Gorwitz R, Fultz-Butts K, et al. Prevention of perinatal group B streptococcal disease. Revised guidelines from CDC. *MMWR Recomm Rep.* 2002;51(RR-11):1–22 PMID: 12211284

80. American Academy of Pediatrics. *Ureaplasma urealyticum* infections. In: Pickering LK, Baker CJ, Kimberlin DW, Long SS, eds. *Red Book: 2012 Report of the Committee on Infectious Diseases.* 29th ed. Elk Grove Village, IL: American Academy of Pediatrics; 2012:772–774

81. American Academy of Pediatrics. *Escherichia coli* and other gram-negative bacilli. In: Pickering LK, Baker CJ, Kimberlin DW, Long SS, eds. *Red Book: 2012 Report of the Committee on Infectious Diseases.* 29th ed. Elk Grove Village, IL: American Academy of Pediatrics; 2012:321–324

82. Venkatesh MP, Garcia-Prats JA. Management of neonatal sepsis by gram-negative pathogens. *Expert Rev Anti Infect Ther.* 2008;6(6):929–938 PMID: 19053905

83. American Academy of Pediatrics. *Listeria monocytogenes* infections (listeriosis). In: Pickering LK, Baker CJ, Kimberlin DW, Long SS, eds. *Red Book: 2012 Report of the Committee on Infectious Diseases.* 29th ed. Elk Grove Village, IL: American Academy of Pediatrics; 2012:471–474

84. Fortunov RM, Hulten KG, Hammerman WA, et al. Community-acquired *Staphylococcus aureus* infections in term and near-term previously healthy neonates. *Pediatrics.* 2006;118(3):874–881 PMID: 16950976

85. Fortunov RM, Hulten KG, Hammerman WA, et al. Evaluation and treatment of community-acquired *Staphylococcus aureus* infections in term and late-preterm previously healthy neonates. *Pediatrics.* 2007;120(5):937–945 PMID: 17974729

86. Stauffer WM, Kamat D. Neonatal mastitis. *Pediatr Emerg Care.* 2003;19(3):165–166 PMID: 12813301

87. Dehority W, Wang E, Vernon PS, et al. Community-associated methicillin-resistant *Staphylococcus aureus* necrotizing fasciitis in a neonate. *Pediatr Infect Dis J.* 2006;25(11):1080–1081 PMID: 17072137

88. American Academy of Pediatrics. Syphilis. In: Pickering LK, Baker CJ, Kimberlin DW, Long SS, eds. *Red Book: 2012 Report of the Committee on Infectious Diseases.* 29th ed. Elk Grove Village, IL: American Academy of Pediatrics; 2012:690–702

89. American Academy of Pediatrics. Tetanus. In: Pickering LK, Baker CJ, Kimberlin DW, Long SS, eds. *Red Book: 2012 Report of the Committee on Infectious Diseases.* 29th ed. Elk Grove Village, IL: American Academy of Pediatrics; 2012:707–712

90. American Academy of Pediatrics. *Toxoplasma gondii* infections. In: Pickering LK, Baker CJ, Kimberlin DW, Long SS, eds. *Red Book: 2012 Report of the Committee on Infectious Diseases.* 29th ed. Elk Grove Village, IL: American Academy of Pediatrics; 2012:720–728

91. Petersen E. Toxoplasmosis. *Semin Fetal Neonatal Med.* 2007;12(3):214–223 PMID: 17321812

92. Beetz R. Evaluation and management of urinary tract infections in the neonate. *Curr Opin Pediatr.* 2012;24(2):205–211 PMID: 22227782

93. Sachs HC; Committee on Drugs. The transfer of drugs and therapeutics into human breast milk: an update on selected topics. *Pediatrics.* 2013;132(3):e796–e809 PMID: 23979084

94. Hale TW. *Medication and Mothers' Milk: A Manual of Lactational Pharmacology.* 15th ed. Amarillo, TX: Hale Publishing; 2012

References

Chapter 6

1. Stevens DL, Bisno AL, Chambers HF, et al. Practice guidelines for the diagnosis and management of skin and soft-tissue infections. *Clin Infect Dis.* 2005;41(10):1373–1406 PMID: 16231249

2. Liu C, Bayer A, Cosgrove SE, et al. Clinical practice guidelines by the Infectious Diseases Society of America for the treatment of methicillin-resistant *Staphylococcus aureus* infections in adults and children. *Clin Infect Dis.* 2011;52(3):e18–e55 PMID: 21208910

3. Elliott DJ, Zaoutis TE, Troxel AB, et al. Empiric antimicrobial therapy for pediatric skin and soft-tissue infections in the era of methicillin-resistant *Staphylococcus aureus. Pediatrics.* 2009;123(6):e959–e966 PMID: 19470525

4. Inman JC, Rowe M, Ghostine M, et al. Pediatric neck abscesses: changing organisms and empiric therapies. *Laryngoscope.* 2008;118(12):2111–2114 PMID: 18948832

5. Martinez-Aguilar G, Hammerman WA, Mason EO Jr, et al. Clindamycin treatment of invasive infections caused by community-acquired, methicillin-resistant and methicillin-susceptible *Staphylococcus aureus* in children. *Pediatr Infect Dis J.* 2003;22(7):593–598 PMID: 12867833

6. American Academy of Pediatrics. Staphylococcal infections. In: Pickering LK, Baker CJ, Kimberlin DW, Long SS, eds. *Red Book: 2012 Report of the Committee on Infectious Diseases.* 29th ed. Elk Grove Village, IL: American Academy of Pediatrics; 2012:653–668

7. American Academy of Pediatrics. Group A streptococcal infections. In: Pickering LK, Baker CJ, Kimberlin DW, Long SS, eds. *Red Book: 2012 Report of the Committee on Infectious Diseases.* 29th ed. Elk Grove Village, IL: American Academy of Pediatrics; 2012:668–675

8. Bass JW, Freitas BC, Freitas AD, et al. Prospective randomized double blind placebo-controlled evaluation of azithromycin for treatment of cat-scratch disease. *Pediatr Infect Dis J.* 1998;17(6):447–452 PMID: 9655532

9. Timmerman MK, Morley AD, Buwalda J. Treatment of non-tuberculous mycobacterial cervicofacial lymphadenitis in children: critical appraisal of the literature. *Clin Otolaryngol.* 2008;33(6):546–552 PMID: 19126128

10. Iversen RH, Illum P. Cervicofacial nontuberculous mycobacterial lymphadenitis in children. *Dan Med J.* 2012;59(1):A4349 PMID: 22239836

11. Griffith DE, Aksamit T, Brown-Elliott BA, et al. An official ATS/IDSA statement: diagnosis, treatment, and prevention of nontuberculous mycobacterial diseases. *Am J Respir Crit Care Med.* 2007;175(4):367–416 PMID: 17277290

12. Lindeboom JA. Conservative wait-and-see therapy versus antibiotic treatment for nontuberculous mycobacterial cervicofacial lymphadenitis in children. *Clin Infect Dis.* 2011;52(2):180–184 PMID: 21288841

13. Treatment of tuberculosis. *MMWR Recomm Rep.* 2003;52(RR-11):1–77 PMID: 12836625

14. American Academy of Pediatrics. Tuberculosis. In: Pickering LK, Baker CJ, Kimberlin DW, Long SS, eds. *Red Book: 2012 Report of the Committee on Infectious Diseases.* 29th ed. Elk Grove Village, IL: American Academy of Pediatrics; 2012:736–759

15. American Academy of Pediatrics, Centers for Disease Control and Prevention. Pediatric anthrax clinical guidance. *Guidance for the Clinician in Rendering Care to Neonates, Infants and Children.* Clinical report. 2014. In press

16. Talan DA, Abrahamian FM, Moran GJ, et al. Clinical presentation and bacteriologic analysis of infected human bites in patients presenting to emergency departments. *Clin Infect Dis.* 2003;37(11):1481–1489 PMID: 14614671

17. Oehler RL, Velez AP, Mizrachi M, et al. Bite-related and septic syndromes caused by cats and dogs. *Lancet Infect Dis.* 2009;9(7):439–447 PMID: 19555903

18. Thomas N, Brook I. Animal bite-associated infections: microbiology and treatment. *Expert Rev Anti Infect Ther.* 2011;9(2):215–226 PMID: 21342069

19. Lion C, Conroy MC, Carpentier AM, et al. Antimicrobial susceptibilities of *Pasteurella* strains isolated from humans. *Int J Antimicrob Agents.* 2006;27(4):290–293 PMID: 16564680

20. American Academy of Pediatrics. Rabies. In: Pickering LK, Baker CJ, Kimberlin DW, Long SS, eds. *Red Book: 2012 Report of the Committee on Infectious Diseases.* 29th ed. Elk Grove Village, IL: American Academy of Pediatrics; 2012:600–607

21. Hyun DY, Mason EO, Forbes A, et al. Trimethoprim-sulfamethoxazole or clindamycin for treatment of community-acquired methicillin-resistant *Staphylococcus aureus* skin and soft tissue infections. *Pediatr Infect Dis J.* 2009;28(1):57–59 PMID: 19057459

22. American Academy of Pediatrics. *Haemophilus influenzae* infections. In: Pickering LK, Baker CJ, Kimberlin DW, Long SS, eds. *Red Book: 2012 Report of the Committee on Infectious Diseases.* 29th ed. Elk Grove Village, IL: American Academy of Pediatrics; 2012:345–352

23. Yang LP, Keam SJ. Spotlight on retapamulin in impetigo and other uncomplicated superficial skin infections. *Am J Clin Dermatol.* 2008;9(6):411–413 PMID: 18973410

24. Bass JW, Chan DS, Creamer KM, et al. Comparison of oral cephalexin, topical mupirocin and topical bacitracin for treatment of impetigo. *Pediatr Infect Dis J.* 1997;16(7):708–710 PMID: 9239775

25. Boscolo-Rizzo P, Da Mosto MC. Submandibular space infection: a potentially lethal infection. *Int J Infect Dis.* 2009;13(3):327–333 PMID: 18952475

26. Pannaraj PS, Hulten KG, Gonzalez BE, et al. Infective pyomyositis and myositis in children in the era of community-acquired, methicillin-resistant *Staphylococcus aureus* infection. *Clin Infect Dis.* 2006;43(8):953–960 PMID: 16983604

27. Smith-Slatas CL, Bourque M, Salazar JC. *Clostridium septicum* infections in children: a case report and review of the literature. *Pediatrics.* 2006;117(4):e796–e805 PMID: 16567392

28. Jamal N, Teach SJ. Necrotizing fasciitis. *Pediatr Emerg Care.* 2011;27(12):1195–1199 PMID: 22158285

29. Stevens DL. Streptococcal toxic shock syndrome associated with necrotizing fasciitis. *Annu Rev Med.* 2000;51:271–288 PMID: 10774464

30. Abuhammour W, Hasan RA, Rogers D. Necrotizing fasciitis caused by *Aeromonas hydrophilia* in an immunocompetent child. *Pediatr Emerg Care.* 2006;22(1):48–51 PMID: 16418613

31. Daum RS. Clinical practice. Skin and soft-tissue infections caused by methicillin-resistant *Staphylococcus aureus*. *N Engl J Med.* 2007;357(4):380–390 PMID: 17652653

32. Lee MC, Rios AM, Aten MF, et al. Management and outcome of children with skin and soft tissue abscesses caused by community-acquired methicillin-resistant *Staphylococcus aureus*. *Pediatr Infect Dis J.* 2004;23(2):123–127 PMID: 14872177

33. Karamatsu ML, Thorp AW, Brown L. Changes in community-associated methicillin-resistant *Staphylococcus aureus* skin and soft tissue infections presenting to the pediatric emergency department: comparing 2003 to 2008. *Pediatr Emerg Care.* 2012;28(2):131–135 PMID: 22270497

34. Elliott SP. Rat bite fever and *Streptobacillus moniliformis*. *Clin Microbiol Rev.* 2007;20(1):13–22 PMID: 17223620

35. Berk DR, Bayliss SJ. MRSA, staphylococcal scalded skin syndrome, and other cutaneous bacterial emergencies. *Pediatr Ann.* 2010;10:627–633 PMID: 20954609

36. Kaplan SL. Challenges in the evaluation and management of bone and joint infections and the role of new antibiotics for gram positive infections. *Adv Exp Med Biol.* 2009;634:111–120 PMID: 19280853

37. Peltola H, Paakkonen M, Kallio P, et al. Prospective, randomized trial of 10 days versus 30 days of antimicrobial treatment, including a short-term course of parenteral therapy, for childhood septic arthritis. *Clin Infect Dis.* 2009;48(9):1201–1210 PMID: 19323633

38. Bradley JS. What is the appropriate treatment course for bacterial arthritis in children? *Clin Infect Dis.* 2009;48(9):1211–1212 PMID: 19323629

39. Saphyakhajon P, Joshi AY, Huskins WC, et al. Empiric antibiotic therapy for acute osteoarticular infections with suspected methicillin-resistant *Staphylococcus aureus* or *Kingella*. *Pediatr Infect Dis J.* 2008;27(8):765–767 PMID: 18600193

40. Faust SN, Clark J, Pallett A, Clarke NM. Managing bone and joint infection in children. *Arch Dis Child.* 2012;97(6):545–553 PMID: 22440930

41. Arnold JC, Cannavino CR, Ross MK, et al. Acute bacterial osteoarticular infections: eight-year analysis of C-reactive protein for oral step-down therapy. *Pediatrics.* 2012;130(4):e821–e828 PMID: 22966033

42. Workowski KA, Berman S. Sexually transmitted diseases treatment guidelines, 2010. *MMWR Recomm Rep.* 2010;59(RR-12):1–110 PMID: 21160459

43. American Academy of Pediatrics. Gonococcal infections. In: Pickering LK, Baker CJ, Kimberlin DW, Long SS, eds. *Red Book: 2012 Report of the Committee on Infectious Diseases.* 29th ed. Elk Grove Village, IL: American Academy of Pediatrics; 2012: 336–344

References

Chapter 6 (cont)

44. Saavedra-Lozano J, Mejias A, Ahmad N, et al. Changing trends in acute osteomyelitis in children: impact of methicillin-resistant *Staphylococcus aureus* infections. *J Pediatr Orthop*. 2008;28(5):569–575 PMID: 18580375

45. Martinez-Aguilar G, Avalos-Mishaan A, Hulten K, et al. Community-acquired, methicillin-resistant and methicillin-susceptible *Staphylococcus aureus* musculoskeletal infections in children. *Pediatr Infect Dis J*. 2004;23(8):701–706 PMID: 15295218

46. Messina AF, Namtu K, Guild M, Dumois JA, Berman DM. Trimethoprim-sulfamethoxazole therapy for children with acute osteomyelitis. *Pediatr Infect Dis J*. 2011;30(12):1019–1021 PMID: 21817950

47. Jagodzinski NA, Kanwar R, Graham K, et al. Prospective evaluation of a shortened regimen of treatment for acute osteomyelitis and septic arthritis in children. *J Pediatr Orthop*. 2009;29(5):518–525 PMID: 19568027

48. Pääkkönen M, Kallio PE, Kallio MJ, Peltola H. Management of osteoarticular infections caused by *Staphylococcus aureus* is similar to that of other etiologies: analysis of 199 staphylococcal bone and joint infections. *Pediatr Infect Dis J*. 2012;31(5):436–438 PMID: 22189524

49. Ceroni D, Cherkaoui A, Ferey S, et al. *Kingella kingae* osteoarticular infections in young children: clinical features and contribution of a new specific real-time PCR assay to the diagnosis. *J Pediatr Orthop*. 2010;30(3):301–304 PMID: 20357599

50. Chen CJ, Chiu CH, Lin TY, et al. Experience with linezolid therapy in children with osteoarticular infections. *Pediatr Infect Dis J*. 2007;26(11):985–988 PMID: 17984803

51. Chachad S, Kamat D. Management of plantar puncture wounds in children. *Clin Pediatr (Phila)*. 2004;43(3):213–216 PMID: 15094944

52. Bradley JS, Jackson MA; American Academy of Pediatrics Committee on Infectious Diseases. The use of systemic and topical fluoroquinolones. *Pediatrics*. 2011;128(4):e1034–e1045 PMID: 21949152

53. Vaska VL, Grimwood K, Gole GA, Nimmo GR, Paterson DL, Nissan MD. Community-associated methicillin-resistant *Staphylococcus aureus* causing orbital cellulitis in Australian children. *Pediatr Infect Dis J*. 2011;30(11):1003–1006 PMID: 21681121

54. Seltz LB, Smith J, Durairaj VD, et al. Microbiology and antibiotic management of orbital cellulitis. *Pediatrics*. 2011;127(3):e566–e572 PMID: 21321025

55. Peña MT, Preciado D, Orestes M, Choi S. Orbital complications of acute sinusitis: changes in the post-pneumococcal vaccine era. *JAMA Otolaryngol Head Neck Surg*. 2013;139(3):223–227 PMID: 23429877

56. Bedwell J, Bauman NM. Management of pediatric orbital cellulitis and abscess. *Curr Opin Otolaryngol Head Neck Surg*. 2011;19(6):467–473 PMID: 22001661

57. Wald ER. Periorbital and orbital infections. *Pediatr Rev*. 2004;25(9):312–320 PMID: 15342822

58. Sheikh A, Hurwitz B. Antibiotics versus placebo for acute bacterial conjunctivitis. *Cochrane Database Syst Rev*. 2006;(2):CD001211 PMID: 16625540

59. Williams L, Malhotra Y, Murante B, et al. A single-blinded randomized clinical trial comparing polymyxin B-trimethoprim and moxifloxacin for treatment of acute conjunctivitis in children. *J Pediatr*. 2013;162(4):857–861 PMID: 23092529

60. Pichichero ME. Bacterial conjunctivitis in children: antibacterial treatment options in an era of increasing drug resistance. *Clin Pediatr (Phila)*. 2011;50(1):7–13 PMID: 20724317

61. Wilhelmus KR. Antiviral treatment and other therapeutic interventions for herpes simplex virus epithelial keratitis. *Cochrane Database Syst Rev*. 2010;(12):CD002898 PMID: 21154352

62. Liu S, Pavan-Langston D, Colby KA. Pediatric herpes simplex of the anterior segment: characteristics, treatment, and outcomes. *Ophthalmology*. 2012;119(10):2003–2008 PMID: 22796308

63. Young RC, Hodge DO, Liesegang TJ, et al. Incidence, recurrence, and outcomes of herpes simplex virus eye disease in Olmsted County, Minnesota, 1976–2007: the effect of oral antiviral prophylaxis. *Arch Ophthalmol*. 2010;128(9):1178–1183 PMID: 20837803

64. Thordsen JE, Harris L, Hubbard GB III. Pediatric endophthalmitis. A 10-year consecutive series. *Retina*. 2008;28(3 suppl):S3–S7 PMID: 18317341

65. Soheilian M, Rafati N, Mohebbi MR, et al. Prophylaxis of acute posttraumatic bacterial endophthalmitis: a multicenter, randomized clinical trial of intraocular antibiotic injection, report 2. *Arch Ophthalmol*. 2007;125(4):460–465 PMID: 17420365

66. Livermore JL, Felton TW, Abbott J, et al. Pharmacokinetics and pharmacodynamics of anidulafungin for experimental *Candida* endophthalmitis: insights into the utility of echinocandins for treatment of a potentially sight-threatening infection. *Antimicrob Agents Chemother*. 2013;57(1):281–288 PMID: 23114778

67. Kedhar SR, Jabs DA. Cytomegalovirus retinitis in the era of highly active antiretroviral therapy. *Herpes*. 2007;14(3):66–71 PMID: 18371289

68. Nassetta L, Kimberlin D, Whitley R. Treatment of congenital cytomegalovirus infection: implications for future therapeutic strategies. *J Antimicrob Chemother*. 2009;63(5):862–867 PMID: 19287011

69. Kimberlin DW, Lin CY, Sanchez PJ, et al. Effect of ganciclovir therapy on hearing in symptomatic congenital cytomegalovirus disease involving the central nervous system: a randomized, controlled trial. *J Pediatr*. 2003;143(1):16–25 PMID: 12915819

70. Rosenfeld RM, Brown L, Cannon CR, et al; American Academy of Otolaryngology—Head and Neck Surgery Foundation. Clinical practice guideline: acute otitis externa. *Otolaryngol Head Neck Surg*. 2006;134(4 Suppl):S4–S23 PMID: 16638473

71. Dohar JE. Evolution of management approaches for otitis externa. *Pediatr Infect Dis J*. 2003;22(4):299–308 PMID: 12690268

72. Carfrae MJ, Kesser BW. Malignant otitis externa. *Otolaryngol Clin North Am*. 2008;41(3):537–549 PMID: 18435997

73. Kaushik V, Malik T, Saeed SR. Interventions for acute otitis externa. *Cochrane Database Syst Rev*. 2010;(1):CD004740 PMID: 20091565

74. Hoberman A, Paradise JL, Rockette HE, et al. Treatment of acute otitis media in children under 2 years of age. *N Engl J Med*. 2011;364(2):105–115 PMID: 21226576

75. Tähtinen PA, Laine MK, Huovinen P, et al. A placebo-controlled trial of antimicrobial treatment for acute otitis media. *N Engl J Med*. 2011;364(2):116–126 PMID: 21226577

76. Lieberthal AS, Carroll AE, Chonmaitree T, et al. The diagnosis and management of acute otitis media. *Pediatrics*. 2013;131(3):e964–e999 PMID: 23439909

77. Rovers MM, Glasziou P, Appelman CL, et al. Antibiotics for acute otitis media: a meta-analysis with individual patient data. *Lancet*. 2006;368(9545):1429–1435 PMID: 17055944

78. Leach AJ, Morris PS. Antibiotics for the prevention of acute and chronic suppurative otitis media in children. *Cochrane Database Syst Rev*. 2006;(4):CD004401 PMID: 17054203

79. Hoberman A, Paradise JL, Shaikh N, et al. Pneumococcal resistance and serotype 19A in Pittsburgh-area children with acute otitis media before and after introduction of 7-valent pneumococcal polysaccharide vaccine. *Clin Pediatr (Phila)*. 2011;50(2):114–120 PMID: 21098526

80. Pichichero ME. Otitis media. *Pediatr Clin North Am*. 2013;60(2):391-407 PMID: 23481107

81. Macfadyen CA, Acuin JM, Gamble C. Systemic antibiotics versus topical treatments for chronically discharging ears with underlying eardrum perforations. *Cochrane Database Syst Rev*. 2006;(1):CD005608 PMID: 16437533

82. Marchisio P, Chonmaitree T, Leibovitz E, et al. Panel 7: treatment and comparative effectiveness research. *Otolaryngol Head Neck Surg*. 2013;148(4 Suppl):e102–e121 PMID: 23536528

83. Haynes DS, Rutka J, Hawke M, et al. Ototoxicity of ototopical drops—an update. *Otolaryngol Clin North Am*. 2007;40(3):669–683 PMID: 17544701

84. Groth A, Enoksson F, Hultcrantz M, Stalfors J, Stenfeldt K, Hermansson A. Acute mastoiditis in children aged 0-16 years—a national study of 678 cases in Sweden comparing different age groups. *Int J Pediatr Otorhinolaryngol*. 2012;76(10):1494–1500 PMID: 22832239

85. Stahelin-Massik J, Podvinec M, Jakscha J, et al. Mastoiditis in children: a prospective, observational study comparing clinical presentation, microbiology, computed tomography, surgical findings and histology. *Eur J Pediatr*. 2008;167(5):541–548 PMID: 17668240

86. Ongkasuwan J, Valdez TA, Hulten KG, et al. Pneumococcal mastoiditis in children and the emergence of multidrug-resistant serotype 19A isolates. *Pediatrics*. 2008;122(1):34–39 PMID: 18595984

87. Wald ER, Nash D, Eickhoff J. Effectiveness of amoxicillin/clavulanate potassium in the treatment of acute bacterial sinusitis in children. *Pediatrics*. 2009;124(1):9–15 PMID: 19564277

References

Chapter 6 (cont)

88. Wald ER, Applegate KE, Bordley C, et al. Clinical practice guideline for the diagnosis and management of acute bacterial sinusitis in children aged 1 to 18 years. *Pediatrics.* 2013;132(1):e262–e280 PMID: 23796742

89. Whitby CR, Kaplan SL, Mason EO Jr, et al. *Staphylococcus aureus* sinus infections in children. *Int J Pediatr Otorhinolaryngol.* 2011;75(1):118–121 PMID: 21074863

90. Chow AW, Benninger MS, Brook I, et al; Infectious Diseases Society of America. IDSA clinical practice guideline for acute bacterial rhinosinusitis in children and adults. *Clin Infect Dis.* 2012;54(8):e72–e112 PMID: 22438350

91. Ellison SJ. The role of phenoxymethylpenicillin, amoxicillin, metronidazole and clindamycin in the management of acute dentoalveolar abscesses—a review. *Br Dent J.* 2009;206(7):357–362 PMID: 19357666

92. Robertson D, Smith AJ. The microbiology of the acute dental abscess. *J Med Microbiol.* 2009;58(pt 2):155–162 PMID: 19141730

93. American Academy of Pediatrics. Diphtheria. In: Pickering LK, Baker CJ, Kimberlin DW, Long SS, eds. *Red Book: 2012 Report of the Committee on Infectious Diseases.* 29th ed. Elk Grove Village, IL: American Academy of Pediatrics; 2012:307–311

94. Wheeler DS, Dauplaise DJ, Giuliano JS Jr. An infant with fever and stridor. *Pediatr Emerg Care.* 2008;24(1):46–49 PMID: 18212612

95. Sobol SE, Zapata S. Epiglottitis and croup. *Otolaryngol Clin North Am.* 2008;41(3):551–566 PMID: 18435998

96. Nasser M, Fedorowicz Z, Khoshnevisan MH, et al. Acyclovir for treating primary herpetic gingivostomatitis. *Cochrane Database Syst Rev.* 2008;(4):CD006700 PMID: 18843726

97. Amir J, Harel L, Smetana Z, et al. Treatment of herpes simplex gingivostomatitis with aciclovir in children: a randomised double blind placebo controlled study. *BMJ.* 1997;314(7097):1800–1803 PMID: 9224082

98. Kimberlin DW, Jacobs RF, Weller S, et al. Pharmacokinetics and safety of extemporaneously compounded valacyclovir oral suspension in pediatric patients from 1 month through 11 years of age. *Clin Infect Dis.* 2010;50(2):221–228 PMID: 20014952

99. Riordan T. Human infection with *Fusobacterium necrophorum* (necrobacillosis), with a focus on Lemierre's syndrome. *Clin Microbiol Rev.* 2007;20(4):622–659 PMID: 17934077

100. Kuppalli K, Livorsi D, Talati NJ, Osborn M. Lemierre's syndrome due to Fusobacterium necrophorum. *Lancet Infect Dis.* 2012;12(10):808–815 PMID: 22633566

101. Baldassari CM, Howell R, Amorn M, et al. Complications in pediatric deep neck space abscesses. *Otolaryngol Head Neck Surg.* 2011;144(4):592–595 PMID: 21493241

102. Shulman ST, Bisno AL, Clegg HW, et al; Infectious Diseases Society of America. Clinical practice guideline for the diagnosis and management of group A streptococcal pharyngitis: 2012 update by the Infectious Diseases Society of America. *Clin Infect Dis.* 2012;55(10):e86–e102 PMID: 22965026

103. Lennon DR, Farrell E, Martin DR, et al. Once-daily amoxicillin versus twice-daily penicillin V in group A beta-haemolytic streptococcal pharyngitis. *Arch Dis Child.* 2008;93(6):474–478 PMID: 18337284

104. Clegg HW, Ryan AG, Dallas SD, et al. Treatment of streptococcal pharyngitis with once-daily compared with twice-daily amoxicillin: a noninferiority trial. *Pediatr Infect Dis J.* 2006;25(9):761–767 PMID: 16940830

105. Casey JR, Pichichero ME. The evidence base for cephalosporin superiority over penicillin in streptococcal pharyngitis. *Diagn Microbiol Infect Dis.* 2007;57(3 suppl):39S–45S PMID: 17292576

106. Altamimi S, Khalil A, Khalaiwi KA, Milner RA, Pusic MV, Al Othman MA. Short-term late-generation antibiotics versus longer term penicillin for acute streptococcal pharyngitis in children. *Cochrane Database Syst Rev.* 2012;8:CD004872 PMID: 22895944

107. Abdel-Haq N, Quezada M, Asmar BI. Retropharyngeal abscess in children: the rising incidence of methicillin-resistant *Staphylococcus aureus.* *Pediatr Infect Dis J.* 2012;31(7):696–699 PMID: 22481424

108. Cheng J, Elden L. Children with deep space neck infections: our experience with 178 children. *Otolaryngol Head Neck Surg.* 2013;148(6):1037–1042 PMID: 23520072

109. Hopkins A, Lahiri T, Salerno R, et al. Changing epidemiology of life-threatening upper airway infections: the reemergence of bacterial tracheitis. *Pediatrics.* 2006;118(4):1418–1421 PMID: 17015531

110. Tebruegge M, Pantazidou A, Thorburn K, et al. Bacterial tracheitis: a multi-centre perspective. *Scand J Infect Dis.* 2009;41(8):548–557 PMID: 19401934

111. Carrillo-Marquez MA, Hulten KG, Hammerman W, Lamberth L, Mason EO, Kaplan SL. *Staphylococcus aureus* pneumonia in children in the era of community-acquired methicillin-resistance at Texas Children's Hospital. *Pediatr Infect Dis J.* 2011;30(7):545–550 PMID: 21407143

112. Bender JM, Ampofo K, Korgenski K, et al. Pneumococcal necrotizing pneumonia in Utah: does serotype matter? *Clin Infect Dis.* 2008;46(9):1346–1352 PMID: 18419434

113. Brook I. Anaerobic infections in children. *Adv Exp Med Biol.* 2011;697:117–152 PMID: 21120724

114. Muszynski JA, Knatz NL, Sargel CL, et al. Timing of correct parenteral antibiotic initiation and outcomes from severe bacterial community-acquired pneumonia in children. *Pediatr Infect Dis J.* 2011;30(4):295–301 PMID: 21030885

115. Schuh S. Update on management of bronchiolitis. *Curr Opin Pediatr.* 2011;23(1):110–114 PMID: 21157348

116. Mogayzel PJ Jr, Naureckas ET, Robinson KA, et al; Pulmonary Clinical Practice Guidelines Committee. Cystic fibrosis pulmonary guidelines. Chronic medications for maintenance of lung health. *Am J Respir Crit Care Med.* 2013;187(7):680–689 PMID: 23540878

117. Plummer A, Wildman M. Duration of intravenous antibiotic therapy in people with cystic fibrosis. *Cochrane Database Syst Rev.* 2013;5:CD006682 PMID: 23728662

118. Montgomery GS, Howenstine M. Cystic fibrosis. *Pediatr Rev.* 2009;30(8):302–310 PMID: 19648261

119. Geller DE, Rubin BK. Respiratory care and cystic fibrosis. *Respir Care.* 2009;54(6):796–800 PMID: 19467166

120. Blumer JL, Saiman L, Konstan MW, et al. The efficacy and safety of meropenem and tobramycin vs ceftazidime and tobramycin in the treatment of acute pulmonary exacerbations in patients with cystic fibrosis. *Chest.* 2005;128(4):2336–2346 PMID: 16236892

121. Ryan G, Jahnke N, Remmington T. Inhaled antibiotics for pulmonary exacerbations in cystic fibrosis. *Cochrane Database Syst Rev.* 2012;12:CD008319 PMID: 23235659

122. Saiman L. Clinical utility of synergy testing for multidrug-resistant *Pseudomonas aeruginosa* isolated from patients with cystic fibrosis: 'the motion for'. *Paediatr Respir Rev.* 2007;8(3):249–255 PMID: 17868923

123. Waters V, Ratjen F. Combination antimicrobial susceptibility testing for acute exacerbations in chronic infection of *Pseudomonas aeruginosa* in cystic fibrosis. *Cochrane Database Syst Rev.* 2008;(3):CD006961 PMID: 18646176

124. Cheer SM, Waugh J, Noble S. Inhaled tobramycin (TOBI): a review of its use in the management of *Pseudomonas aeruginosa* infections in patients with cystic fibrosis. *Drugs.* 2003;63(22):2501–2520 PMID: 14609360

125. Plosker GL. Aztreonam lysine for inhalation solution: in cystic fibrosis. *Drugs.* 2010;70(14):1843–1855 PMID: 20836577

126. Döring G, Flume P, Heijerman H, Elborn JS; Consensus Study Group. Treatment of lung infection in patients with cystic fibrosis: current and future strategies. *J Cyst Fibros.* 2012;11(6):461–479 PMID: 23137712

127. Southern KW, Barker PM, Solis-Moya A, Patel L. Macrolide antibiotics for cystic fibrosis. *Cochrane Database Syst Rev.* 2012;11:CD002203 PMID: 23152214

128. Moskowitz SM, Silva SJ, Mayer-Hamblett N, et al. Shifting patterns of inhaled antibiotic use in cystic fibrosis. *Pediatr Pulmonol.* 2008;43(9):874–881 PMID: 18668689

129. American Academy of Pediatrics. Pertussis. In: Pickering LK, Baker CJ, Kimberlin DW, Long SS, eds. *Red Book: 2012 Report of the Committee on Infectious Diseases.* 29th ed. Elk Grove Village, IL: American Academy of Pediatrics; 2012:553–566

References

Chapter 6 (cont)

130. Altunaiji S, Kukuruzovic R, Curtis N, et al. Antibiotics for whooping cough (pertussis). *Cochrane Database Syst Rev.* 2007;(3):CD004404 PMID: 17636756

131. Pavia AT. Viral infections of the lower respiratory tract: old viruses, new viruses, and the role of diagnosis. *Clin Infect Dis.* 2011;52(suppl 4):S284–S289 PMID: 21460286

132. Bradley JS, Byington CL, Shah SS, et al. The management of community-acquired pneumonia in infants and children older than 3 months of age: clinical practice guidelines by the Pediatric Infectious Diseases Society and the Infectious Diseases Society of America. *Clin Infect Dis.* 2011;53(7):e25–e76 PMID: 21880587

133. Esposito S, Cohen R, Domingo JD, et al. Antibiotic therapy for pediatric community-acquired pneumonia: do we know when, what and for how long to treat? *Pediatr Infect Dis J.* 2012;31(6): e78–e85 PMID: 22466326

134. Durbin WJ, Stille C. Pneumonia. *Pediatr Rev.* 2008;29(5):147–160 PMID: 18450836

135. Ambroggio L, Taylor JA, Tabb LP, Newschaffer CJ, Evans AA, Shah SS. Comparative effectiveness of empiric β-lactam monotherapy and β-lactam-macrolide combination therapy in children hospitalized with community-acquired pneumonia. *J Pediatr.* 2012;161(6):1097–1103 PMID: 22901738

136. Bradley JS, Arguedas A, Blumer JL, et al. Comparative study of levofloxacin in the treatment of children with community-acquired pneumonia. *Pediatr Infect Dis J.* 2007;26(10):868–878 PMID: 17901791

137. Hidron AI, Low CE, Honig EG, et al. Emergence of community-acquired methicillin-resistant *Staphylococcus aureus* strain USA300 as a cause of necrotising community-onset pneumonia. *Lancet Infect Dis.* 2009;9(6):384–392 PMID: 19467478

138. Finelli L, Fiore A, Dhara R, et al. Influenza-associated pediatric mortality in the United States: increase of *Staphylococcus aureus* coinfection. *Pediatrics.* 2008;122(4):805–811 PMID: 18829805

139. St Peter SD, Tsao K, Spilde TL, et al. Thoracoscopic decortication vs tube thoracostomy with fibrinolysis for empyema in children: a prospective, randomized trial. *J Pediatr Surg.* 2009;44(1): 106–111 PMID: 19159726

140. Islam S, Calkins CM, Goldin AB, et al; APSA Outcomes and Clinical Trials Committee, 2011-2012. The diagnosis and management of empyema in children: a comprehensive review from the APSA Outcomes and Clinical Trials Committee. *J Pediatr Surg.* 2012;47(11):2101–2110 PMID: 23164006

141. Aziz A, Healey JM, Qureshi F, et al. Comparative analysis of chest tube thoracostomy and video-assisted thoracoscopic surgery in empyema and parapneumonic effusion associated with pneumonia in children. *Surg Infect (Larchmt).* 2008;9(3):317–323 PMID: 18570573

142. Sonnappa S, Cohen G, Owens CM, et al. Comparison of urokinase and video-assisted thoracoscopic surgery for treatment of childhood empyema. *Am J Respir Crit Care Med.* 2006;174(2):221–227 PMID: 16675783

143. Freifeld AG, Bow EJ, Sepkowitz KA, et al; Infectious Diseases Society of America. Clinical practice guideline for the use of antimicrobial agents in neutropenic patients with cancer: 2010 update by the Infectious Diseases Society of America. *Clin Infect Dis.* 2011;52(4):e56–e93 PMID: 21258094

144. Guidelines for the management of adults with hospital-acquired, ventilator-associated, and healthcare-associated pneumonia. *Am J Respir Crit Care Med.* 2005;171(4):388–416 PMID: 15699079

145. Foglia E, Meier MD, Elward A. Ventilator-associated pneumonia in neonatal and pediatric intensive care unit patients. *Clin Microbiol Rev.* 2007;20(3):409–425 PMID: 17630332

146. Srinivasan R, Asselin J, Gildengorin G, et al. A prospective study of ventilator-associated pneumonia in children. *Pediatrics.* 2009;123(4):1108–1115 PMID: 19336369

147. Boselli E, Breilh D, Djabarouti S, et al. Reliability of mini-bronchoalveolar lavage for the measurement of epithelial lining fluid concentrations of tobramycin in critically ill patients. *Intensive Care Med.* 2007;33(9):1519–1523 PMID: 17530217

148. Arnold HM, Sawyer AM, Kollef MH. Use of adjunctive aerosolized antimicrobial therapy in the treatment of Pseudomonas aeruginosa and Acinetobacter baumannii ventilator-associated pneumonia. *Respir Care.* 2012;57(8):1226–1233 PMID: 22349038

149. American Academy of Pediatrics. Chlamydial infections. In: Pickering LK, Baker CJ, Kimberlin DW, Long SS, eds. *Red Book: 2012 Report of the Committee on Infectious Diseases.* 29th ed. Elk Grove Village, IL: American Academy of Pediatrics; 2012:272–281

150. American Academy of Pediatrics. Cytomegalovirus infection. In: Pickering LK, Baker CJ, Kimberlin DW, Long SS, eds. *Red Book: 2012 Report of the Committee on Infectious Diseases.* 29th ed. Elk Grove Village, IL: American Academy of Pediatrics; 2012:300–305

151. American Academy of Pediatrics. Tularemia. In: Pickering LK, Baker CJ, Kimberlin DW, Long SS, eds. *Red Book: 2012 Report of the Committee on Infectious Diseases.* 29th ed. Elk Grove Village, IL: American Academy of Pediatrics; 2012:768–769

152. Nigrovic LE, Wingerter SL. Tularemia. *Infect Dis Clin North Am.* 2008;22(3):489–504 PMID: 18755386

153. Thompson GR 3rd. Pulmonary coccidioidomycosis. *Semin Respir Crit Care Med.* 2011;32(6):754–763 PMID: 22167403

154. American Academy of Pediatrics. Coccidioidomycosis. In: Pickering LK, Baker CJ, Kimberlin DW, Long SS, eds. *Red Book: 2012 Report of the Committee on Infectious Diseases.* 29th ed. Elk Grove Village, IL: American Academy of Pediatrics; 2012:289–291

155. American Academy of Pediatrics. Histoplasmosis. In: Pickering LK, Baker CJ, Kimberlin DW, Long SS, eds. *Red Book: 2012 Report of the Committee on Infectious Diseases.* 29th ed. Elk Grove Village, IL: American Academy of Pediatrics; 2012:409–411

156. Wheat LJ, Freifeld AG, Kleiman MB, et al. Clinical practice guidelines for the management of patients with histoplasmosis: 2007 update by the Infectious Diseases Society of America. *Clin Infect Dis.* 2007;45(7):807–825 PMID: 17806045

157. American Academy of Pediatrics Committee on Infectious Diseases. Antiviral therapy and prophylaxis for influenza in children. *Pediatrics.* 2007;119(4):852–860 PMID: 17403862

158. American Academy of Academy Committee on Infectious Diseases. Recommendations for prevention and control of influenza in children, 2013–2014. *Pediatrics.* 2013;132(4):e1089–e1104 PMID: 23999962

159. Kimberlin DW, Acosta EP, Prichard MN, et al; National Institute of Allergy and Infectious Diseases Collaborative Antiviral Study Group. Oseltamivir pharmacokinetics, dosing, and resistance among children aged <2 years with influenza. *J Infect Dis.* 2013;207(5):709–720 PMID: 23230059

160. Yang K, Guglielmo BJ. Diagnosis and treatment of extended-spectrum and AmpC beta-lactamase-producing organisms. *Ann Pharmacother.* 2007;41(9):1427–1435 PMID: 17666573

161. Mandell LA, Wunderink RG, Anzueto A, et al. Infectious Diseases Society of America/American Thoracic Society consensus guidelines on the management of community-acquired pneumonia in adults. *Clin Infect Dis.* 2007;44(Suppl 2):S27–S72 PMID: 17278083

162. Mulholland S, Gavranich JB, Gillies MB, Chang AB. Antibiotics for community-acquired lower respiratory tract infections secondary to Mycoplasma pneumoniae in children. *Cochrane Database Syst Rev.* 2012;9:CD004875 PMID: 22972079

163. Cardinale F, Chironna M, Chinellato I, Principi N, Esposito S. Clinical relevance of Mycoplasma pneumoniae macrolide resistance in children. *J Clin Microbiol.* 2013;51(2):723–724 PMID: 23224091

164. Mofenson LM, Brady MT, Danner SP, et al; Centers for Disease Control and Prevention; National Institutes of Health; HIV Medicine Association of the Infectious Diseases Society of America; Pediatric Infectious Diseases Society; American Academy of Pediatrics. Guidelines for the prevention and treatment of opportunistic infections among HIV-exposed and HIV-infected children: recommendations from CDC, the National Institutes of Health, the HIV Medicine Association of the Infectious Diseases Society of America, the Pediatric Infectious Diseases Society, and the American Academy of Pediatrics. *MMWR Recomm Rep.* 2009;58(RR-11):1–166 PMID: 19730409

165. Saltzman RW, Albin S, Russo P, Sullivan KE. Clinical conditions associated with PCP in children. *Pediatr Pulmonol.* 2012;47(5):510–516 PMID: 22009851

166. Michalopoulos A, Falagas ME. Colistin and polymyxin B in critical care. *Crit Care Clin.* 2008;24(2):377–391 PMID: 18361952

167. Micek ST, Reichley RM, Kollef MH. Health care-associated pneumonia (HCAP): empiric antibiotics targeting methicillin-resistant *Staphylococcus aureus* (MRSA) and *Pseudomonas aeruginosa* predict optimal outcome. *Medicine (Baltimore).* 2011;90(6):390–395 PMID: 22033455

References

Chapter 6 (cont)

168. American Academy of Pediatrics. Respiratory syncytial virus. In: Pickering LK, Baker CJ, Kimberlin DW, Long SS, eds. *Red Book: 2012 Report of the Committee on Infectious Diseases.* 29th ed. Elk Grove Village, IL: American Academy of Pediatrics; 2012:609–619

169. Centers for Disease Control and Prevention. Recommendations for use of an isoniazid-rifapentine regimen with direct observation to treat latent Mycobacterium tuberculosis infection. *MMWR Morb Mortal Wkly Rep.* 2011;60(48):1650–1653 PMID: 22157884

170. Meehan WP III, Fleegler E, Bachur RG. Adherence to guidelines for managing the well-appearing febrile infant: assessment using a case-based, interactive survey. *Pediatr Emerg Care.* 2010;26(12):875–880 PMID: 21088637

171. Greenhow TL, Hung YY, Herz AM. Changing epidemiology of bacteremia in infants aged 1 week to 3 months. *Pediatrics.* 2012;129(3):e590–e596 PMID: 22371459

172. Byington CL, Rittichier KK, Bassett KE, et al. Serious bacterial infections in febrile infants younger than 90 days of age: the importance of ampicillin-resistant pathogens. *Pediatrics.* 2003;111(5 pt 1):964–968 PMID: 12728072

173. Lee GM, Fleisher GR, Harper MB. Management of febrile children in the age of the conjugate pneumococcal vaccine: a cost-effectiveness analysis. *Pediatrics.* 2001;108(4):835–844 PMID: 11581433

174. Ishimine P. The evolving approach to the young child who has fever and no obvious source. *Emerg Med Clin North Am.* 2007;25(4):1087–1115 PMID: 17950137

175. Joffe MD, Alpern ER. Occult pneumococcal bacteremia: a review. *Pediatr Emerg Care.* 2010;26(6):448–457 PMID: 20531134

176. Hakim H, Mylotte JM, Faden H. Morbidity and mortality of staphylococcal bacteremia in children. *Am J Infect Control.* 2007;35(2):102–105 PMID: 17327189

177. Luthander J, Bennet R, Giske CG, Nilsson A, Eriksson M. Age and risk factors influence the microbial aetiology of bloodstream infection in children. *Acta Paediatr.* 2013;102(2):182–186 PMID: 23121094

178. Ross AC, Toltzis P, O'Riordan MA, et al. Frequency and risk factors for deep focus of infection in children with *Staphylococcus aureus* bacteremia. *Pediatr Infect Dis J.* 2008;27(5):396–399 PMID: 18398384

179. Carrillo-Marquez MA, Hulten KG, Mason EO, et al. Clinical and molecular epidemiology of *Staphylococcus aureus* catheter-related bacteremia in children. *Pediatr Infect Dis J.* 2010;29(5): 410–414 PMID: 20431380

180. Baddour LM, Wilson WR, Bayer AS, et al. Infective endocarditis: diagnosis, antimicrobial therapy, and management of complications: a statement for healthcare professionals from the Committee on Rheumatic Fever, Endocarditis, and Kawasaki Disease, Council on Cardiovascular Disease in the Young, and the Councils on Clinical Cardiology, Stroke, and Cardiovascular Surgery and Anesthesia, American Heart Association: endorsed by the Infectious Diseases Society of America. *Circulation.* 2005;111(23):e394–e434 PMID: 15956145

181. Johnson JA, Boyce TG, Cetta F, Steckelberg JM, Johnson JN. Infective endocarditis in the pediatric patient: a 60-year single-institution review. *Mayo Clin Proc.* 2012;87(7):629–635 PMID: 22766082

182. Pasquali SK, He X, Mohamad Z, et al. Trends in infective endocarditis hospitalizations at US children's hospitals: impact of the 2007 American Heart Association Antibiotic Prophylaxis Guidelines. *Am Heart J.* 2012;163(5):894–899 PMID: 22607869

183. Wilson W, Taubert KA, Gewitz M, et al. Prevention of infective endocarditis: guidelines from the American Heart Association: a guideline from the American Heart Association Rheumatic Fever, Endocarditis, and Kawasaki Disease Committee, Council on Cardiovascular Disease in the Young, and the Council on Clinical Cardiology, Council on Cardiovascular Surgery and Anesthesia, and the Quality of Care and Outcomes Research Interdisciplinary Working Group. *Circulation.* 2007;116(15):1736–1754 PMID: 17446442

184. Silberbach M. Update: infective endocarditis prophylaxis: reckoning with the evidence. *Pediatr Rev.* 2008;29(5):169–170 PMID: 18450838

185. Ridgway JM, Parikh DA, Wright R, et al. Lemierre syndrome: a pediatric case series and review of literature. *Am J Otolaryngol.* 2010;31(1):38–45 PMID: 19944898

186. Goldenberg NA, Knapp-Clevenger R, Hays T, et al. Lemierre's and Lemierre's-like syndromes in children: survival and thromboembolic outcomes. *Pediatrics.* 2005;116(4):e543–e548 PMID: 16147971

187. Parikh SV, Memon N, Echols M, et al. Purulent pericarditis: report of 2 cases and review of the literature. *Medicine (Baltimore).* 2009;88(1):52–65 PMID: 19352300

188. Demmler GJ. Infectious pericarditis in children. *Pediatr Infect Dis J.* 2006;25(2):165–166 PMID: 16462296

189. Klein EJ, Boster DR, Stapp JR, et al. Diarrhea etiology in a children's hospital emergency department: a prospective cohort study. *Clin Infect Dis.* 2006;43(7):807–813 PMID: 16941358

190. Vernacchio L, Vezina RM, Mitchell AA, et al. Diarrhea in American infants and young children in the community setting: incidence, clinical presentation and microbiology. *Pediatr Infect Dis J.* 2006;25(1):2–7 PMID: 16395094

191. Goldwater PN. Treatment and prevention of enterohemorrhagic *Escherichia coli* infection and hemolytic uremic syndrome. *Expert Rev Anti Infect Ther.* 2007;5(4):653–663 PMID: 17678428

192. Bennish ML, Khan WA, Begum M, et al. Low risk of hemolytic uremic syndrome after early effective antimicrobial therapy for *Shigella dysenteriae* type 1 infection in Bangladesh. *Clin Infect Dis.* 2006;42(3):356–362 PMID: 16392080

193. Smith KE, Wilker PR, Reiter PL, Hedican EB, Bender JB, Hedberg CW. Antibiotic treatment of *Escherichia coli* O157 infection and the risk of hemolytic uremic syndrome, Minnesota. *Pediatr Infect Dis J.* 2012;31(1):37–41 PMID: 21892124

194. Tribble DR, Sanders JW, Pang LW, et al. Traveler's diarrhea in Thailand: randomized, double-blind trial comparing single-dose and 3-day azithromycin-based regimens with a 3-day levofloxacin regimen. *Clin Infect Dis.* 2007;44(3):338–346 PMID: 17205438

195. Ang JY, Mathur A. Traveler's diarrhea: updates for pediatricians. *Pediatr Ann.* 2008;37(12):814–820 PMID: 19143332

196. Paredes-Paredes M, Flores-Figueroa J, Dupont HL. Advances in the treatment of travelers' diarrhea. *Curr Gastroenterol Rep.* 2011;13(5):402–407 PMID: 21773708

197. DuPont HL. Azithromycin for the self-treatment of traveler's diarrhea. *Clin Infect Dis.* 2007;44(3):347–349 PMID: 17205439

198. DuPont HL, Ericsson CD, Farthing MJ, et al. Expert review of the evidence base for prevention of travelers' diarrhea. *J Travel Med.* 2009;16(3):149–160 PMID: 19538575

199. Ouyang-Latimer J, Jafri S, VanTassel A, et al. In vitro antimicrobial susceptibility of bacterial enteropathogens from international travelers to Mexico, Guatemala, and India from 2006 to 2008. *Antimicrob Agents Chemother.* 2011;55(2):874–878 PMID: 21115800

200. O'Ryan M, Lucero Y, O'Ryan-Soriano MA, et al. An update on management of severe acute infectious gastroenteritis in children. *Expert Rev Anti Infect Ther.* 2010;8(6):671–682 PMID: 20521895

201. Koo HL, DuPont HL. Rifaximin: a unique gastrointestinal-selective antibiotic for enteric diseases. *Curr Opin Gastroenterol.* 2010;26(1):17–25 PMID: 19881343

202. Riddle MS, Arnold S, Tribble DR. Effect of adjunctive loperamide in combination with antibiotics on treatment outcomes in traveler's diarrhea: a systematic review and meta-analysis. *Clin Infect Dis.* 2008;47(8):1007–1014 PMID: 18781873

203. Butler T. Loperamide for the treatment of traveler's diarrhea: broad or narrow usefulness? *Clin Infect Dis.* 2008;47(8):1015–1016 PMID: 18781871

204. Janda JM, Abbott SL. The genus *Aeromonas:* taxonomy, pathogenicity, and infection. *Clin Microbiol Rev.* 2010;23(1):35–73 PMID: 20065325

205. American Academy of Pediatrics. *Campylobacter* infections. In: Pickering LK, Baker CJ, Kimberlin DW, Long SS, eds. *Red Book: 2012 Report of the Committee on Infectious Diseases.* 29th ed. Elk Grove Village, IL: American Academy of Pediatrics; 2012:262–264

206. Fullerton KE, Ingram LA, Jones TF, et al. Sporadic campylobacter infection in infants: a population-based surveillance case-control study. *Pediatr Infect Dis J.* 2007;26(1):19–24 PMID: 17195700

207. Kirkpatrick BD, Tribble DR. Update on human Campylobacter jejuni infections. *Curr Opin Gastroenterol.* 2011;27(1):1–7 PMID: 21124212

References

Chapter 6 (cont)

208. Kaushik JS, Gupta P, Faridi MM, et al. Single dose azithromycin versus ciprofloxacin for cholera in children: a randomized controlled trial. *Indian Pediatr.* 2010;47(4):309–315 PMID: 19578229

209. Cohen MB. *Clostridium difficile* infections: emerging epidemiology and new treatments. *J Pediatr Gastroenterol Nutr.* 2009;48(suppl 2):S63–S65 PMID: 19300129

210. American Academy of Pediatrics. *Clostridium difficile.* In: Pickering LK, Baker CJ, Kimberlin DW, Long SS, eds. *Red Book: 2012 Report of the Committee on Infectious Diseases.* 29th ed. Elk Grove Village, IL: American Academy of Pediatrics; 2012:285–287

211. Kelly CP, LaMont JT. *Clostridium difficile*—more difficult than ever. *N Engl J Med.* 2008;359(18):1932–1940 PMID: 18971494

212. Hill DR, Beeching NJ. Travelers' diarrhea. *Curr Opin Infect Dis.* 2010;23(5):481–487 PMID: 20683261

213. Rimbara E, Fischbach LA, Graham DY. Optimal therapy for *Helicobacter pylori* infections. *Nat Rev Gastroenterol Hepatol.* 2011;8(2):79–88 PMID: 21293508

214. McColl KE. Clinical practice. *Helicobacter pylori* infection. *N Engl J Med.* 2010;362(17):1597–1604 PMID: 20427808

215. Bontems P, Kalach N, Oderda G, et al. Sequential therapy versus tailored triple therapies for *Helicobacter pylori* infection in children. *J Pediatr Gastroenterol Nutr.* 2011;53(6):646–650 PMID: 21701406

216. American Academy of Pediatrics. *Helicobacter pylori* infections. In: Pickering LK, Baker CJ, Kimberlin DW, Long SS, eds. *Red Book: 2012 Report of the Committee on Infectious Diseases.* 29th ed. Elk Grove Village, IL: American Academy of Pediatrics; 2012:354–356

217. Chiu CH, Lin TY, Ou JT. A clinical trial comparing oral azithromycin, cefixime and no antibiotics in the treatment of acute uncomplicated *Salmonella* enteritis in children. *J Paediatr Child Health.* 1999;35(4):372–374 PMID: 10457295

218. Onwuezobe IA, Oshun PO, Odigwe CC. Antimicrobials for treating symptomatic non-typhoidal Salmonella infection. *Cochrane Database Syst Rev.* 2012;11:CD001167 PMID: 23152205

219. Girgis NI, Sultan Y, Hammad O, et al. Comparison of the efficacy, safety and cost of cefixime, ceftriaxone and aztreonam in the treatment of multidrug-resistant *Salmonella typhi* septicemia in children. *Pediatr Infect Dis J.* 1995;14(7):603–605 PMID: 7567290

220. Frenck RW Jr, Mansour A, Nakhla I, et al. Short-course azithromycin for the treatment of uncomplicated typhoid fever in children and adolescents. *Clin Infect Dis.* 2004;38(7):951–957 PMID: 15034826

221. Effa EE, Bukirwa H. Azithromycin for treating uncomplicated typhoid and paratyphoid fever (enteric fever). *Cochrane Database Syst Rev.* 2008;(4):CD006083 PMID: 18843701

222. Effa EE, Lassi ZS, Critchley JA, et al. Fluoroquinolones for treating typhoid and paratyphoid fever (enteric fever). *Cochrane Database Syst Rev.* 2011;(10):CD004530 PMID: 21975746

223. Martin JM, Pitetti R, Maffei F, et al. Treatment of shigellosis with cefixime: two days vs five days. *Pediatr Infect Dis J.* 2000;19(6):522–526 PMID: 10877166

224. Basualdo W, Arbo A. Randomized comparison of azithromycin versus cefixime for treatment of shigellosis in children. *Pediatr Infect Dis J.* 2003;22(4):374–377 PMID: 12712971

225. American Academy of Pediatrics. *Shigella* infections. In: Pickering LK, Baker CJ, Kimberlin DW, Long SS, eds. *Red Book: 2012 Report of the Committee on Infectious Diseases.* 29th ed. Elk Grove Village, IL: American Academy of Pediatrics; 2012:645–647

226. Vinh H, Anh VT, Anh ND, et al. A multi-center randomized trial to assess the efficacy of gatifloxacin versus ciprofloxacin for the treatment of shigellosis in Vietnamese children. *PLoS Negl Trop Dis.* 2011;5(8):e1264 PMID: 21829747

227. Abdel-Haq NM, Asmar BI, Abuhammour WM, et al. *Yersinia enterocolitica* infection in children. *Pediatr Infect Dis J.* 2000;19(10):954–958 PMID: 11055595

228. Abdel-Haq NM, Papadopol R, Asmar BI, Brown WJ. Antibiotic susceptibilities of *Yersinia enterocolitica* recovered from children over a 12-year period. *Int J Antimicrob Agents.* 2006;27(5):449–452 PMID: 16621458

229. Lee SL, Islam S, Cassidy LD, et al. Antibiotics and appendicitis in the pediatric population: an American Pediatric Surgical Association Outcomes and Clinical Trials Committee systematic review. *J Pediatr Surg.* 2010;45(11):2181–2185 PMID: 21034941

230. Guillet-Caruba C, Cheikhelard A, Guillet M, et al. Bacteriologic epidemiology and empirical treatment of pediatric complicated appendicitis. *Diagn Microbiol Infect Dis.* 2011;69(4):376–381 PMID: 21396532

231. Solomkin JS, Mazuski JE, Bradley JS, et al. Diagnosis and management of complicated intra-abdominal infection in adults and children: guidelines by the Surgical Infection Society and the Infectious Diseases Society of America. *Clin Infect Dis.* 2010;50(2):133–164 PMID: 20034345

232. Bradley JS, Behrendt CE, Arrieta AC, et al. Convalescent phase outpatient parenteral antiinfective therapy for children with complicated appendicitis. *Pediatr Infect Dis J.* 2001;20(1):19–24 PMID: 11176562

233. Fraser JD, Aguayo P, Leys CM, et al. A complete course of intravenous antibiotics vs a combination of intravenous and oral antibiotics for perforated appendicitis in children: a prospective, randomized trial. *J Pediatr Surg.* 2010;45(6):1198–1202 PMID: 20620320

234. Lin YS, Huang YC, Lin TY. Abdominal tuberculosis in children: a diagnostic challenge. *J Microbiol Immunol Infect.* 2010;43(3):188–193 PMID: 21291845

235. Hlavsa MC, Moonan PK, Cowan LS, et al. Human tuberculosis due to *Mycobacterium bovis* in the United States, 1995–2005. *Clin Infect Dis.* 2008;47(2):168–175 PMID: 18532886

236. Brook I, Frazier EH. The aerobic and anaerobic bacteriology of perirectal abscesses. *J Clin Microbiol.* 1997;35(11):2974–2976 PMID: 9350771

237. Chadha V, Schaefer FS, Warady BA. Dialysis-associated peritonitis in children. *Pediatr Nephrol.* 2010;25(3):425–440 PMID: 19190935

238. Warady BA, Bakkaloglu S, Newland J, et al. Consensus guidelines for the prevention and treatment of catheter-related infections and peritonitis in pediatric patients receiving peritoneal dialysis: 2012 update. *Perit Dial Int.* 2012;32(Suppl 2):S32–S86 PMID: 22851742

239. Preece ER, Athan E, Watters DA, Gyorki DE. Spontaneous bacterial peritonitis: a rare mimic of acute appendicitis. *ANZ J Surg.* 2012;82(4):283–284 PMID: 22510192

240. Workowski K. In the clinic. Chlamydia and gonorrhea. *Ann Intern Med.* 2013;158(3):ITC2-1. Erratum in: *Ann Intern Med.* 2013;158(6):504 PMID: 23381058

241. Santillanes G, Gausche-Hill M, Lewis RJ. Are antibiotics necessary for pediatric epididymitis? *Pediatr Emerg Care.* 2011;27(3):174–178 PMID: 21346680

242. Klin B, Zlotkevich L, Horne T, et al. Epididymitis in childhood: a clinical retrospective study over 5 years. *Isr Med Assoc J.* 2001;3(11):833–835 PMID: 11729579

243. Smith JC, Mailman T, MacDonald NE. How to get and get rid of gonorrhea. *Adv Exp Med Biol.* 2013;764:219–239 PMID: 23654071

244. Centers for Disease Control and Prevention. Update to CDC's sexually transmitted diseases treatment guidelines, 2010: oral cephalosporins no longer a recommended treatment for gonococcal infections. *MMWR Morb Mortal Wkly Rep.* 2012;61(31):590–594 PMID: 22874837

245. Update to CDC's sexually transmitted diseases treatment guidelines, 2006: fluoroquinolones no longer recommended for treatment of gonococcal infections. *MMWR Morb Mortal Wkly Rep.* 2007;56(14):332–336 PMID: 17431378

246. James SH, Whitley RJ. Treatment of herpes simplex virus infections in pediatric patients: current status and future needs. *Clin Pharmacol Ther.* 2010;88(5):720–724 PMID: 20881952

247. Fife KH, Warren TJ, Justus SE, et al. An international, randomized, double-blind, placebo-controlled, study of valacyclovir for the suppression of herpes simplex virus type 2 genital herpes in newly diagnosed patients. *Sex Transm Dis.* 2008;35(7):668–673 PMID: 18461016

248. Chappell CA, Wiesenfeld HC. Pathogenesis, diagnosis, and management of severe pelvic inflammatory disease and tuboovarian abscess. *Clin Obstet Gynecol.* 2012;55(4):893–903 PMID: 23090458

249. Kingston M, French P, Goh B, et al. UK national guidelines on the management of syphilis 2008. *Int J STD AIDS.* 2008;19(11):729–740 PMID: 18931264

250. O'Brien G. Bacterial vaginosis. *Pediatr Rev.* 2008;29(6):209–211 PMID: 18515339

251. das Neves J, Pinto E, Teixeira B, et al. Local treatment of vulvovaginal candidosis: general and practical considerations. *Drugs.* 2008;68(13):1787–1802 PMID: 18729533

References

Chapter 6 (cont)

252. Jasper JM, Ward MA. *Shigella* vulvovaginitis in a prepubertal child. *Pediatr Emerg Care.* 2006;22(8):585–586 PMID: 16912629

253. Hansen MT, Sanchez VT, Eyster K, et al. *Streptococcus pyogenes* pharyngeal colonization resulting in recurrent, prepubertal vulvovaginitis. *J Pediatr Adolesc Gynecol.* 2007;20(5):315–317 PMID: 17868900

254. Yogev R, Bar-Meir M. Management of brain abscesses in children. *Pediatr Infect Dis J.* 2004;23(2):157–159 PMID: 14872183

255. Sheehan JP, Jane JA, Ray DK, et al. Brain abscess in children. *Neurosurg Focus.* 2008;24(6):e6 PMID: 18518751

256. Frazier JL, Ahn ES, Jallo GI. Management of brain abscesses in children. *Neurosurg Focus.* 2008;24(6):e8 PMID: 18518753

257. Tunkel AR, Glaser CA, Bloch KC, et al. The management of encephalitis: clinical practice guidelines by the Infectious Diseases Society of America. *Clin Infect Dis.* 2008;47(3):303–327 PMID: 18582201

258. Long SS. Encephalitis diagnosis and management in the real world. *Adv Exp Med Biol.* 2011;697:153–173 PMID: 21120725

259. Kotton CN, Kumar D, Caliendo AM, et al; Transplantation Society International CMV Consensus Group. International consensus guidelines on the management of cytomegalovirus in solid organ transplantation. *Transplantation.* 2010;89(7):779–795 PMID: 20224515

260. Doja A, Bitnun A, Ford Jones EL, et al. Pediatric Epstein-Barr virus-associated encephalitis: 10-year review. *J Child Neurol.* 2006;21(5):384–391 PMID: 16901443

261. Whitley RJ. Therapy of herpes virus infections in children. *Adv Exp Med Biol.* 2008;609:216–232 PMID: 18193668

262. Brouwer MC, McIntyre P, de Gans J, et al. Corticosteroids for acute bacterial meningitis. *Cochrane Database Syst Rev.* 2010;(9):CD004405 PMID: 20824838

263. Fritz D, Brouwer MC, van de Beek D. Dexamethasone and long-term survival in bacterial meningitis. *Neurology.* 2012;79(22):2177–2179 PMID: 23152589

264. Peltola H, Roine I, Fernandez J, et al. Adjuvant glycerol and/or dexamethasone to improve the outcomes of childhood bacterial meningitis: a prospective, randomized, double-blind, placebo-controlled trial. *Clin Infect Dis.* 2007;45(10):1277–1286 PMID: 17968821

265. Wall EC, Ajdukiewicz KM, Heyderman RS, Garner P. Osmotic therapies added to antibiotics for acute bacterial meningitis. *Cochrane Database Syst Rev.* 2013;3:CD008806 PMID: 23543568

266. Tunkel AR, Hartman BJ, Kaplan SL, et al. Practice guidelines for the management of bacterial meningitis. *Clin Infect Dis.* 2004;39(9):1267–1284 PMID: 15494903

267. Prasad K, Singh MB. Corticosteroids for managing tuberculous meningitis. *Cochrane Database Syst Rev.* 2008;(1):CD002244 PMID: 18254003

268. Kandasamy J, Dwan K, Hartley JC, et al. Antibiotic-impregnated ventriculoperitoneal shunts—a multi-centre British paediatric neurosurgery group (BPNG) study using historical controls. *Childs Nerv Syst.* 2011;27(4):575–581 PMID: 20953871

269. Al-Dabbagh M, Dobson S. Management of shunt related infections. *Adv Exp Med Biol.* 2011;719:105–115 PMID: 22125038

270. National Institute for Health and Clinical Excellence. Urinary tract infection in children: diagnosis, treatment and long-term management, clinical guideline. 2007. http://www.nice.org.uk/nicemedia/pdf/CG54fullguideline.pdf. Accessed November 14, 2013

271. Montini G, Tullus K, Hewitt I. Febrile urinary tract infections in children. *N Engl J Med.* 2011;365(3):239–250 PMID: 21774712

272. Yang CC, Shao PL, Lu CY, et al. Comparison of acute lobar nephronia and uncomplicated urinary tract infection in children. *J Microbiol Immunol Infect.* 2010;43(3):207–214 PMID: 21291848

273. Cheng CH, Tsau YK, Chang CJ, et al. Acute lobar nephronia is associated with a high incidence of renal scarring in childhood urinary tract infections. *Pediatr Infect Dis J.* 2010;29(7):624–628 PMID: 20234330

274. Hodson EM, Willis NS, Craig JC. Antibiotics for acute pyelonephritis in children. *Cochrane Database Syst Rev.* 2007;(4):CD003772 PMID: 17943796

275. Bocquet N, Sergent Alaoui A, Jais JP, et al. Randomized trial of oral versus sequential IV/oral antibiotic for acute pyelonephritis in children. *Pediatrics.* 2012;129(2):e269–e275 PMID: 22291112

276. American Academy of Pediatrics Subcommittee on Urinary Tract Infection, Steering Committee on Quality Improvement and Management. Urinary tract infection: clinical practice guideline for the diagnosis and management of the initial UTI in febrile infants and children 2 to 24 months. *Pediatrics.* 2011;128(3):595–610 PMID: 21873693

277. Craig JC, Simpson JM, Williams GJ, et al. Antibiotic prophylaxis and recurrent urinary tract infection in children. *N Engl J Med.* 2009;361(18):1748–1759 PMID: 19864673

278. Williams G, Craig JC. Long-term antibiotics for preventing recurrent urinary tract infection in children. *Cochrane Database Syst Rev.* 2011;(3):CD001534 PMID: 21412822

279. Brandstrom P, Esbjorner E, Herthelius M, et al. The Swedish reflux trial in children: I. Study design and study population characteristics. *J Urol.* 2010;184(1):274–279 PMID: 20478580

280. American Academy of Pediatrics. Actinomycosis. In: Pickering LK, Baker CJ, Kimberlin DW, Long SS, eds. *Red Book: 2012 Report of the Committee on Infectious Diseases.* 29th ed. Elk Grove Village, IL: American Academy of Pediatrics; 2012:219–220

281. Brook I. Actinomycosis: diagnosis and management. *South Med J.* 2008;101(10):1019–1023 PMID: 18791528

282. American Academy of Pediatrics, Centers for Disease Control and Prevention. AAP/CDC guidance for the clinician in management of anthrax in neonates, infants, and children following a bioterror exposure. *Pediatrics.* In press

283. Sweeney DA, Hicks CW, Cui X, et al. Anthrax infection. *Am J Respir Crit Care Med.* 2011;184(12):1333–1341 PMID: 21852539

284. American Academy of Pediatrics. Brucellosis. In: Pickering LK, Baker CJ, Kimberlin DW, Long SS, eds. *Red Book: Red Book: 2012 Report of the Committee on Infectious Diseases.* 29th ed. Elk Grove Village, IL: American Academy of Pediatrics; 2012:256–258

285. Shen MW. Diagnostic and therapeutic challenges of childhood brucellosis in a nonendemic country. *Pediatrics.* 2008;121(5):e1178–e1183 PMID: 18450861

286. Mile B, Valerija K, Krsto G, Ivan V, Ilir D, Nikola L. Doxycycline-rifampin versus doxycycline-rifampin-gentamicin in treatment of human brucellosis. *Trop Doct.* 2012;42(1):13–17 PMID: 22290107

287. Franco MP, Mulder M, Gilman RH, et al. Human brucellosis. *Lancet Infect Dis.* 2007;7(12):775–786 PMID: 18045560

288. Florin TA, Zaoutis TE, Zaoutis LB. Beyond cat scratch disease: widening spectrum of *Bartonella henselae* infection. *Pediatrics.* 2008;121(5):e1413–e1425 PMID: 18443019

289. Massei F, Gori L, Macchia P, et al. The expanded spectrum of bartonellosis in children. *Infect Dis Clin North Am.* 2005;19(3):691–711 PMID: 16102656

290. Klassen TP, Hartling L, Wiebe N, et al. Acyclovir for treating varicella in otherwise healthy children and adolescents. *Cochrane Database Syst Rev.* 2005;(4):CD002980 PMID: 16235308

291. Kimberlin DW, Jacobs RF, Weller S, et al. Pharmacokinetics and safety of extemporaneously compounded valacyclovir oral suspension in pediatric patients from 1 month through 11 years of age. *Clin Infect Dis.* 2010;50(2):221–228 PMID: 20014952

292. Saez-Llorens X, Yogev R, Arguedas A, et al. Pharmacokinetics and safety of famciclovir in children with herpes simplex or varicella-zoster virus infection. *Antimicrob Agents Chemother.* 2009;53(5):1912–1920 PMID: 19273678

293. Ismail N, Bloch KC, McBride JW. Human ehrlichiosis and anaplasmosis. *Clin Lab Med.* 2010;30(1):261–292 PMID: 20513551

294. Schutze GE, Buckingham SC, Marshall GS, et al. Human monocytic ehrlichiosis in children. *Pediatr Infect Dis J.* 2007;26(6):475–479 PMID: 17529862

295. Wormser GP, Dattwyler RJ, Shapiro ED, et al. The clinical assessment, treatment, and prevention of lyme disease, human granulocytic anaplasmosis, and babesiosis: clinical practice guidelines by the Infectious Diseases Society of America. *Clin Infect Dis.* 2006;43(9):1089–1134 PMID: 17029130

296. Thomas RJ, Dumler JS, Carlyon JA. Current management of human granulocytic anaplasmosis, human monocytic ehrlichiosis and *Ehrlichia ewingii* ehrlichiosis. *Expert Rev Anti Infect Ther.* 2009;7(6):709–722 PMID: 19681699

References

Chapter 6 (cont)

297. Freifeld AG, Bow EJ, Sepkowitz KA, et al. Clinical practice guideline for the use of antimicrobial agents in neutropenic patients with cancer: 2010 update by the Infectious Diseases Society of America. *Clin Infect Dis.* 2011;52(4):e56–e93 PMID: 21258094

298. Arnon SS. Creation and development of the public service orphan drug human botulism immune globulin. *Pediatrics.* 2007;119(4):785–789 PMID: 17403850

299. Newburger JW, Takahashi M, Gerber MA, et al. Diagnosis, treatment, and long-term management of Kawasaki disease: a statement for health professionals from the Committee on Rheumatic Fever, Endocarditis and Kawasaki Disease, Council on Cardiovascular Disease in the Young, American Heart Association. *Circulation.* 2004;110(17):2747–2771 PMID: 15505111

300. Newburger JW, Sleeper LA, McCrindle BW, et al. Randomized trial of pulsed corticosteroid therapy for primary treatment of Kawasaki disease. *N Engl J Med.* 2007;356(7):663–675 PMID: 17301297

301. Kobayashi T, Saji T, Otani T, et al; RAISE study group investigators. Efficacy of immunoglobulin plus prednisolone for prevention of coronary artery abnormalities in severe Kawasaki disease (RAISE study): a randomised, open-label, blinded-endpoints trial. *Lancet.* 2012;379(9826): 1613–1620 PMID: 22405251

302. Son MB, Gauvreau K, Burns JC, et al. Infliximab for intravenous immunoglobulin resistance in Kawasaki disease: a retrospective study. *J Pediatr.* 2011;158(4):644–649 PMID: 21129756

303. American Academy of Pediatrics. Kawasaki disease. In: Pickering LK, Baker CJ, Kimberlin DW, Long SS, eds. *Red Book: 2012 Report of the Committee on Infectious Diseases.* 29th ed. Elk Grove Village, IL: American Academy of Pediatrics; 2012:454–460

304. American Academy of Pediatrics. Leprosy. In: Pickering LK, Baker CJ, Kimberlin DW, Long SS, eds. *Red Book: 2012 Report of the Committee on Infectious Diseases.* 29th ed. Elk Grove Village, IL: American Academy of Pediatrics; 2012:466–469

305. Griffith ME, Hospenthal DR, Murray CK. Antimicrobial therapy of leptospirosis. *Curr Opin Infect Dis.* 2006;19(6):533–537 PMID: 17075327

306. American Academy of Pediatrics. Leptospirosis. In: Pickering LK, Baker CJ, Kimberlin DW, Long SS, eds. *Red Book: 2012 Report of the Committee on Infectious Diseases.* 29th ed. Elk Grove Village, IL: American Academy of Pediatrics; 2012:469–471

307. American Academy of Pediatrics. Lyme disease. In: Pickering LK, Baker CJ, Kimberlin DW, Long SS, eds. *Red Book: 2012 Report of the Committee on Infectious Diseases.* 29th ed. Elk Grove Village, IL: American Academy of Pediatrics; 2012:474–479

308. Wiersinga WJ, Currie BJ, Peacock SJ. Melioidosis. *N Engl J Med.* 2012;367(11):1035–1044 PMID: 22970946

309. Cheng AC, Chierakul W, Chaowagul W, et al. Consensus guidelines for dosing of amoxicillin-clavulanate in melioidosis. *Am J Trop Med Hyg.* 2008;78(2):208–209 PMID: 18256414

310. Cheng AC, McBryde ES, Wuthiekanun V, et al. Dosing regimens of cotrimoxazole (trimethoprim-sulfamethoxazole) for melioidosis. *Antimicrob Agents Chemother.* 2009;53(10):4193–4199 PMID: 19620336

311. Cruz AT, Ong LT, Starke JR. Mycobacterial infections in Texas children: a 5-year case series. *Pediatr Infect Dis J.* 2010;29(8):772–774 PMID: 20661106

312. Wilson JW. Nocardiosis: updates and clinical overview. *Mayo Clin Proc.* 2012;87(4):403–407 PMID: 22469352

313. American Academy of Pediatrics. Nocardiosis. In: Pickering LK, Baker CJ, Kimberlin DW, Long SS, eds. *Red Book: 2012 Report of the Committee on Infectious Diseases.* 29th ed. Elk Grove Village, IL: American Academy of Pediatrics; 2012:521–522

314. Koirala J. Plague: disease, management, and recognition of act of terrorism. *Infect Dis Clin North Am.* 2006;20(2):273–287 PMID: 16762739

315. Stenseth NC, Atshabar BB, Begon M, et al. Plague: past, present, and future. *PLoS Med.* 2008;5(1):e3 PMID: 18198939

316. American Academy of Pediatrics. Plague. In: Pickering LK, Baker CJ, Kimberlin DW, Long SS, eds. *Red Book: 2012 Report of the Committee on Infectious Diseases.* 29th ed. Elk Grove Village, IL: American Academy of Pediatrics; 2012:569–571

317. Gikas A, Kokkini S, Tsioutis C. Q fever: clinical manifestations and treatment. *Expert Rev Anti Infect Ther.* 2010;8(5):529–539 PMID: 20455682
318. Anderson A, Bijlmer H, Fournier PE, et al. Diagnosis and management of Q fever—United States, 2013: recommendations from CDC and the Q Fever Working Group. *MMWR Recomm Rep.* 2013;62(RR-03):1–30 PMID: 23535757
319. Woods CR. Rocky Mountain spotted fever in children. *Pediatr Clin North Am.* 2013;60(2):455–470 PMID: 23481111
320. American Academy of Pediatrics. Rocky Mountain spotted fever. In: Pickering LK, Baker CJ, Kimberlin DW, Long SS, eds. *Red Book: 2012 Report of the Committee on Infectious Diseases.* 29th ed. Elk Grove Village, IL: American Academy of Pediatrics; 2012:623–625
321. American Academy of Pediatrics. Tetanus. In: Pickering LK, Baker CJ, Kimberlin DW, Long SS, eds. *Red Book: 2012 Report of the Committee on Infectious Diseases.* 29th ed. Elk Grove Village, IL: American Academy of Pediatrics; 2012:707–712
322. Brook I. Current concepts in the management of Clostridium tetani infection. *Expert Rev Anti Infect Ther.* 2008;6(3):327–336 PMID: 18588497
323. Lappin E, Ferguson AJ. Gram-positive toxic shock syndromes. *Lancet Infect Dis.* 2009;9(5):281–290 PMID: 19393958
324. Dellinger RP, Levy MM, Rhodes A, et al; Surviving Sepsis Campaign Guidelines Committee including the Pediatric Subgroup. Surviving sepsis campaign: international guidelines for management of severe sepsis and septic shock: 2012. *Crit Care Med.* 2013;41(2):580–637 PMID: 23353941

Chapter 7

1. Vila J, Pachón J. Therapeutic options for Acinetobacter baumannii infections: an update. *Expert Opin Pharmacother.* 2012;13(16):2319–2336 PMID: 23035697
2. Fishbain J, Peleg AY. Treatment of *Acinetobacter* infections. *Clin Infect Dis.* 2010;51(1):79–84 PMID: 20504234
3. Segal SC, Zaoutis TE, Kagen J, et al. Epidemiology of and risk factors for *Acinetobacter* species bloodstream infection in children. *Pediatr Infect Dis J.* 2007;26(10):920–926 PMID: 17901798
4. Brook I. Actinomycosis: diagnosis and management. *South Med J.* 2008;101(10):1019–1023 PMID: 18791528
5. Janda JM, Abbott SL. The genus *Aeromonas*: taxonomy, pathogenicity, and infection. *Clin Microbiol Rev.* 2010;23(1):35–73 PMID: 20065325
6. Aravena-Román M, Inglis TJ, Henderson B, Riley TV, Chang BJ. Antimicrobial susceptibilities of Aeromonas strains isolated from clinical and environmental sources to 26 antimicrobial agents. *Antimicrob Agents Chemother.* 2012;56(2):1110–1112 PMID: 22123695
7. Paturel L, Casalta JP, Habib G, et al. *Actinobacillus actinomycetemcomitans* endocarditis. *Clin Microbiol Infect.* 2004;10(2):98–118 PMID: 14759235
8. Dumler JS, Madigan JE, Pusterla N, et al. Ehrlichioses in humans: epidemiology, clinical presentation, diagnosis, and treatment. *Clin Infect Dis.* 2007;45(suppl 1):S45–S51 PMID: 17582569
9. Ismail N, Bloch KC, McBride JW. Human ehrlichiosis and anaplasmosis. *Clin Lab Med.* 2010;30(1):261–292 PMID: 20513551
10. Therriault BL, Daniels LM, Carter YL, et al. Severe sepsis caused by *Arcanobacterium haemolyticum:* a case report and review of the literature. *Ann Pharmacother.* 2008;42(11):1697–1702 PMID: 18812563
11. American Academy of Pediatrics and Centers for Disease Control and Prevention. Pediatric anthrax clinical guidance. *Guidance for the Clinician in Rendering Care to Neonates, Infants, and Children.* Clinical report. 2014. In press
12. American Academy of Pediatrics. *Bacillus cereus* infections. In: Pickering LK, Baker CJ, Kimberlin DW, Long SS, eds. *Red Book: 2012 Report of the Committee on Infectious Diseases.* 29th ed. Elk Grove Village, IL: American Academy of Pediatrics; 2012:245–247
13. Bottone EJ. Bacillus cereus, a volatile human pathogen. *Clin Microbiol Rev.* 2010;23(2):382–398 PMID: 20375358

Chapter 7 (cont)

14. Wexler HM. Bacteroides: the good, the bad, and the nitty-gritty. *Clin Microbiol Rev.* 2007;20(4): 593–621 PMID: 17934076

15. Snydman DR, Jacobus NV, McDermott LA, et al. Lessons learned from the anaerobe survey: historical perspective and review of the most recent data (2005-2007). *Clin Infect Dis.* 2010;50(Suppl 1):S26–S33 PMID: 20067390

16. Florin TA, Zaoutis TE, Zaoutis LB. Beyond cat scratch disease: widening spectrum of *Bartonella henselae* infection. *Pediatrics.* 2008;121(5):e1413–e1425 PMID: 18443019

17. Massei F, Gori L, Macchia P, et al. The expanded spectrum of bartonellosis in children. *Infect Dis Clin North Am.* 2005;19(3):691–711 PMID: 16102656

18. Foucault C, Brouqui P, Raoult D. *Bartonella quintana* characteristics and clinical management. *Emerg Infect Dis.* 2006;12(2):217–223 PMID: 16494745

19. Tiwari T, Murphy TV, Moran J. Recommended antimicrobial agents for the treatment and postexposure prophylaxis of pertussis: 2005 CDC Guidelines. *MMWR Recomm Rep.* 2005;54(RR-14):1–16 PMID: 16340941

20. American Academy of Pediatrics. Pertussis. In: Pickering LK, Baker CJ, Kimberlin DW, Long SS, eds. *Red Book: 2012 Report of the Committee on Infectious Diseases.* 29th ed. Elk Grove Village, IL: American Academy of Pediatrics; 2012:553–566

21. Feder HM Jr. Lyme disease in children. *Infect Dis Clin North Am.* 2008;22(2):315–326 PMID: 18452804

22. American Academy of Pediatrics. Lyme disease. In: Pickering LK, Baker CJ, Kimberlin DW, Long SS, eds. *Red Book: 2012 Report of the Committee on Infectious Diseases.* 29th ed. Elk Grove Village, IL: American Academy of Pediatrics; 2012:474–479

23. Wormser GP, Dattwyler RJ, Shapiro ED, et al. The clinical assessment, treatment, and prevention of Lyme disease, human granulocytic anaplasmosis, and babesiosis: clinical practice guidelines by the Infectious Diseases Society of America. *Clin Infect Dis.* 2006;43(9):1089–1134 PMID: 17029130

24. American Academy of Pediatrics. *Borrelia* infections. In: Pickering LK, Baker CJ, Kimberlin DW, Long SS, eds. *Red Book: 2012 Report of the Committee on Infectious Diseases.* 29th ed. Elk Grove Village, IL: American Academy of Pediatrics; 2012:254–256

25. Dworkin MS, Schwan TG, Anderson DE Jr, et al. Tick-borne relapsing fever. *Infect Dis Clin North Am.* 2008;22(3):449–468 PMID: 18755384

26. American Academy of Pediatrics. Brucellosis. In: Pickering LK, Baker CJ, Kimberlin DW, Long SS, eds. *Red Book: 2012 Report of the Committee on Infectious Diseases.* 29th ed. Elk Grove Village, IL: American Academy of Pediatrics; 2012:256–258

27. Shen MW. Diagnostic and therapeutic challenges of childhood brucellosis in a nonendemic country. *Pediatrics.* 2008;121(5):e1178–e1183 PMID: 18450861

28. Mile B, Valerija K, Krsto G, Ivan V, Ilir D, Nikola L. Doxycycline-rifampin versus doxycycline-rifampin-gentamicin in treatment of human brucellosis. *Trop Doct.* 2012;42(1):13–17 PMID: 22290107

29. American Academy of Pediatrics. *Burkholderia* infections. In: Pickering LK, Baker CJ, Kimberlin DW, Long SS, eds. *Red Book: 2012 Report of the Committee on Infectious Diseases.* 29th ed. Elk Grove Village, IL: American Academy of Pediatrics; 2012:258–260

30. Waters V, Ratjen F. Multidrug-resistant organisms in cystic fibrosis: management and infection-control issues. *Expert Rev Anti Infect Ther.* 2006;4(5):807–819 PMID: 17140357

31. King P, Lomovskaya O, Griffith DC, et al. In vitro pharmacodynamics of levofloxacin and other aerosolized antibiotics under multiple conditions relevant to chronic pulmonary infection in cystic fibrosis. *Antimicrob Agents Chemother.* 2010;54(1):143–148 PMID: 19805554

32. Horsley A, Jones AM. Antibiotic treatment for Burkholderia cepacia complex in people with cystic fibrosis experiencing a pulmonary exacerbation. *Cochrane Database Syst Rev.* 2012;10:CD009529 PMID: 23076960

33. Wiersinga WJ, Currie BJ, Peacock SJ. Melioidosis. *N Engl J Med.* 2012;367(11):1035–1044 PMID: 22970946

34. Cheng AC, Chierakul W, Chaowagul W, et al. Consensus guidelines for dosing of amoxicillin-clavulanate in melioidosis. *Am J Trop Med Hyg.* 2008;78(2):208–209 PMID: 18256414

35. Cheng AC, McBryde ES, Wuthiekanun V, et al. Dosing regimens of cotrimoxazole (trimethoprim-sulfamethoxazole) for melioidosis. *Antimicrob Agents Chemother.* 2009;53(10):4193–4199 PMID: 19620336

36. Fujihara N, Takakura S, Saito T, et al. A case of perinatal sepsis by *Campylobacter fetus* subsp *fetus* infection successfully treated with carbapenem—case report and literature review. *J Infect.* 2006;53(5):e199–e202 PMID: 16542730

37. American Academy of Pediatrics. *Campylobacter* infections. In: Pickering LK, Baker CJ, Kimberlin DW, Long SS, eds. *Red Book: 2012 Report of the Committee on Infectious Diseases.* 29th ed. Elk Grove Village, IL: American Academy of Pediatrics; 2012:262–264

38. Ternhag A, Asikainen T, Giesecke J, et al. A meta-analysis on the effects of antibiotic treatment on duration of symptoms caused by infection with *Campylobacter* species. *Clin Infect Dis.* 2007;44(5):696–700 PMID: 17278062

39. Kirkpatrick BD, Tribble DR. Update on human *Campylobacter jejuni* infections. *Curr Opin Gastroenterol.* 2011;27(1):1–7 PMID: 21124212

40. Oehler RL, Velez AP, Mizrachi M, et al. Bite-related and septic syndromes caused by cats and dogs. *Lancet Infect Dis.* 2009;9(7):439–447 PMID: 19555903

41. Jolivet-Gougeon A, Sixou JL, Tamanai-Shacoori Z, Bonnaure-Mallet M. Antimicrobial treatment of Capnocytophaga infections. *Int J Antimicrob Agents.* 2007;29(4):367–373 PMID: 17250994

42. Wang HK, Chen YC, Teng LJ, et al. Brain abscess associated with multidrug-resistant *Capnocytophaga ochracea* infection. *J Clin Microbiol.* 2007;45(2):645–647 PMID: 17135428

43. Blasi F, Tarsia P, Aliberti S. *Chlamydophila pneumoniae.* *Clin Microbiol Infect.* 2009;15(1):29–35 PMID: 19220337

44. Burillo A, Bouza E. *Chlamydophila pneumoniae.* *Infect Dis Clin North Am.* 2010;24(1):61–71 PMID: 20171546

45. Beeckman DS, Vanrompay DC. Zoonotic *Chlamydophila psittaci* infections from a clinical perspective. *Clin Microbiol Infect.* 2009;15(1):11–17 PMID: 19220335

46. Darville T. *Chlamydia trachomatis* infections in neonates and young children. *Semin Pediatr Infect Dis.* 2005;16(4):235–244 PMID: 16210104

47. American Academy of Pediatrics. Chlamydial infections. In: Pickering LK, Baker CJ, Kimberlin DW, Long SS, eds. *Red Book: 2012 Report of the Committee on Infectious Diseases.* 29th ed. Elk Grove Village, IL: American Academy of Pediatrics; 2012:272–281

48. Workowski KA, Berman S. Sexually transmitted diseases treatment guidelines, 2010. *MMWR Recomm Rep.* 2010;59(RR-12):1–110 PMID: 21160459

49. Campbell JI, Lan NP, Qui PT, Dung le T, Farrar JJ, Baker S. A successful antimicrobial regime for Chromobacterium violaceum induced bacteremia. *BMC Infect Dis.* 2013;13:4 PMID: 23286235

50. Sirinavin S, Techasaensiri C, Benjaponpitak S, et al. Invasive *Chromobacterium violaceum* infection in children: case report and review. *Pediatr Infect Dis J.* 2005;24(6):559–561 PMID: 15933571

51. Chowdhry SA, Cohen AR. Citrobacter brain abscesses in neonates: early surgical intervention and review of the literature. *Childs Nerv Syst.* 2012;28(10):1715–1722 PMID: 22526440

52. Doran TI. The role of *Citrobacter* in clinical disease of children: review. *Clin Infect Dis.* 1999;28(2):384–394 PMID: 10064257

53. Jacoby GA. AmpC beta-lactamases. *Clin Microbiol Rev.* 2009;22(1):161–182 PMID: 19136439

54. Sobel J. Botulism. *Clin Infect Dis.* 2005;41(8):1167–1173 PMID: 16163636

55. American Academy of Pediatrics. Botulism and infant botulism. In: Pickering LK, Baker CJ, Kimberlin DW, Long SS, eds. *Red Book: 2012 Report of the Committee on Infectious Diseases.* 29th ed. Elk Grove Village, IL: American Academy of Pediatrics; 2012:281–284

56. Hill SE, Iqbal R, Cadiz CL, Le J. Foodborne botulism treated with heptavalent botulism antitoxin. *Ann Pharmacother.* 2013;47(2):e12 PMID: 23362041

57. Cohen MB. *Clostridium difficile* infections: emerging epidemiology and new treatments. *J Pediatr Gastroenterol Nutr.* 2009;48(suppl 2):S63–S65 PMID: 19300129

58. American Academy of Pediatrics. *Clostridium difficile.* In: Pickering LK, Baker CJ, Kimberlin DW, Long SS, eds. *Red Book: 2012 Report of the Committee on Infectious Diseases.* 29th ed. Elk Grove Village, IL: American Academy of Pediatrics; 2012:285–287

References

Chapter 7 (cont)

59. American Academy of Pediatrics. Clostridial myonecrosis. In: Pickering LK, Baker CJ, Kimberlin DW, Long SS, eds. *Red Book: 2012 Report of the Committee on Infectious Diseases.* 29th ed. Elk Grove Village, IL: American Academy of Pediatrics; 2012:284–285

60. American Academy of Pediatrics. *Clostridium perfringens* food poisoning. In: Pickering LK, Baker CJ, Kimberlin DW, Long SS, eds. *Red Book: 2012 Report of the Committee on Infectious Diseases.* 29th ed. Elk Grove Village, IL: American Academy of Pediatrics; 2012:288–289

61. American Academy of Pediatrics. Tetanus. In: Pickering LK, Baker CJ, Kimberlin DW, Long SS, eds. *Red Book: 2012 Report of the Committee on Infectious Diseases.* 29th ed. Elk Grove Village, IL: American Academy of Pediatrics; 2012:707–712

62. Brook I. Current concepts in the management of *Clostridium tetani* infection. *Expert Rev Anti Infect Ther.* 2008;6(3):327–336 PMID: 18588497

63. American Academy of Pediatrics. Diphtheria. In: Pickering LK, Baker CJ, Kimberlin DW, Long SS, eds. *Red Book: 2012 Report of the Committee on Infectious Diseases.* 29th ed. Elk Grove Village, IL: American Academy of Pediatrics; 2012:307–311

64. Fernandez-Roblas R, Adames H, Martín-de-Hijas NZ, Almeida DG, Gadea I, Esteban J. In vitro activity of tigecycline and 10 other antimicrobials against clinical isolates of the genus Corynebacterium. *Int J Antimicrob Agents.* 2009;33(5):453–455 PMID: 19153032

65. Holdiness MR. Management of cutaneous erythrasma. *Drugs.* 2002;62(8):1131–1141 PMID: 12010076

66. Dalal A, Likhi R. *Corynebacterium minutissimum* bacteremia and meningitis: a case report and review of literature. *J Infect.* 2008;56(1):77–79 PMID: 18036665

67. Anderson A, Bijlmer H, Fournier PE, et al. Diagnosis and management of Q fever—United States, 2013: recommendations from CDC and the Q Fever Working Group. *MMWR Recomm Rep.* 2013;62(RR-03):1–30 PMID: 23535757

68. Parker NR, Barralet JH, Bell AM. Q fever. *Lancet.* 2006;367(9511):679–688 PMID: 16503466

69. Pritt BS, Sloan LM, Johnson DK, et al. Emergence of a new pathogenic Ehrlichia species, Wisconsin and Minnesota, 2009. *N Engl J Med.* 2011;365(5):422–429 PMID: 21812671

70. Paul K, Patel SS. *Eikenella corrodens* infections in children and adolescents: case reports and review of the literature. *Clin Infect Dis.* 2001;33(1):54–61 PMID: 11389495

71. Ceyhan M, Celik M. Elizabethkingia meningosepticum (Chryseobacterium meningosepticum) infections in children. *Int J Pediatr.* 2011;2011:215–237 PMID: 22046191

72. Hsu MS, Liao CH, Huang YT, et al. Clinical features, antimicrobial susceptibilities, and outcomes of *Elizabethkingia meningoseptica (Chryseobacterium meningosepticum)* bacteremia at a medical center in Taiwan, 1999–2006. *Eur J Clin Microbiol Infect Dis.* 2011;30(10):1271–1278 PMID: 21461847

73. Detection of Enterobacteriaceae isolates carrying metallo-beta-lactamase—United States, 2010. *MMWR Morb Mortal Wkly Rep.* 2010;59(24):750 PMID: 20577157

74. Dowzicky MJ, Park CH. Update on antimicrobial susceptibility rates among gram-negative and gram-positive organisms in the United States: results from the Tigecycline Evaluation and Surveillance Trial (TEST) 2005 to 2007. *Clin Ther.* 2008;30(11):2040–2050 PMID: 19108792

75. Livermore DM, Warner M, Mushtaq S, Doumith M, Zhang J, Woodford N. What remains against carbapenem-resistant Enterobacteriaceae? Evaluation of chloramphenicol, ciprofloxacin, colistin, fosfomycin, minocycline, nitrofurantoin, temocillin and tigecycline. *Int J Antimicrob Agents.* 2011;37(5):415–419 PMID: 21429716

76. Arias CA, Murray BE. Emergence and management of drug-resistant enterococcal infections. *Expert Rev Anti Infect Ther.* 2008;6(5):637–655 PMID: 18847403

77. American Academy of Pediatrics. Non-group A or B streptococcal and enterococcal infections. In: Pickering LK, Baker CJ, Kimberlin DW, Long SS, eds. *Red Book: 2012 Report of the Committee on Infectious Diseases.* 29th ed. Elk Grove Village, IL: American Academy of Pediatrics; 2012:686–688

78. Hollenbeck BL, Rice LB. Intrinsic and acquired resistance mechanisms in enterococcus. *Virulence.* 2012;3(5):421–433 PMID: 23076243

79. Veraldi S, Girgenti V, Dassoni F, et al. Erysipeloid: a review. *Clin Exp Dermatol.* 2009;34(8):859–862 PMID: 19663854

80. Pitout JD. Extraintestinal pathogenic Escherichia coli: an update on antimicrobial resistance, laboratory diagnosis and treatment. *Expert Rev Anti Infect Ther.* 2012;10(10):1165–1176 PMID: 23199402

81. Hepburn MJ, Simpson AJ. Tularemia: current diagnosis and treatment options. *Expert Rev Anti Infect Ther.* 2008;6(2):231–240 PMID: 18380605

82. Huggan PJ, Murdoch DR. Fusobacterial infections: clinical spectrum and incidence of invasive disease. *J Infect.* 2008;57(4):283–239 PMID: 18805588

83. Riordan T. Human infection with *Fusobacterium necrophorum* (necrobacillosis), with a focus on Lemierre's syndrome. *Clin Microbiol Rev.* 2007;20(4):622–659 PMID: 17934077

84. Donders G. Diagnosis and management of bacterial vaginosis and other types of abnormal vaginal bacterial flora: a review. *Obstet Gynecol Surv.* 2010;65(7):462–473 PMID: 20723268

85. Huang ST, Lee HC, Lee NY, et al. Clinical characteristics of invasive *Haemophilus aphrophilus* infections. *J Microbiol Immunol Infect.* 2005;38(4):271–276 PMID: 16118675

86. Tristram S, Jacobs MR, Appelbaum PC. Antimicrobial resistance in *Haemophilus influenzae*. *Clin Microbiol Rev.* 2007;20(2):368–389 PMID: 17428889

87. Rimbara E, Fischbach LA, Graham DY. Optimal therapy for *Helicobacter pylori* infections. *Nat Rev Gastroenterol Hepatol.* 2011;8(2):79–88 PMID: 21293508

88. McColl KE. Clinical practice. *Helicobacter pylori* infection. *N Engl J Med.* 2010;362(17):1597–1604 PMID: 20427808

89. Georgopoulos SD, Papastergiou V, Karatapanis S. Current options for the treatment of Helicobacter pylori. *Expert Opin Pharmacother.* 2013;14(2):211–223 PMID: 23331077

90. Petrosillo N, Giannella M, Lewis R, Viale P. Treatment of carbapenem-resistant Klebsiella pneumoniae: the state of the art. *Expert Rev Anti Infect Ther.* 2013;11(2):159–177 PMID: 23409822

91. Nordmann P, Cuzon G, Naas T. The real threat of *Klebsiella pneumoniae* carbapenemase-producing bacteria. *Lancet Infect Dis.* 2009;9(4):228–236 PMID: 19324295

92. Bergen PJ, Landersdorfer CB, Lee HJ, Li J, Nation RL. 'Old' antibiotics for emerging multidrug-resistant bacteria. *Curr Opin Infect Dis.* 2012;25(6):626–633 PMID: 23041772

93. Yagupsky P, Porsch E, St Geme JW 3rd. *Kingella kingae:* an emerging pathogen in young children. *Pediatrics.* 2011;127(3):557–565 PMID: 21321033

94. Yagupsky P. Antibiotic susceptibility of Kingella kingae isolates from children with skeletal system infections. *Pediatr Infect Dis J.* 2012;31(2):212 PMID: 22252209

95. Viasus D, Di Yacovo S, Garcia-Vidal C, et al. Community-acquired Legionella pneumophila pneumonia: a single-center experience with 214 hospitalized sporadic cases over 15 years. *Medicine (Baltimore).* 2013;92(1):51–60 PMID: 23266795

96. Griffith ME, Hospenthal DR, Murray CK. Antimicrobial therapy of leptospirosis. *Curr Opin Infect Dis.* 2006;19(6):533–537 PMID: 17075327

97. Florescu D, Hill L, Sudan D, et al. Leuconostoc bacteremia in pediatric patients with short bowel syndrome: case series and review. *Pediatr Infect Dis J.* 2008;27(11):1013–1019 PMID: 18833028

98. Bortolussi R. Listeriosis: a primer. *CMAJ.* 2008;179(8):795–797 PMID: 18787096

99. Murphy TF, Parameswaran GI. *Moraxella catarrhalis,* a human respiratory tract pathogen. *Clin Infect Dis.* 2009;49(1):124–131 PMID: 19480579

100. Falagas ME, Kavvadia PK, Mantadakis E, et al. *Morganella morganii* infections in a general tertiary hospital. *Infection.* 2006;34(6):315–321 PMID: 17180585

101. Sinha AK, Kempley ST, Price E, et al. Early onset *Morganella morganii* sepsis in a newborn infant with emergence of cephalosporin resistance caused by depression of AMPC beta-lactamase production. *Pediatr Infect Dis J.* 2006;25(4):376–377 PMID: 16567997

102. American Academy of Pediatrics. Diseases caused by nontuberculous mycobacteria. In: Pickering LK, Baker CJ, Kimberlin DW, Long SS, eds. *Red Book: 2012 Report of the Committee on Infectious Diseases.* 29th ed. Elk Grove Village, IL: American Academy of Pediatrics; 2012:759–767

103. Petrini B. *Mycobacterium abscessus:* an emerging rapid-growing potential pathogen. *APMIS.* 2006;114(5):319–328 PMID: 16725007

104. Griffith DE, Aksamit T, Brown-Elliott BA, et al. An official ATS/IDSA statement: diagnosis, treatment, and prevention of nontuberculous mycobacterial diseases. *Am J Respir Crit Care Med.* 2007;175(4):367–416 PMID: 17277290

Chapter 7 (cont)

105. American Academy of Pediatrics. Tuberculosis. In: Pickering LK, Baker CJ, Kimberlin DW, Long SS, eds. *Red Book: 2012 Report of the Committee on Infectious Diseases.* 29th ed. Elk Grove Village, IL: American Academy of Pediatrics; 2012:736–759

106. Hlavsa MC, Moonan PK, Cowan LS, et al. Human tuberculosis due to *Mycobacterium bovis* in the United States, 1995–2005. *Clin Infect Dis.* 2008;47(2):168–175 PMID: 18532886

107. Hay RJ. *Mycobacterium chelonae*—a growing problem in soft tissue infection. *Curr Opin Infect Dis.* 2009;22(2):99–101 PMID: 19276876

108. Uslan DZ, Kowalski TJ, Wengenack NL, et al. Skin and soft tissue infections due to rapidly growing mycobacteria: comparison of clinical features, treatment, and susceptibility. *Arch Dermatol.* 2006;142(10):1287–1292 PMID: 17043183

109. American Academy of Pediatrics. Leprosy. In: Pickering LK, Baker CJ, Kimberlin DW, Long SS, eds. *Red Book: 2012 Report of the Committee on Infectious Diseases.* 29th ed. Elk Grove Village, IL: American Academy of Pediatrics; 2012:466–469

110. Doedens RA, van der Sar AM, Bitter W, et al. Transmission of *Mycobacterium marinum* from fish to a very young child. *Pediatr Infect Dis J.* 2008;27(1):81–83 PMID: 18162949

111. Treatment of tuberculosis. *MMWR Recomm Rep.* 2003;52(RR-11):1–77 PMID: 12836625

112. Waites KB, Crabb DM, Duffy LB. Comparative in vitro activities of the investigational fluoroquinolone DC-159a and other antimicrobial agents against human mycoplasmas and ureaplasmas. *Antimicrob Agents Chemother.* 2008;52(10):3776–3778 PMID: 18663020

113. Watt KM, Massaro MM, Smith B, Cohen-Wolkowiez M, Benjamin DK Jr, Laughon MM. Pharmacokinetics of moxifloxacin in an infant with Mycoplasma hominis meningitis. *Pediatr Infect Dis J.* 2012;31(2):197–199 PMID: 22016080

114. Bradley JS, Byington CL, Shah SS, et al. The management of community-acquired pneumonia in infants and children older than 3 months of age: clinical practice guidelines by the Pediatric Infectious Diseases Society and the Infectious Diseases Society of America. *Clin Infect Dis.* 2011;53(7):e25–e76 PMID: 21880587

115. Akaike H, Miyashita N, Kubo M, et al; Atypical Pathogen Study Group. In vitro activities of 11 antimicrobial agents against macrolide-resistant Mycoplasma pneumoniae isolates from pediatric patients: results from a multicenter surveillance study. *Jpn J Infect Dis.* 2012;65(6): 535–538 PMID: 23183207

116. Centers for Disease Control and Prevention. Update to CDC's sexually transmitted diseases treatment guidelines, 2010: oral cephalosporins no longer a recommended treatment for gonococcal infections. *MMWR Morb Mortal Wkly Rep.* 2012;61(31):590–594

117. Wu HM, Harcourt BH, Hatcher CP, et al. Emergence of ciprofloxacin-resistant *Neisseria meningitidis* in North America. *N Engl J Med.* 2009;360(9):886–892 PMID: 19246360

118. Glikman D, Matushek SM, Kahana MD, Daum RS. Pneumonia and empyema caused by penicillin-resistant Neisseria meningitidis: a case report and literature review. *Pediatrics.* 2006;117(5):e1061–e1066 PMID: 16606681

119. Wilson JW. Nocardiosis: updates and clinical overview. *Mayo Clin Proc.* 2012;87(4):403–407 PMID: 22469352

120. American Academy of Pediatrics. Nocardiosis. In: Pickering LK, Baker CJ, Kimberlin DW, Long SS, eds. *Red Book: 2012 Report of the Committee on Infectious Diseases.* 29th ed. Elk Grove Village, IL: American Academy of Pediatrics; 2012:521–522

121. Rowlinson MC, Bruckner DA, Hinnebusch C, et al. Clearance of *Cellulosimicrobium cellulans* bacteremia in a child without central venous catheter removal. *J Clin Microbiol.* 2006;44(7): 2650–2654 PMID: 16825406

122. Goldstein EJ, Citron DM, Merriam CV, Tyrrell KL. Ceftaroline versus isolates from animal bite wounds: comparative in vitro activities against 243 isolates, including 156 Pasteurella species isolates. *Antimicrob Agents Chemother.* 2012;56(12):6319–6323 PMID: 23027193

123. Brazier J, Chmelar D, Dubreuil L, et al. European surveillance study on antimicrobial susceptibility of Gram-positive anaerobic cocci. *Int J Antimicrob Agents.* 2008;31(4):316–320 PMID: 18180149

124. Ozdemir O, Sari S, Terzioglu S, Zenciroglu A. Plesiomonas shigelloides sepsis and meningoencephalitis in a surviving neonate. *J Microbiol Immunol Infect.* 2010;43(4):344–346 PMID: 20688296

125. Stock I, Wiedemann B. Natural antimicrobial susceptibilities of *Plesiomonas shigelloides* strains. *J Antimicrob Chemother.* 2001;48(6):803–811 PMID: 11733464

126. Kommedal O, Nystad TW, Bolstad B, et al. Antibiotic susceptibility of blood culture isolates of anaerobic bacteria at a Norwegian university hospital. *APMIS.* 2007;115(8):956–961 PMID: 17696952

127. Nisbet M, Briggs S, Ellis-Pegler R, et al. *Propionibacterium acnes:* an under-appreciated cause of post-neurosurgical infection. *J Antimicrob Chemother.* 2007;60(5):1097–1103 PMID: 17875606

128. Perry A, Lambert P. Propionibacterium acnes: infection beyond the skin. *Expert Rev Anti Infect Ther.* 2011;9(12):1149–1156 PMID: 22114965

129. Karlowsky JA, Lagacé-Wiens PR, Simner PJ, et al. Antimicrobial resistance in urinary tract pathogens in Canada from 2007 to 2009: CANWARD surveillance study. *Antimicrob Agents Chemother.* 2011;55(7):3169–3175 PMID: 21537027

130. Harris PN, Ferguson JK. Antibiotic therapy for inducible AmpC β-lactamase-producing Gram-negative bacilli: what are the alternatives to carbapenems, quinolones and aminoglycosides? *Int J Antimicrob Agents.* 2012;40(4):297–305 PMID: 22824371

131. Tumbarello M, Citton R, Spanu T, et al. ESBL-producing multidrug-resistant *Providencia stuartii* infections in a university hospital. *J Antimicrob Chemother.* 2004;53(2):277–282 PMID: 14688041

132. Grgurich PE, Hudcova J, Lei Y, Sarwar A, Craven DE. Management and prevention of ventilator-associated pneumonia caused by multidrug-resistant pathogens. *Expert Rev Respir Med.* 2012;6(5):533–555 PMID: 23134248

133. Tam VH, Chang KT, Abdelraouf K, et al. Prevalence, resistance mechanisms, and susceptibility of multidrug-resistant bloodstream isolates of *Pseudomonas aeruginosa. Antimicrob Agents Chemother.* 2010;54(3):1160–1164 PMID: 20086165

134. Freifeld AG, Bow EJ, Sepkowitz KA, et al. Clinical practice guideline for the use of antimicrobial agents in neutropenic patients with cancer: 2010 update by the Infectious Diseases Society of America. *Clin Infect Dis.* 2011;52(4):e56–e93 PMID: 21258094

135. Bergen PJ, Landersdorfer CB, Lee HJ, Li J, Nation RL. 'Old' antibiotics for emerging multidrug-resistant bacteria. *Curr Opin Infect Dis.* 2012;25(6):626–633 PMID: 23041772

136. Döring G, Flume P, Heijerman H, Elborn JS; Consensus Study Group. Treatment of lung infection in patients with cystic fibrosis: current and future strategies. *J Cyst Fibros.* 2012;11(6):   461–479 PMID: 23137712

137. Mogayzel PJ Jr, Naureckas ET, Robinson KA, et al; Pulmonary Clinical Practice Guidelines Committee. Cystic fibrosis pulmonary guidelines. Chronic medications for maintenance of lung health. *Am J Respir Crit Care Med.* 2013;187(7):680–689 PMID: 23540878

138. Saiman L. Clinical utility of synergy testing for multidrug-resistant *Pseudomonas aeruginosa* isolated from patients with cystic fibrosis: 'the motion for'. *Paediatr Respir Rev.* 2007;8(3):249–255 PMID: 17868923

139. Yamshchikov AV, Schuetz A, Lyon GM. *Rhodococcus equi* infection. *Lancet Infect Dis.* 2010;10(5):350–359 PMID: 20417417

140. American Academy of Pediatrics. Rickettsial diseases. In: Pickering LK, Baker CJ, Kimberlin DW, Long SS, eds. *Red Book: 2012 Report of the Committee on Infectious Diseases.* 29th ed. Elk Grove Village, IL: American Academy of Pediatrics; 2012:620–625

141. Buckingham SC, Marshall GS, Schutze GE, et al. Clinical and laboratory features, hospital course, and outcome of Rocky Mountain spotted fever in children. *J Pediatr.* 2007;150(2):180–184 PMID: 17236987

142. American Academy of Pediatrics. *Salmonella* infections. In: Pickering LK, Baker CJ, Kimberlin DW, Long SS, eds. *Red Book: 2012 Report of the Committee on Infectious Diseases.* 29th ed. Elk Grove Village, IL: American Academy of Pediatrics; 2012:635–640

143. Chimalizeni Y, Kawaza K, Molyneux E. The epidemiology and management of non typhoidal salmonella infections. *Adv Exp Med Biol.* 2010;659:33–46 PMID: 20204753

References

Chapter 7 (cont)

144. Onwuezobe IA, Oshun PO, Odigwe CC. Antimicrobials for treating symptomatic non-typhoidal Salmonella infection. *Cochrane Database Syst Rev.* 2012;11:CD001167 PMID: 23152205

145. Kato Y, Fukayama M, Adachi T, et al. Multidrug-resistant typhoid fever outbreak in travelers returning from Bangladesh. *Emerg Infect Dis.* 2007;13(12):1954–1955 PMID: 18258058

146. To KK, Wong SS, Cheng VC, et al. Epidemiology and clinical features of Shewanella infection over an eight-year period. *Scand J Infect Dis.* 2010;42(10):757–762 PMID: 20524786

147. Sivapalasingam S, Nelson JM, Joyce K, et al. High prevalence of antimicrobial resistance among *Shigella* isolates in the United States tested by the National Antimicrobial Resistance Monitoring System from 1999 to 2002. *Antimicrob Agents Chemother.* 2006;50(1):49–54 PMID: 16377666

148. American Academy of Pediatrics. *Shigella* infections. In: Pickering LK, Baker CJ, Kimberlin DW, Long SS, eds. *Red Book: 2012 Report of the Committee on Infectious Diseases.* 29th ed. Elk Grove Village, IL: American Academy of Pediatrics; 2012:645–647

149. Sjölund Karlsson M, Bowen A, Reporter R, et al. Outbreak of infections caused by Shigella sonnei with reduced susceptibility to azithromycin in the United States. *Antimicrob Agents Chemother.* 2013;57(3):1559–1560 PMID: 23274665

150. Vinh H, Anh VT, Anh ND, Campbell JI, et al. A multi-center randomized trial to assess the efficacy of gatifloxacin versus ciprofloxacin for the treatment of shigellosis in Vietnamese children. *PLoS Negl Trop Dis.* 2011;5(8):e1264 PMID: 21829747

151. Gaastra W, Boot R, Ho HT, et al. Rat bite fever. *Vet Microbiol.* 2009;133(3):211–228 PMID: 19008054

152. American Academy of Pediatrics. Rat bite fever. In: Pickering LK, Baker CJ, Kimberlin DW, Long SS, eds. *Red Book: 2012 Report of the Committee on Infectious Diseases.* 29th ed. Elk Grove Village, IL: American Academy of Pediatrics; 2012:608–609

153. Liu C, Bayer A, Cosgrove SE, et al. Clinical practice guidelines by the Infectious Diseases Society of America for the treatment of methicillin-resistant *Staphylococcus aureus* infections in adults and children. *Clin Infect Dis.* 2011;52(3):e18–e55 PMID: 21208910

154. Long CB, Madan RP, Herold BC. Diagnosis and management of community-associated MRSA infections in children. *Expert Rev Anti Infect Ther.* 2010;8(2):183–195 PMID: 20109048

155. Hidron AI, Edwards JR, Patel J, et al. NHSN annual update: antimicrobial-resistant pathogens associated with healthcare-associated infections: annual summary of data reported to the National Healthcare Safety Network at the Centers for Disease Control and Prevention, 2006–2007. *Infect Control Hosp Epidemiol.* 2008;29(11):996–1011 PMID: 18947320

156. Cheung GY, Otto M. Understanding the significance of Staphylococcus epidermidis bacteremia in babies and children. *Curr Opin Infect Dis.* 2010;23(3):208–216 PMID: 20179594

157. Falagas ME, Valkimadi PE, Huang YT, Matthaiou DK, Hsueh PR. Therapeutic options for Stenotrophomonas maltophilia infections beyond co-trimoxazole: a systematic review. *J Antimicrob Chemother.* 2008;62(5):889–894 PMID: 1866294

158. Looney WJ, Narita M, Muhlemann K. *Stenotrophomonas maltophilia:* an emerging opportunist human pathogen. *Lancet Infect Dis.* 2009;9(5):312–323 PMID: 19393961

159. American Academy of Pediatrics. Group A streptococcal infections. In: Pickering LK, Baker CJ, Kimberlin DW, Long SS, eds. *Red Book: 2012 Report of the Committee on Infectious Diseases.* 29th ed. Elk Grove Village, IL: American Academy of Pediatrics; 2012:668–680

160. American Academy of Pediatrics. Group B streptococcal infections. In: Pickering LK, Baker CJ, Kimberlin DW, Long SS, eds. *Red Book: 2012 Report of the Committee on Infectious Diseases.* 29th ed. Elk Grove Village, IL: American Academy of Pediatrics; 2012:680–688

161. Belko J, Goldmann DA, Macone A, et al. Clinically significant infections with organisms of the *Streptococcus milleri* group. *Pediatr Infect Dis J.* 2002;21(8):715–723 PMID: 12192158

162. Broyles LN, Van Beneden C, Beall B, et al. Population-based study of invasive disease due to beta-hemolytic streptococci of groups other than A and B. *Clin Infect Dis.* 2009;48(6):706–712 PMID: 19187026

163. Stelzmueller I, Fille M, Hager J, et al. Group *milleri* streptococci in paediatric infections. *Eur J Pediatr Surg.* 2009;19(1):21–24 PMID: 19221948

164. Deutschmann MW, Livingstone D, Cho JJ, Vanderkooi OG, Brookes JT. The significance of Streptococcus anginosus group in intracranial complications of pediatric rhinosinusitis. *JAMA Otolaryngol Head Neck Surg.* 2013;139(2):157–160 PMID: 23429946

165. Jacobs MR. Antimicrobial-resistant *Streptococcus pneumoniae:* trends and management. *Expert Rev Anti Infect Ther.* 2008;6(5):619–635 PMID: 18847402

166. American Academy of Pediatrics. Pneumococcal infections. In: Pickering LK, Baker CJ, Kimberlin DW, Long SS, eds. *Red Book: 2012 Report of the Committee on Infectious Diseases.* 29th ed. Elk Grove Village, IL: American Academy of Pediatrics; 2012:571–582

167. Jones RN, Jacobs MR, Sader HS. Evolving trends in *Streptococcus pneumoniae* resistance: implications for therapy of community-acquired bacterial pneumonia. *Int J Antimicrob Agents.* 2010;36(3):197–204 PMID: 20558045

168. Baddour LM, Wilson WR, Bayer AS, et al. Infective endocarditis: diagnosis, antimicrobial therapy, and management of complications: a statement for healthcare professionals from the Committee on Rheumatic Fever, Endocarditis, and Kawasaki Disease, Council on Cardiovascular Disease in the Young, and the Councils on Clinical Cardiology, Stroke, and Cardiovascular Surgery and Anesthesia, American Heart Association: endorsed by the Infectious Diseases Society of America. *Circulation.* 2005;111(23):e394–e434 PMID: 15956145

169. Kaplan SL, Mason EO Jr, Wald ER, et al. Decrease of invasive pneumococcal infections in children among 8 children's hospitals in the United States after the introduction of the 7-valent pneumococcal conjugate vaccine. *Pediatrics.* 2004;113(3 Pt1):443–449 PMID: 14993532

170. American Academy of Pediatrics. Syphilis. In: Pickering LK, Baker CJ, Kimberlin DW, Long SS, eds. *Red Book: 2012 Report of the Committee on Infectious Diseases.* 29th ed. Elk Grove Village, IL: American Academy of Pediatrics; 2012:690–703

171. Schelonka RL, Waites KB. *Ureaplasma* infection and neonatal lung disease. *Semin Perinatol.* 2007;31(1):2–9 PMID: 17317421

172. American Academy of Pediatrics. Cholera. In: Pickering LK, Baker CJ, Kimberlin DW, Long SS, eds. *Red Book: 2012 Report of the Committee on Infectious Diseases.* 29th ed. Elk Grove Village, IL: American Academy of Pediatrics; 2012:789–791

173. Charles RC, Ryan ET. Cholera in the 21st century. *Curr Opin Infect Dis.* 2011;24(5):472–477 PMID: 21799407

174. Dechet AM, Yu PA, Koram N, et al. Nonfoodborne *Vibrio* infections: an important cause of morbidity and mortality in the United States, 1997–2006. *Clin Infect Dis.* 2008;46(7):970–976 PMID: 18444811

175. Daniels NA. Vibrio vulnificus oysters: pearls and perils. *Clin Infect Dis.* 2011;52(6):788–792 PMID: 21367733

176. Fàbrega A, Vila J. Yersinia enterocolitica: pathogenesis, virulence and antimicrobial resistance. *Enferm Infecc Microbiol Clin.* 2012;30(1):24–32 PMID: 22019131

177. American Academy of Pediatrics. *Yersinia enterocolitica* and *Yersina pseudotuberculosis.* In: Pickering LK, Baker CJ, Kimberlin DW, Long SS, eds. *Red Book: 2012 Report of the Committee on Infectious Diseases.* 29th ed. Elk Grove Village, IL: American Academy of Pediatrics; 2012:795–797

178. American Academy of Pediatrics. Plague. In: Pickering LK, Baker CJ, Kimberlin DW, Long SS, eds. *Red Book: 2012 Report of the Committee on Infectious Diseases.* 29th ed. Elk Grove Village, IL: American Academy of Pediatrics; 2012:569–571

179. Butler T. Plague into the 21st century. *Clin Infect Dis.* 2009;49(5):736–742 PMID: 19606935

180. Tauxe RV. Salad and pseudoappendicitis: *Yersinia pseudotuberculosis* as a foodborne pathogen. *J Infect Dis.* 2004;189(5):761–763 PMID: 14976590

References

Chapter 8

1. Cornely OA, Bohme A, Buchheidt D, et al. Primary prophylaxis of invasive fungal infections in patients with hematologic malignancies. Recommendations of the Infectious Diseases Working Party of the German Society for Haematology and Oncology. *Haematologica.* 2009;94(1):113–122 PMID: 19066334

2. Almyroudis NG, Segal BH. Prevention and treatment of invasive fungal diseases in neutropenic patients. *Curr Opin Infect Dis.* 2009;22(4):385–393 PMID: 19506476

3. Maschmeyer G. The changing face of febrile neutropenia-from monotherapy to moulds to mucositis. Prevention of mould infections. *J Antimicrob Chemother.* 2009;63(suppl 1):i27–i30 PMID: 19372178

4. Freifeld AG, Bow EJ, Sepkowitz KA, et al. Clinical practice guideline for the use of antimicrobial agents in neutropenic patients with cancer: 2010 update by the Infectious Diseases Society of America. *Clin Infect Dis.* 2011;52(4):e56–e93 PMID: 21258094

5. De Pauw BE, Donnelly JP. Prophylaxis and aspergillosis—has the principle been proven? *N Engl J Med.* 2007;356(4):409–411 PMID: 17251538

6. Playford EG, Webster AC, Sorell TC, et al. Antifungal agents for preventing fungal infections in solid organ transplant recipients. *Cochrane Database Syst Rev.* 2004;(3):CD004291 PMID: 15266524

7. Salavert M. Prophylaxis, pre-emptive or empirical antifungal therapy: which is best in non-lung transplant recipients? *Int J Antimicrob Agents.* 2008;32(suppl 2):S149–S153 PMID: 19013340

8. Eschenauer GA, Lam SW, Carver PL. Antifungal prophylaxis in liver transplant recipients. *Liver Transpl.* 2009;15(8):842–858 PMID: 19642130

9. Walsh TJ, Anaissie EJ, Denning DW, et al. Treatment of aspergillosis: clinical practice guidelines of the Infectious Diseases Society of America. *Clin Infect Dis.* 2008;46(3):327–360 PMID: 18177225

10. Thomas L, Baggen L, Chisholm J, et al. Diagnosis and treatment of aspergillosis in children. *Expert Rev Anti Infect Ther.* 2009;7(4):461–472 PMID: 19400765

11. Friberg LE, Ravva P, Karlsson MO, et al. Integrated population pharmacokinetic analysis of voriconazole in children, adolescents, and adults. *Antimicrob Agents Chemother.* 2012;56(6): 3032–3042 PMID: 22430956

12. Cornely OA, Maertens J, Bresnik M, et al. Liposomal amphotericin B as initial therapy for invasive mold infection: a randomized trial comparing a high-loading dose regimen with standard dosing (AmBiLoad trial). *Clin Infect Dis.* 2007;44(10):1289–1297 PMID: 17443465

13. Bartelink IH, Wolfs T, Jonker M, et al. Highly variable plasma concentrations of voriconazole in pediatric hematopoietic stem cell transplantation patients. *Antimicrob Agents Chemother.* 2013;57(1):235–240 PMID: 23114771

14. Marr KA, Schlamm H, Rottinghaus ST, et al. A randomised, double-bind study of combination antifungal therapy with voriconazole and anidulafungin versus voriconazole monotherpay for primary treatment of invasive aspergillosis; Abstract LB2812. 22nd European Congress of Clinical Microbiology and Infectious Diseases (ECCMID), March 31–April 3, 2012; London

15. Ashouri N, Singh J, Arrieta A. Micafungin in pediatrics: when one size does not fit all. *Expert Opin Drug Metab Toxicol.* 2008;4(4):463–469 PMID: 18433348

16. Chapman SW, Dismukes WE, Proia LA, et al. Clinical practice guidelines for the management of blastomycosis: 2008 update by the Infectious Diseases Society of America. *Clin Infect Dis.* 2008;46(12):1801–1812 PMID: 18462107

17. McKinnell JA, Pappas PG. Blastomycosis: new insights into diagnosis, prevention, and treatment. *Clin Chest Med.* 2009;30(2):227–239 PMID: 19375630

18. Walsh CM, Morris SK, Brophy JC, et al. Disseminated blastomycosis in an infant. *Pediatr Infect Dis J.* 2006;25(7):656–658 PMID: 16804444

19. Pappas PG, Kauffman CA, Andes D, et al. Clinical practice guidelines for the management of candidiasis: 2009 update by the Infectious Diseases Society of America. *Clin Infect Dis.* 2009;48(5):503–535 PMID: 19191635

20. Goins RA, Ascher D, Waecker N, et al. Comparison of fluconazole and nystatin oral suspensions for treatment of oral candidiasis in infants. *Pediatr Infect Dis J.* 2002;21(12):1165–1167 PMID: 12506950

21. Piper L, Smith PB, Hornik CP, et al. Fluconazole loading dose pharmacokinetics and safety in infants. *Pediatr Infect Dis J.* 2011;30(5):375–378 PMID: 21085048

22. Prasad N, Gupta A. Fungal peritonitis in peritoneal dialysis patients. *Perit Dial Int.* 2005;25(3):207–222 PMID: 15981767

23. Sobel JD. Vulvovaginal candidosis. *Lancet.* 2007;369(9577):1961–1971 PMID: 17560449

24. Lopez Martinez R, Mendez Tovar LJ. Chromoblastomycosis. *Clin Dermatol.* 2007;25(2):188–194 PMID: 17350498

25. Ameen M. Chromoblastomycosis: clinical presentation and management. *Clin Exp Dermatol.* 2009;34(8):849–854 PMID: 19575735

26. Galgiani JN, Ampel NM, Blair JE, et al. Coccidioidomycosis. *Clin Infect Dis.* 2005;41(9):1217–1223 PMID: 16206093

27. Anstead GM, Graybill JR. Coccidioidomycosis. *Infect Dis Clin North Am.* 2006;20(3):621–643 PMID: 16984872

28. Williams PL. Coccidioidal meningitis. *Ann N Y Acad Sci.* 2007;1111:377–384 PMID: 17363442

29. American Academy of Pediatrics. Coccidioidomycosis. In: Pickering LK, Baker CJ, Kimberlin DW, Long SS, eds. *Red Book: 2012 Report of the Committee on Infectious Diseases.* 29th ed. Elk Grove Village, IL: American Academy of Pediatrics; 2012:289–291

30. Homans JD, Spencer L. Itraconazole treatment of nonmeningeal coccidioidomycosis in children: two case reports and review of the literature. *Pediatr Infect Dis J.* 2010;29(1):65–67 PMID: 19884875

31. Chayakulkeeree M, Perfect JR. Cryptococcosis. *Infect Dis Clin North Am.* 2006;20(3):507–544 PMID: 16984867

32. Jarvis JN, Harrison TS. Pulmonary cryptococcosis. *Semin Respir Crit Care Med.* 2008;29(2):141–150 PMID: 18365996

33. American Academy of Pediatrics. *Cryptococcus neoformans* infections (cryptococcosis). In: Pickering LK, Baker CJ, Kimberlin DW, Long SS, eds. *Red Book: 2012 Report of the Committee on Infectious Diseases.* 29th ed. Elk Grove Village, IL: American Academy of Pediatrics; 2012:294–296

34. Perfect JR, Dismukes WE, Dromer F, et al. Clinical practice guidelines for the management of cryptococcal disease: 2010 update by the Infectious Diseases Society of America. *Clin Infect Dis.* 2010;50(3):291–322 PMID: 20047480

35. Naggie S, Perfect JR. Molds: hyalohyphomycosis, phaeohyphomycosis, and zygomycosis. *Clin Chest Med.* 2009;30(2):337–353 PMID: 19375639

36. Cortez KJ, Roilides E, Quiroz-Telles F, et al. Infections caused by *Scedosporium* spp. *Clin Microbiol Rev.* 2008;21(1):157–197 PMID: 18202441

37. Wheat LJ, Freifeld AG, Kleiman MB, et al. Clinical practice guidelines for the management of patients with histoplasmosis: 2007 update by the Infectious Diseases Society of America. *Clin Infect Dis.* 2007;45(7):807–825 PMID: 17806045

38. American Academy of Pediatrics. *Borrelia* infections (relapsing fever). In: Pickering LK, Baker CJ, Kimberlin DW, Long SS, eds. *Red Book: 2012 Report of the Committee on Infectious Diseases.* 29th ed. Elk Grove Village, IL: American Academy of Pediatrics; 2012:254–256

39. Queiroz-Telles F, Goldani LZ, Schlamm HT, et al. An open-label comparative pilot study of oral voriconazole and itraconazole for long-term treatment of paracoccidioidomycosis. *Clin Infect Dis.* 2007;45(11):1462–1469 PMID: 17990229

40. Menezes VM, Soares BG, Fontes CJ. Drugs for treating paracoccidioidomycosis. *Cochrane Database Syst Rev.* 2006;(2):CD004967 PMID: 16625617

41. American Academy of Pediatrics. Paracoccidioidomycosis (South American blastomycosis). In: Pickering LK, Baker CJ, Kimberlin DW, Long SS, eds. *Red Book: 2012 Report of the Committee on Infectious Diseases.* 29th ed. Elk Grove Village, IL: American Academy of Pediatrics; 2012:530–531

42. Li DM, de Hoog GS. Cerebral phaeohyphomycosis—a cure at what lengths? *Lancet Infect Dis.* 2009;9(6):376–383 PMID: 19467477

43. Panel on Opportunistic Infections in HIV-Exposed and HIV-Infected Children. Guidelines for the prevention and treatment of opportunistic infections in HIV-exposed and HIV-infected children. http://aidsinfo.nih.gov/contentfiles/lvguidelines/oi_guidelines_pediatrics.pdf. Accessed November 14, 2013

References

Chapter 8 (cont)

44. Kauffman CA, Bustamante B, Chapman SW, et al. Clinical practice guidelines for the management of sporotrichosis: 2007 update by the Infectious Diseases Society of America. *Clin Infect Dis.* 2007;45(10):1255–1265 PMID: 17968818

45. Walsh TJ, Kontoyiannis DP. Editorial commentary: what is the role of combination therapy in management of zygomycosis? *Clin Infect Dis.* 2008;47(3):372–374 PMID: 18558877

46. Chayakulkeeree M, Ghannoum MA, Perfect JR. Zygomycosis: the re-emerging fungal infection. *Eur J Clin Microbiol Infect Dis.* 2006;25(4):215–229 PMID: 16568297

47. Spellberg B, Walsh TJ, Kontoyiannis DP, et al. Recent advances in the management of mucormycosis: from bench to bedside. *Clin Infect Dis.* 2009;48(12):1743–1751 PMID: 19435437

48. Reed C, Bryant R, Ibrahim AS, et al. Combination polyene-caspofungin treatment of rhino-orbital-cerebral mucormycosis. *Clin Infect Dis.* 2008;47(3):364–371 PMID: 18558882

49. Ali S, Graham TA, Forgie SE. The assessment and management of tinea capitis in children. *Pediatr Emerg Care.* 2007;23(9):662–668 PMID: 17876261

50. Shy R. Tinea corporis and tinea capitis. *Pediatr Rev.* 2007;28(5):164–174 PMID: 17473121

51. Andrews MD, Burns M. Common tinea infections in children. *Am Fam Physician.* 2008;77(10):1415–1420 PMID: 18533375

52. de Berker D. Clinical practice. Fungal nail disease. *N Engl J Med.* 2009;360(20):2108–2116 PMID: 19439745

53. Pantazidou A, Tebruegge M. Recurrent tinea versicolor: treatment with itraconazole or fluconazole? *Arch Dis Child.* 2007;92(11):1040–1042 PMID: 17954488

Chapter 9

1. Lenaerts L, De Clercq E, Naesens L. Clinical features and treatment of adenovirus infections. *Rev Med Virol.* 2008;18(6):357–374 PMID: 18655013

2. Michaels MG. Treatment of congenital cytomegalovirus: where are we now? *Expert Rev Anti Infect Ther.* 2007;5(3):441–448 PMID: 17547508

3. Biron KK. Antiviral drugs for cytomegalovirus diseases. *Antiviral Res.* 2006;71(2–3):154–163 PMID: 16765457

4. Boeckh M, Ljungman P. How we treat cytomegalovirus in hematopoietic cell transplant recipients. *Blood.* 2009;113(23):5711–5719 PMID: 19299333

5. Vaudry W, Ettenger R, Jara P, et al. Valganciclovir dosing according to body surface area and renal function in pediatric solid organ transplant recipients. *Am J Transplant.* 2009;9(3):636–643 PMID: 19260840

6. Emanuel D, Cunningham I, Jules-Elysee K, et al. Cytomegalovirus pneumonia after bone marrow transplantation successfully treated with the combination of ganciclovir and high-dose intravenous immune globulin. *Ann Intern Med.* 1988;109(10):777–782 PMID: 2847609

7. Reed EC, Bowden RA, Dandliker PS, et al. Treatment of cytomegalovirus pneumonia with ganciclovir and intravenous cytomegalovirus immunoglobulin in patients with bone marrow transplants. *Ann Intern Med.* 1988;109(10):783–788 PMID: 2847610

8. Foscarnet-Ganciclovir Cytomegalovirus Retinitis Trial. 4. Visual outcomes. Studies of Ocular Complications of AIDS Research Group in collaboration with the AIDS Clinical Trials Group. *Ophthalmology.* 1994;101(7):1250–1261 PMID: 8035989

9. Musch DC, Martin DF, Gordon JF, Davis MD, Kuppermann BD. Treatment of cytomegalovirus retinitis with a sustained-release ganciclovir implant. The Ganciclovir Implant Study Group. *N Engl J Med.* 1997;337(2):83–90 PMID: 9211677

10. Martin DF, Sierra-Madero J, Walmsley S, et al. A controlled trial of valganciclovir as induction therapy for cytomegalovirus retinitis. *N Engl J Med.* 2002;346(15):1119–1126 PMID: 11948271

11. Kempen JH, Jabs DA, Wilson LA, Dunn JP, West SK, Tonascia JA. Risk of vision loss in patients with cytomegalovirus retinitis and the acquired immunodeficiency syndrome. *Arch Ophthalmol.* 2003;121(4):466–476 PMID: 12695243

12. Studies of Ocular Complications of AIDS Research Group. The AIDS Clinical Trials Group. The ganciclovir implant plus oral ganciclovir versus parenteral cidofovir for the treatment of cytomegalovirus retinitis in patients with acquired immunodeficiency syndrome: the Ganciclovir Cidofovir Cytomegalovirus Retinitis Trial. *Am J Ophthalmol.* 2001;131(4):457–467 PMID: 11292409

13. Dieterich DT, Kotler DP, Busch DF, et al. Ganciclovir treatment of cytomegalovirus colitis in AIDS: a randomized, double-blind, placebo-controlled multicenter study. *J Infect Dis.* 1993;167(2):278–282 PMID: 8380610

14. Gerna G, Sarasini A, Baldanti F, Percivalle E, Zella D, Revello MG. Quantitative systemic and local evaluation of the antiviral effect of ganciclovir and foscarnet induction treatment on human cytomegalovirus gastrointestinal disease of patients with AIDS. Italian Foscarnet GID Study Group. *Antiviral Res.* 1997;34(1):39–50 PMID: 9107384

15. Markham A, Faulds D. Ganciclovir. An update of its therapeutic use in cytomegalovirus infection. *Drugs.* 1994;48(3):455–484 PMID: 7527763

16. Kimberlin DW, Acosta EP, Sanchez PJ, et al. Pharmacokinetic and pharmacodynamic assessment of oral valganciclovir in the treatment of symptomatic congenital cytomegalovirus disease. *J Infect Dis.* 2008;197(6):836–845 PMID: 18279073

17. Kimberlin DW, Jester PM, Sanchez PJ, et al. Six months versus six weeks of oral valganciclovir for infants with symptomatic congenital cytomegalovirus (CMV) disease with and without central nervous system (CNS) involvement: results of a Phase III, randomized, double-blind, placebo-controlled, multinational study. IDWeek 2013 (annual meeting of the Pediatric Infectious Diseases Society, the Infectious Diseases Society of America, the HIV Medical Association, and the Society for Healthcare Epidemiology of America), San Francisco, CA, October 5, 2013; Late-Breaker Abstract #43178

18. Griffiths P, Whitley R, Snydman DR, et al. Contemporary management of cytomegalovirus infection in transplant recipients: guidelines from an IHMF workshop, 2007. *Herpes.* 2008;15(1):4–12 PMID: 18983762

19. Panel on Opportunistic Infections in HIV-Exposed and HIV-Infected Children. Guidelines for the prevention and treatment of opportunistic infections in HIV-exposed and HIV-infected children. http://aidsinfo.nih.gov/contentfiles/lvguidelines/oi_guidelines_pediatrics.pdf. Accessed November 14, 2013

20. Biebl A, Webersinke C, Traxler B, et al. Fatal Epstein-Barr virus encephalitis in a 12-year-old child: an underappreciated neurological complication? *Nat Clin Pract Neurol.* 2009;5(3):171–174 PMID: 19262593

21. Chadaide Z, Voros E, Horvath S. Epstein-Barr virus encephalitis mimicking clinical and electroencephalographic characteristics of herpes simplex encephalitis. *J Med Virol.* 2008;80(11):1930–1932 PMID: 18814244

22. American Academy of Pediatrics. Epstein-Barr virus infections (infectious mononucleosis). In: Pickering LK, Baker CJ, Kimberlin DW, Long SS, eds. *Red Book: 2012 Report of the Committee on Infectious Diseases.* 29th ed. Elk Grove Village, IL: American Academy of Pediatrics; 2012:318–321

23. Gross TG. Treatment for Epstein-Barr virus-associated PTLD. *Herpes.* 2009;15(3):64–67 PMID: 19306606

24. Styczynski J, Reusser P, Einsele H, et al. Management of HSV, VZV and EBV infections in patients with hematological malignancies and after SCT: guidelines from the Second European Conference on Infections in Leukemia. *Bone Marrow Transplant.* 2009;43(10):757–770 PMID: 19043458

25. Kurbegov AC, Sokol RJ. Hepatitis B therapy in children. *Expert Rev Gastroenterol Hepatol.* 2009;3(1):39–49 PMID: 19210112

26. Jonas MM, Kelly D, Pollack H, et al. Safety, efficacy, and pharmacokinetics of adefovir dipivoxil in children and adolescents (age 2 to <18 years) with chronic hepatitis B. *Hepatology.* 2008;47(6):1863–1871 PMID: 18433023

27. Lai CL, Rosmawati M, Lao J, et al. Entecavir is superior to lamivudine in reducing hepatitis B virus DNA in patients with chronic hepatitis B infection. *Gastroenterology.* 2002;123(6):1831–1838 PMID: 12454840

28. Honkoop P, De Man RA. Entecavir: a potent new antiviral drug for hepatitis B. *Expert Opin Investig Drugs.* 2003;12(4):683–688 PMID: 12665423

References

Chapter 9 (cont)

29. Shaw T, Locarnini S. Entecavir for the treatment of chronic hepatitis B. *Expert Rev Anti Infect Ther.* 2004;2(6):853–871 PMID: 15566330

30. Elisofon SA, Jonas MM. Hepatitis B and C in children: current treatment and future strategies. *Clin Liver Dis.* 2006;10(1):133–148 PMID: 16376798

31. Jonas MM, Block JM, Haber BA, et al. Treatment of children with chronic hepatitis B virus infection in the United States: patient selection and therapeutic options. *Hepatology.* 2010;52(6):2192–2205 PMID: 20890947

32. Haber BA, Block JM, Jonas MM, et al. Recommendations for screening, monitoring, and referral of pediatric chronic hepatitis B. *Pediatrics.* 2009;124(5):e1007–1013 PMID: 19805457

33. Shneider BL, Gonzàlez-Peralta R, Roberts EA. Controversies in the management of pediatric liver disease: hepatitis B, C and NAFLD: summary of a single topic conference. *Hepatology.* 2006;44(5):1344–1354 PMID: 17058223

34. Jain MK, Comanor L, White C, et al. Treatment of hepatitis B with lamivudine and tenofovir in HIV/HBV-coinfected patients: factors associated with response. *J Viral Hepat.* 2007;14(3):176–182 PMID: 17305883

35. Sokal EM, Conjeevaram HS, Roberts EA, et al. Interferon alfa therapy for chronic hepatitis B in children: a multinational randomized controlled trial. *Gastroenterology.* 1998;114(5):988–995 PMID: 9558288

36. Jonas MM, Mizerski J, Badia IB, et al. Clinical trial of lamivudine in children with chronic hepatitis B. *N Engl J Med.* 2002;346(22):1706–1713 PMID: 12037150

37. Chang TT, Gish RG, de Man R, et al. A comparison of entecavir and lamivudine for HBeAg-positive chronic hepatitis B. *N Engl J Med.* 2006;354(10):1001–1010 PMID: 16525137

38. Liaw YF, Gane E, Leung N, et al. 2-Year GLOBE trial results: telbivudine is superior to lamivudine in patients with chronic hepatitis B. *Gastroenterology.* 2009;136(2):486–495 PMID: 19027013

39. Keam SJ, Cvetkovic RS. Peginterferon-alpha-2a (40 kD) plus ribavirin: a review of its use in the management of chronic hepatitis C mono-infection. *Drugs.* 2008;68(9):1273–1317 PMID: 18547135

40. Marcellin P, Forns X, Goeser T, et al. Telaprevir is effective given every 8 or 12 hours with ribavirin and peginterferon alfa-2a or -2b to patients with chronic hepatitis C. *Gastroenterology.* 2011;140(2):459–468 PMID: 21034744

41. Poordad F, McCone J Jr, Bacon BR, et al. Boceprevir for untreated chronic HCV genotype 1 infection. *N Engl J Med.* 2011;364(13):1195–1206 PMID: 21449783

42. Schwarz KB, Gonzalez-Peralta RP, Murray KF, et al. The combination of ribavirin and peginterferon is superior to peginterferon and placebo for children and adolescents with chronic hepatitis C. *Gastroenterology.* 2011;140(2):450–458 PMID: 21036173

43. Nelson DR. The role of triple therapy with protease inhibitors in hepatitis C virus genotype 1 naïve patients. *Liver Int.* 2011;31(Suppl 1):53–57 PMID: 21205138

44. Strader DB, Wright T, Thomas DL, Seeff LB; American Association for the Study of Liver Diseases. Diagnosis, management, and treatment of hepatitis C. *Hepatology.* 2004;39(4):1147–1171 PMID: 15057920

45. Soriano V, Puoti M, Sulkowski M, et al. Care of patients coinfected with HIV and hepatitis C virus: 2007 updated recommendations from the HCV-HIV International Panel. *AIDS.* 2007;21(9):1073–1089 PMID: 17502718

46. Hollier LM, Wendel GD. Third trimester antiviral prophylaxis for preventing maternal genital herpes simplex virus (HSV) recurrences and neonatal infection. *Cochrane Database Syst Rev.* 2008;(1):CD004946 PMID: 18254066

47. Pinninti SG, Feja KN, Kimberlin DW, et al. Neonatal herpes disease despite maternal antenatal antiviral suppressive therapy: a multicenter case series of the first such infants reported. Presented at: 48th Annual Meeting of The Infectious Diseases Society of America; October 22, 2010; Vancouver, British Columbia

48. Pinninti SG, Angara R, Feja KN, et al. Neonatal herpes disease despite maternal antenatal antiviral suppressive therapy: a multicenter case series. *J Pediatr.* 2012;161(1):134–138 PMID: 22336576

49. Kimberlin DW, Jacobs RF, Weller S, et al. Pharmacokinetics and safety of extemporaneously compounded valacyclovir oral suspension in pediatric patients from 1 month to 12 years of age. *Clin Infect Dis.* 2010;50(2):221–228 PMID: 20014952

50. Abdel Massih RC, Razonable RR. Human herpesvirus 6 infections after liver transplantation. *World J Gastroenterol.* 2009;15(21):2561–2569 PMID: 19496184

51. Mofenson LM, Brady MT, Danner SP, et al. Guidelines for the prevention and treatment of opportunistic infections among HIV-exposed and HIV-infected children: recommendations from CDC, the National Institutes of Health, the HIV Medicine Association of the Infectious Diseases Society of America, the Pediatric Infectious Diseases Society, and the American Academy of Pediatrics. *MMWR Recomm Rep.* 2009;58(RR-11):1–166 PMID: 19730409

52. Violari A, Cotton MF, Gibb DM, et al. Early antiretroviral therapy and mortality among HIV-infected infants. *N Engl J Med.* 2008;359(21):2233–2244 PMID: 19020325

53. Acosta EP, Jester P, Gal P, et al, for the NIAID Collaborative Antiviral Study Group. Oseltamivir dosing for influenza infection in premature neonates. *J Infect Dis.* 2010;202(4):563–566 PMID: 20594104

54. Kimberlin DW, Acosta EP, Prichard MN, et al; NIAID Collaborative Antiviral Study Group. Oseltamivir pharmacokinetics, dosing, and resistance among children aged <2 years with influenza. *J Infect Dis.* 2013;207(5):709–720 PMID: 23230059

55. American Academy of Pediatrics. Measles. In: Pickering LK, Baker CJ, Kimberlin DW, Long SS, eds. *Red Book: 2012 Report of the Committee on Infectious Diseases.* 29th ed. Elk Grove Village, IL: American Academy of Pediatrics; 2012:489–499

56. American Academy of Pediatrics. Respiratory syncytial virus. In: Pickering LK, Baker CJ, Kimberlin DW, Long SS, eds. *Red Book: 2012 Report of the Committee on Infectious Diseases.* 29th ed. Elk Grove Village, IL: American Academy of Pediatrics; 2012:609–618

57. Whitley RJ. Therapy of herpes virus infections in children. *Adv Exp Med Biol.* 2008;609:216–232 PMID: 18193668

Chapter 10

1. Blessmann J, Ali IK, Nu PA, et al. Longitudinal study of intestinal *Entamoeba histolytica* infections in asymptomatic adult carriers. *J Clin Microbiol.* 2003;41(10):4745–4750 PMID: 14532214

2. Haque R, Huston CD, Hughes M, et al. Amebiasis. *N Engl J Med.* 2003;348(16):1565–1573 PMID: 1270037

3. Parasitic infections. In: Abramowicz M, ed. *Handbook of Antimicrobial Therapy.* New Rochelle, NY: The Medical Letter, Inc; 2011:221–277

4. Stanley SL Jr. Amoebiasis. *Lancet.* 2003;361(9362):1025–1034 PMID: 12660071

5. Barnett ND, Kaplan AM, Hopkin RJ, et al. Primary amoebic meningoencephalitis with *Naegleria fowleri*: clinical review. *Pediatr Neurol.* 1996;15(3):230–234 PMID: 8916161

6. Vargas-Zepeda J, Gomez-Alcala AV, Vasquez-Morales JA, et al. Successful treatment of *Naegleria fowleri* meningoencephalitis by using intravenous amphotericin B, fluconazole and rifampicin. *Arch Med Res.* 2005;36(1):83–86 PMID: 15900627

7. Goswick SM, Brenner GM. Activities of azithromycin and amphotericin B against *Naegleria fowleri* in vitro and in a mouse model of primary amebic meningoencephalitis. *Antimicrob Agents Chemother.* 2003;47(2):524–528 PMID: 12543653

8. Slater CA, Sickel JZ, Visvesvara GS, et al. Brief report: successful treatment of disseminated acanthamoeba infection in an immunocompromised patient. *N Engl J Med.* 1994;331(2):85–87 PMID: 8208270

9. Deetz TR, Sawyer MH, Billman G, et al. Successful treatment of *Balamuthia* amoebic encephalitis: presentation of 2 cases. *Clin Infect Dis.* 2003;37(10):1304–1012 PMID: 14583863

10. Chotmongkol V, Sawadpanitch K, Sawanyawisuth K, et al. Treatment of eosinophilic meningitis with a combination of prednisolone and mebendazole. *Am J Trop Med Hyg.* 2006;74(6):1122–1124 PMID: 16760531

11. Lo Re V III, Gluckman SJ. Eosinophilic meningitis. *Am J Med.* 2003;114(3):217–223 PMID: 12637136

References

Chapter 10 (cont)

12. Jitpimolmard S, Sawanyawisuth K, Morakote N, et al. Albendazole therapy for eosinophilic meningitis caused by *Angiostrongylus cantonensis. Parasitol Res.* 2007;100(6):1293–1296 PMID: 17177056

13. Checkley AM, Chiodini PL, Dockrell DH, et al. Eosinophilia in returning travelers and migrants from the tropics: UK recommendations for investigation and initial management. *J Infect.* 2010; 60(1):1–20 PMID: 19931558

14. Centers for Disease Control and Prevention. Refugee health guidelines: intestinal parasites overseas recommendations. Recommendations for overseas presumptive treatment of intestinal parasites for refugees destined for the United States. http://www.cdc.gov/immigrantrefugeehealth/guidelines/ domestic/intestinal-parasites-domestic.html. Accessed November 14, 2013

15. American Academy of Pediatrics. *Ascaris lumbricoides.* In: Pickering LK, Baker CJ, Kimberlin DW, Long SS, eds. *Red Book: 2012 Report of the Committee on Infectious Diseases.* 29th ed. Elk Grove Village, IL: American Academy of Pediatrics; 2012:239–240

16. Vannier E, Gewurz BE, Krause PJ. Human babesiosis. *Infect Dis Clin North Am.* 2008;22(3): 469–488 PMID: 18755385

17. Wormser GP, Dattwyler RJ, Shapiro ED, et al. The clinical assessment, treatment, and prevention of Lyme disease, human granulocytic anaplasmosis, and babesiosis: clinical practice guidelines by the Infectious Diseases Society of America. *Clin Infect Dis.* 2006;43(9):1089–1134 PMID: 17029130

18. Boustani MR, Gelfand JA. Babesiosis. *Clin Infect Dis.* 1996;22(4):611–615 PMID: 8729197

19. Fisk T, Keystone J, Kozarsky P. *Cyclospora cayetanensis, Isospora belli, Sarcocystis* species, *Balantidium coli,* and *Blastocystis hominis.* In: Mandell GL, Bennet JE, Dolin R, eds. *Principles and Practice of Infectious Diseases.* Philadelphia, PA: Elsevier Churchill Livingstone; 2005:3228–3237

20. American Academy of Pediatrics. *Baylisascaris* infections. In: Pickering LK, Baker CJ, Kimberlin DW, Long SS, eds. *Red Book: 2012 Report of the Committee on Infectious Diseases.* 29th ed. Elk Grove Village, IL: American Academy of Pediatrics; 2012:251–252

21. Park SY, Glaser C, Murray WJ, et al. Raccoon roundworm *(Baylisascaris procyonis)* encephalitis: case report and field investigation. *Pediatrics.* 2000;106(4):e56 PMID: 11015551

22. Shlim DR, Hoge CW, Rajah R, et al. Is *Blastocystis hominis* a cause of diarrhea in travelers? A prospective controlled study in Nepal. *Clin Infect Dis.* 1995;21(1):97–101 PMID: 7578767

23. Udkow MP, Markell EK. *Blastocystis hominis:* prevalence in asymptomatic versus symptomatic hosts. *J Infect Dis.* 1993;168(1):242–244 PMID: 8515120

24. Bern C, Montgomery SP, Herwaldt BL, et al. Evaluation and treatment of Chagas disease in the United States: a systematic review. *JAMA.* 2007;298(18):2171–2181 PMID: 18000201

25. Maguire JH. Trypanosoma. In: Gorbach SL, Bartlett JG, Blacklow NR, eds. *Infectious Diseases.* 3rd ed. Philadelphia, PA: Lippincott Williams & Wilkins; 2004:2327–2334

26. Amadi B, Mwiya M, Musuku J, et al. Effect of nitazoxanide on morbidity and mortality in Zambian children with cryptosporidiosis: a randomised controlled trial. *Lancet.* 2002;360(9343):1375–1380 PMID: 12423984

27. Kosek M, Alcantara C, Lima AA, et al. Cryptosporidiosis: an update. *Lancet Infect Dis.* 2001;1(4):262–269 PMID: 11871513

28. Davies AP, Chalmers RM. Cryptosporidiosis. *BMJ.* 2009;339:b4168 PMID: 19841008

29. Bushen OY, Lima AA, Guerrant RL. Cryptosporidiosis. In: Guerrant RL, Walker DH, Weller PF, eds. *Tropical Infectious Diseases.* Philadelphia, PA: Elsevier-Churchill Livingstone; 2006:1003–1014

30. Derouin F, Lagrange-Xelot M. Treatment of parasitic diarrhea in HIV-infected patients. *Expert Rev Anti Infect Ther.* 2008;6(3):337–349 PMID: 18588498

31. Jelinek T, Maiwald H, Nothdurft HD, et al. Cutaneous larva migrans in travelers: synopsis of histories, symptoms, and treatment of 98 patients. *Clin Infect Dis.* 1994;19(6):1062–1066 PMID: 7534125

32. Prociv P, Croese J. Human enteric infection with *Ancylostoma caninum:* hookworms reappraised in the light of a "new" zoonosis. *Acta Trop.* 1996;62(1):23–44 PMID: 8971276

33. Eberhard ML, Arrowood MJ. *Cyclospora* spp. *Curr Opin Infect Dis.* 2002;15(5):519–522 PMID: 12686886

34. Ortega YR, Sanchez R. Update on *Cyclospora cayetanensis*, a food-borne and waterborne parasite. *Clin Microbiol Rev.* 2010;23(1):218–234 PMID: 20065331

35. Garcia HH, Pretell EJ, Gilman RH, et al. A trial of antiparasitic treatment to reduce the rate of seizures due to cerebral cysticercosis. *N Engl J Med.* 2004;350(3):249–258 PMID: 14724304

36. Garcia HH, Evans CA, Nash TE, et al. Current consensus guidelines for treatment of neurocysticercosis. *Clin Microbiol Rev.* 2002;15(4):747–756 PMID: 12364377

37. Lillie P, McGann H. Empiric albendazole therapy and new onset seizures—a cautionary note. *J Infect.* 2010;60(5):403–404 PMID: 20153773

38. Stark DJ, Beebe N, Marriott D, et al. Dientamoebiasis: clinical importance and recent advances. *Trends Parasitol.* 2006;22(2):92–96 PMID: 16380293

39. Johnson EH, Windsor JJ, Clark CG. Emerging from obscurity: biological, clinical, and diagnostic aspects of *Dientamoeba fragilis*. *Clin Microbiol Rev.* 2004;17(3):553–570 PMID: 15258093

40. Smego RA Jr, Bhatti S, Khaliq AA, et al. Percutaneous aspiration-injection-reaspiration drainage plus albendazole or mebendazole for hepatic cystic echinococcosis: a meta-analysis. *Clin Infect Dis.* 2003;37(8):1073–1083 PMID: 14523772

41. Franchi C, Di Vico B, Teggi A. Long-term evaluation of patients with hydatidosis treated with benzimidazole carbamates. *Clin Infect Dis.* 1999;29(2):304–309 PMID: 10476732

42. Grencis RK, Cooper ES. Enterobius, trichuris, capillaria, and hookworm including ancylostoma caninum. *Gastroenterol Clin North Am.* 1996;25(3):579–597 PMID: 8863041

43. Tisch DJ, Michael E, Kazura JW. Mass chemotherapy options to control lymphatic filariasis: a systematic review. *Lancet Infect Dis.* 2005;5(8):514–523 PMID: 16048720

44. Ottesen EA, Nutman TB. Tropical pulmonary eosinophilia. *Annu Rev Med.* 1992;43:417–424 PMID: 1580599

45. Jong EC, Wasserheit JN, Johnson RJ, et al. Praziquantel for the treatment of *Clonorchis/Opisthorchis* infections: report of a double-blind, placebo-controlled trial. *J Infect Dis.* 1985;152(3):637–640 PMID: 3897401

46. Calvopina M, Guderian RH, Paredes W, et al. Treatment of human pulmonary paragonimiasis with triclabendazole: clinical tolerance and drug efficacy. *Trans R Soc Trop Med Hyg.* 1998;92(5):566–569 PMID: 9861383

47. Johnson RJ, Jong EC, Dunning SB, et al. Paragonimiasis: diagnosis and the use of praziquantel in treatment. *Rev Infect Dis.* 1985;7(2):200–206 PMID: 4001715

48. Graham CS, Brodie SB, Weller PF. Imported *Fasciola hepatica* infection in the United States and treatment with triclabendazole. *Clin Infect Dis.* 2001;33(1):1–5 PMID: 11389487

49. Gardner TB, Hill DR. Treatment of giardiasis. *Clin Microbiol Rev.* 2001;14(1):114–128 PMID: 11148005

50. Ross AG, Olds GR, Cripps AW, Farrar JJ, McManus DP. Enteropathogens and chronic illness in returning travelers. *New Engl J Med.* 2013;368(19):1817–1825 PMID: 23656647

51. Abboud P, Lemee V, Gargala G, et al. Successful treatment of metronidazole- and albendazole-resistant giardiasis with nitazoxanide in a patient with acquired immunodeficiency syndrome. *Clin Infect Dis.* 2001;32(12):1792–1794 PMID: 11360222

52. Hotez PJ, Brooker S, Bethony JM, et al. Hookworm infection. *N Engl J Med.* 2004;351(8):799–807 PMID: 15317893

53. World Health Organization, Technical Report Series 949. Control of the leishmaniases. Report of a meeting of the WHO Expert Committee on the Control of Leishmaniases, Geneva, 22–26 March 2010

54. Alrajhi AA, Ibrahim EA, De Vol EB, et al. Fluconazole for the treatment of cutaneous leishmaniasis caused by *Leishmania* major. *N Engl J Med.* 2002;346(12):891–895 PMID: 11907288

55. Bern C, Adler-Moore J, Berenguer J, et al. Liposomal amphotericin B for the treatment of visceral leishmaniasis. *Clin Infect Dis.* 2006;43(7):917–924 PMID: 16941377

56. Ritmeijer K, Dejenie A, Assefa Y, et al. A comparison of miltefosine and sodium stibogluconate for treatment of visceral leishmaniasis in an Ethiopian population with high prevalence of HIV infection. *Clin Infect Dis.* 2006;43(3):357–364 PMID: 16804852

57. Sundar S, Jha TK, Thakur CP, et al. Oral miltefosine for Indian visceral leishmaniasis. *N Engl J Med.* 2002;347(22):1739–1746 PMID: 12456849

Chapter 10 (cont)

58. Sundar S, Jha TK, Thakur CP, et al. Injectable paromomycin for visceral leishmaniasis in India. *N Engl J Med.* 2007;356(25):2571–2581 PMID: 17582067

59. American Academy of Pediatrics. Pediculosis. In: Pickering LK, Baker CJ, Kimberlin DW, Long SS, eds. *Red Book: 2012 Report of the Committee on Infectious Diseases.* 29th ed. Elk Grove Village, IL: American Academy of Pediatrics; 2012:543–547

60. Foucault C, Ranque S, Badiaga S, et al. Oral ivermectin in the treatment of body lice. *J Infect Dis.* 2006;193(3):474–476 PMID: 16388498

61. Fischer PR, Bialek R. Prevention of malaria in children. *Clin Infect Dis.* 2002;34(4):493–498 PMID: 11797176

62. Freedman DO. Clinical practice. Malaria prevention in short-term travelers. *N Engl J Med.* 2008;359(6):603–612 PMID: 18687641

63. Kain KC, Shanks GD, Keystone JS. Malaria chemoprophylaxis in the age of drug resistance. I. Currently recommended drug regimens. *Clin Infect Dis.* 2001;33(2):226–234 PMID: 11418883

64. Kain KC, Keystone JS. Malaria in travelers. Epidemiology, disease, and prevention. *Infect Dis Clin North Am.* 1998;12(2):267–284 PMID: 9658245

65. Overbosch D, Schilthuis H, Bienzle U, et al. Atovaquone-proguanil versus mefloquine for malaria prophylaxis in nonimmune travelers: results from a randomized, double-blind study. *Clin Infect Dis.* 2001;33(7):1015–1021 PMID: 11528574

66. Centers for Disease Control and Prevention. Malaria. In: Brunette GW, ed. *CDC Health Information for International Travel 2014: The Yellow Book.* New York, NY: Oxford University Press; 2014:228–245. http://wwwnc.cdc.gov/travel/yellowbook/2014/chapter-3-infectious-diseases-related-to-travel/malaria. Accessed November 15, 2013

67. American Academy of Pediatrics. Pinworm infection. In: Pickering LK, Baker CJ, Kimberlin DW, Long SS, eds. *Red Book: 2012 Report of the Committee on Infectious Diseases.* 29th ed. Elk Grove Village, IL: American Academy of Pediatrics; 2012:566–567

68. American Academy of Pediatrics. Scabies. In: Pickering LK, Baker CJ, Kimberlin DW, Long SS, eds. *Red Book: 2012 Report of the Committee on Infectious Diseases.* 29th ed. Elk Grove Village, IL: American Academy of Pediatrics; 2012:641–643

69. Usha V, Gopalakrishnan Nair TV. A comparative study of oral ivermectin and topical permethrin cream in the treatment of scabies. *J Am Acad Dermatol.* 2000;42(2 pt 1):236–240 PMID: 10642678

70. Brodine SK, Thomas A, Huang R, et al. Community based parasitic screening and treatment of Sudanese refugees: application and assessment of Centers for Disease Control guidelines. *Am J Trop Med Hyg.* 2009;80(3):425–430 PMID: 19270293

71. Doenhoff MJ, Pica-Mattoccia L. Praziquantel for the treatment of schistosomiasis: its use for control in areas with endemic disease and prospects for drug resistance. *Expert Rev Anti Infect Ther.* 2006;4(2):199–210 PMID: 16597202

72. Fenwick A, Webster JP. Schistosomiasis: challenges for control, treatment and drug resistance. *Curr Opin Infect Dis.* 2006;19(6):577–582 PMID: 17075334

73. Centers for Disease Control and Prevention. Parasites—schistosomiasis. Resources for health professionals. http://www.cdc.gov/parasites/schistosomiasis/health_professionals/index.html#tx. Accessed November 15, 2013

74. Marti H, Haji HJ, Savioli L, et al. A comparative trial of a single-dose ivermectin versus three days of albendazole for treatment of *Strongyloides stercoralis* and other soil-transmitted helminth infections in children. *Am J Trop Med Hyg.* 1996;55(5):477–481 PMID: 8940976

75. Segarra-Newnham M. Manifestations, diagnosis, and treatment of *Strongyloides stercoralis* infection. *Ann Pharmacother.* 2007;41(12):1992–2001 PMID: 17940124

76. Schaffel R, Nucci M, Portugal R, et al. Thiabendazole for the treatment of strongyloidiasis in patients with hematologic malignancies. *Clin Infect Dis.* 2000;31(3):821–822 PMID: 11017840

77. McAuley JB. Toxoplasmosis in children. *Pediatr Infect Dis J.* 2008;27(2):161–162 PMID: 18227714

78. McLeod R, Boyer K, Karrison T, et al. Outcome of treatment for congenital toxoplasmosis, 1981–2004: the National Collaborative Chicago-Based, Congenital Toxoplasmosis Study. *Clin Infect Dis.* 2006;42(10):1383–1394 PMID: 16619149

79. Petersen E. Prevention and treatment of congenital toxoplasmosis. *Expert Rev Anti Infect Ther.* 2007;5(2):285–293 PMID: 17402843

80. Adachi JA, Ericsson CD, Jiang ZD, et al. Azithromycin found to be comparable to levofloxacin for the treatment of US travelers with acute diarrhea acquired in Mexico. *Clin Infect Dis.* 2003;37(9):1165–1171 PMID: 14557959

81. Diemert DJ. Prevention and self-treatment of traveler's diarrhea. *Clin Microbiol Rev.* 2006;19(3):583–594 PMID: 16847088

82. DuPont HL. Therapy for and prevention of traveler's diarrhea. *Clin Infect Dis.* 2007;45(suppl 1):S78–S84 PMID: 17582576

83. Gottstein B, Pozio E, Nöckler K. Epidemiology, diagnosis, treatment, and control of trichinellosis. *Clin Microbiol Rev.* 2009;22(1):127–145 PMID: 19136437

84. American Academy of Pediatrics. *Trichomonas vaginalis* (trichomoniasis). In: Pickering LK, Baker CJ, Kimberlin DW, Long SS, eds. *Red Book: 2012 Report of the Committee on Infectious Diseases.* 29th ed. Elk Grove Village, IL: American Academy of Pediatrics; 2012:729–731

85. Bern C, Montgomery SP, Herwaldt BL, et al. Evaluation and treatment of chagas disease in the United States: a systematic review. *JAMA.* 2007;298(18):2171–2181 PMID: 18000201

86. Fairlamb AH. Chemotherapy of human African trypanosomiasis: current and future prospects. *Trends Parasitol.* 2003;19(11):488–494 PMID: 14580959

87. Pépin J, Milord F. The treatment of human African trypanosomiasis. *Adv Parasitol.* 1994;33:1–47 PMID: 8122565

88. Bisser S, N'Siesi FX, Lejon V, et al. Equivalence trial of melarsoprol and nifurtimox monotherapy and combination therapy for the treatment of second-stage Trypanosoma brucei gambiense sleeping sickness. *J Infect Dis.* 2007;195(3):322–329 PMID: 17205469

89. Sahlas DJ, MacLean JD, Janevski J, et al. Clinical problem-solving. Out of Africa. *N Engl J Med.* 2002;347(10):749–753 PMID: 12213947

90. American Academy of Pediatrics. Trichuriasis (whipworm infection). In: Pickering LK, Baker CJ, Kimberlin DW, Long SS, eds. *Red Book: 2012 Report of the Committee on Infectious Diseases.* 29th ed. Elk Grove Village, IL: American Academy of Pediatrics; 2012:731–732

Chapter 11

1. Acosta EP, Jester P, Gal P, et al, for the NIAID Collaborative Antiviral Study Group. Oseltamivir dosing for influenza infection in premature neonates. *J Infect Dis.* 2010;202(4):563–566 PMID: 20594104

2. Kimberlin DW, Acosta EP, Prichard MN, et al, for the NIAID Collaborative Antiviral Study Group. Oseltamivir pharmacokinetics, dosing, and resistance among children aged <2 years with influenza. *J Infect Dis.* 2013;207(5):709–720 PMID: 23230059

Chapter 13

1. Schwartz GJ, Muñoz A, Schneider MF, et al. New equations to estimate GFR in children with CKD. *J Am Soc Nephrol.* 2009;20(3):629–637 PMID: 19158356

2. Staples A, LeBlond R, Watkins S, Wong C, Brandt J. Validation of the revised Schwartz estimating equation in a predominantly non-CKD population. *Pediatr Nephrol.* 2010;25(11):2321–2326 PMID: 20652327

Chapter 14

1. Oehler RL, Velez AP, Mizrachi M, et al. Bite-related and septic syndromes caused by cats and dogs. *Lancet Infect Dis.* 2009;9(7):439–447 PMID: 19555903

2. Lion C, Conroy MC, Carpentier AM, et al. Antimicrobial susceptibilities of *Pasteurella* strains isolated from humans. *Int J Antimicrob Agents.* 2006;27(4):290–293 PMID: 16564680

3. Stevens DL, Bisno AL, Chambers HF, et al. Practice guidelines for the diagnosis and management of skin and soft-tissue infections. *Clin Infect Dis.* 2005;41(10):1373–1406 PMID: 16231249

Chapter 14 (cont)

4. Talan DA, Abrahamian FM, Moran GJ, et al. Clinical presentation and bacteriologic analysis of infected human bites in patients presenting to emergency departments. *Clin Infect Dis.* 2003;37(11):1481–1489 PMID: 14614671

5. Wilson W, Taubert KA, Gewitz M, et al. Prevention of infective endocarditis: guidelines from the American Heart Association: a guideline from the American Heart Association Rheumatic Fever, Endocarditis, and Kawasaki Disease Committee, Council on Cardiovascular Disease in the Young, and the Council on Clinical Cardiology, Council on Cardiovascular Surgery and Anesthesia, and the Quality of Care and Outcomes Research Interdisciplinary Working Group. *Circulation.* 2007;116(15):1736–1754 PMID: 17446442

6. Pasquali SK, He X, Mohamad Z, et al. Trends in endocarditis hospitalizations at US children's hospitals: impact of the 2007 American Heart Association antibiotic prophylaxis guidelines. *Am Heart J.* 2012;163(5):894–899 PMID: 22607869

7. Cohn AC, MacNeil JR, Clark TA, et al; Centers for Disease Control and Prevention. Prevention and control of meningococcal disease: recommendations of the Advisory Committee on Immunization Practices (ACIP). *MMWR Recomm Rep.* 2013;62(RR-2):1–28 PMID: 23515099

8. American Academy of Pediatrics. Pertussis. In: Pickering LK, Baker CJ, Kimberlin DW, Long SS, eds. *Red Book: 2012 Report of the Committee on Infectious Diseases.* 29th ed. Elk Grove Village, IL: American Academy of Pediatrics; 2012:553–566

9. Tiwari T, Murphy TV, Moran J. Recommended antimicrobial agents for the treatment and postexposure prophylaxis of pertussis: 2005 CDC guidelines. *MMWR Recomm Rep.* 2005;54(RR-14):1–16 PMID: 16340941

10. Brook I. Current concepts in the management of *Clostridium tetani* infection. *Expert Rev Anti Infect Ther.* 2008;6(3):327–336 PMID: 18588497

11. American Academy of Pediatrics. Tetanus (lockjaw). In: Pickering LK, Baker CJ, Kimberlin DW, Long SS, eds. *Red Book: 2012 Report of the Committee on Infectious Diseases.* 29th ed. Elk Grove Village, IL: American Academy of Pediatrics; 2012:707–712

12. Treatment of tuberculosis. *MMWR Recomm Rep.* 2003;52(RR-11):1–77 PMID: 12836625

13. American Academy of Pediatrics. Tuberculosis. In: Pickering LK, Baker CJ, Kimberlin DW, Long SS, eds. *Red Book: 2012 Report of the Committee on Infectious Diseases.* 29th ed. Elk Grove Village, IL: American Academy of Pediatrics; 2012:736–759

14. Pinninti SG, Angara R, Feja KN, et al. Neonatal herpes disease despite maternal antenatal antiviral suppressive therapy: a multicenter case series. *J Pediatr.* 2012;161(1):134–138 PMID: 22336576

15. American Academy of Academy Committee on Infectious Diseases. Recommendations for prevention and control of influenza in children, 2013–2014. *Pediatrics.* 2013;132(4):e1089–e1104

16. Kimberlin DW, Acosta EP, Prichard MN, et al, for the NIAID Collaborative Antiviral Study Group. Oseltamivir pharmacokinetics, dosing, and resistance among children aged <2 years with influenza. *J Infect Dis.* 2013;207(5):709–720 PMID: 23230059

17. American Academy of Pediatrics. Rabies. In: Pickering LK, Baker CJ, Kimberlin DW, Long SS, eds. *Red Book: 2012 Report of the Committee on Infectious Diseases.* 29th ed. Elk Grove Village, IL: American Academy of Pediatrics; 2012:600–607

18. American Academy of Pediatrics. *Pneumocystis jirovecii* infections. In: Pickering LK, Baker CJ, Kimberlin DW, Long SS, eds. *Red Book: 2012 Report of the Committee on Infectious Diseases.* 29th ed. Elk Grove Village, IL: American Academy of Pediatrics; 2012:582–587

19. Mofenson LM, Brady MT, Danner SP, et al; Centers for Disease Control and Prevention; National Institutes of Health; HIV Medicine Association of the Infectious Diseases Society of America; Pediatric Infectious Diseases Society; American Academy of Pediatrics. Guidelines for the prevention and treatment of opportunistic infections among HIV-exposed and HIV-infected children: recommendations from CDC, the National Institutes of Health, the HIV Medicine Association of the Infectious Diseases Society of America, the Pediatric Infectious Diseases Society, and the American Academy of Pediatrics. *MMWR Recomm Rep.* 2009;58(RR-11):1–166 PMID: 19730409

20. Leach AJ, Morris PS. Antibiotics for the prevention of acute and chronic suppurative otitis media in children. *Cochrane Database Syst Rev.* 2006;(4):CD004401 PMID: 17054203

21. McDonald S, Langton Hewer CD, Nunez DA. Grommets (ventilation tubes) for recurrent acute otitis media in children. *Cochrane Database Syst Rev.* 2008;(4):CD004741 PMID: 18843668

22. Williams GJ, Craig JC, Carapetis JR. Preventing urinary tract infections in early childhood. *Adv Exp Med Biol.* 2013;764:211–218 PMID: 23654070

23. Craig JC, Simpson JM, Williams GJ, et al. Antibiotic prophylaxis and recurrent urinary tract infection in children. *N Engl J Med.* 2009;361(18):1748–1759 PMID: 19864673

24. Williams G, Craig JC. Long-term antibiotics for preventing recurrent urinary tract infection in children. *Cochrane Database Syst Rev.* 2011;(3):CD001534 PMID: 21412872

25. American Academy of Pediatrics Subcommittee on Urinary Tract Infection and Steering Committee on Quality Improvement and Management. Urinary tract infection: clinical practice guideline for the diagnosis and management of the initial UTI in febrile infants and children 2 to 24 months. *Pediatrics.* 2011;128(3):595–610 PMID: 21873693

26. Antimicrobial prophylaxis for surgery. *Treat Guidel Med Lett.* 2012;10(122):73–80 PMID: 22996382

27. Mangram AJ, Horan TC, Pearson ML, et al. Guideline for prevention of surgical site infection, 1999. Hospital Infection Control Practices Advisory Committee. *Infect Control Hosp Epidemiol.* 1999;20(4):250–280 PMID: 10219875

28. Edwards FH, Engelman RM, Houck P, et al. The Society of Thoracic Surgeons practice guideline series: antibiotic prophylaxis in cardiac surgery, part I: duration. *Ann Thorac Surg.* 2006;81(1):397–404 PMID: 16368422

29. Engelman R, Shahian D, Shemin R, et al. The Society of Thoracic Surgeons practice guideline series: antibiotic prophylaxis in cardiac surgery, part II: antibiotic choice. *Ann Thorac Surg.* 2007;83(4):1569–1576 PMID: 17383396

30. Kirby JP, Mazuski JE. Prevention of surgical site infection. *Surg Clin North Am.* 2009;89(2):365–389 PMID: 19281889

31. Haley RW, Culver DH, Morgan WM, et al. Identifying patients at high risk of surgical wound infection. A simple multivariate index of patient susceptibility and wound contamination. *Am J Epidemiol.* 1985;121(2):206–215 PMID: 4014116

32. Dellinger EP. What is the ideal time for administration of antimicrobial prophylaxis for a surgical procedure? *Ann Surg.* 2008;247(6):927–928 PMID: 18520218

Chapter 15

1. Tetzlaff TR, McCracken GH Jr, Nelson JD. Oral antibiotic therapy for skeletal infections of children. II. Therapy of osteomyelitis and suppurative arthritis. *J Pediatr.* 1978;92(3):485–490 PMID: 632997

2. Weichert S, Sharland M, Clarke NM, et al. Acute haematogenous osteomyelitis in children: is there any evidence for how long we should treat? *Curr Opin Infect Dis.* 2008;21(3):258–262 PMID: 18448970

3. Paakkonen M, Peltola H. Antibiotic treatment for acute haematogenous osteomyelitis of childhood: moving towards shorter courses and oral administration. *Int J Antimicrob Agents.* 2011;38(4):273–280 PMID: 21640559

4. Rice HE, Brown RL, Gollin G, et al. Results of a pilot trial comparing prolonged intravenous antibiotics with sequential intravenous/oral antibiotics for children with perforated appendicitis. *Arch Surg.* 2001;136(12):1391–1395 PMID: 11735866

5. Fraser JD, Aguayo P, Leys CM, et al. A complete course of intravenous antibiotics vs a combination of intravenous and oral antibiotics for perforated appendicitis in children: a prospective, randomized trial. *J Pediatr Surg.* 2010;45(6):1198–1202 PMID: 20620320

6. Hoberman A, Wald ER, Hickey RW, et al. Oral versus initial intravenous therapy for urinary tract infections in young febrile children. *Pediatrics.* 1999;104(1 pt 1):79–86 PMID: 10390264

7. Bradley JS, Jackson MA; American Academy of Pediatrics Committee on Infectious Diseases. The use of systemic and topical fluoroquinolones. *Pediatrics.* 2011;128(4):e1034–e1045 PMID: 21949152

Chapter 15 (cont)

8. Arnold JC, Cannavino CR, Ross MK, et al. Acute bacterial osteoarticular infections: eight-year analysis of C-reactive protein for oral step-down therapy. *Pediatrics.* 2012;130(4):e821–e828 PMID: 22966033

9. Kaplan SL, Mason EO Jr, Feigin RD. Clindamycin versus nafcillin or methicillin in the treatment of Staphylococcus aureus osteomyelitis in children. *South Med J.* 1982;75(2):138–142 PMID: 7036354

Chapter 16

1. Best EJ, Gazarian M, Cohn R, Wilkinson M, Palasanthiran P. Once-daily gentamicin in infants and children: a prospective cohort study evaluating safety and the role of therapeutic drug monitoring in minimizing toxicity. *Pediatr Infect Dis J.* 2011;30(10):827–832 PMID: 21577177

2. Smyth AR, Bhatt J. Once-daily versus multiple-daily dosing with intravenous aminoglycosides for cystic fibrosis. *Cochrane Database Syst Rev.* 2012;2:CD002009 PMID: 22336782

3. Gruchalla RS, Pirmohamed M. Clinical practice. Antibiotic allergy. *N Engl J Med.* 2006;354(6):601–609 PMID: 16467547

4. Solensky R. Allergy to β-lactam antibiotics. *J Allergy Clin Immunol.* 2012;130(6):1442–1442 PMID: 23195529

5. Cephalosporins for patients with penicillin allergy. *Med Lett Drugs Ther.* 2012;54(1406):101 PMID: 23282790

6. Bradley JS, Wassel RT, Lee L, Nambiar S. Intravenous ceftriaxone and calcium in the neonate: assessing the risk for cardiopulmonary adverse events. *Pediatrics.* 2009;123(4):e609–e613 PMID: 19289450

7. Wong VK, Wright HT Jr, Ross LA, Mason WH, Inderlied CB, Kim KS. Imipenem/cilastatin treatment of bacterial meningitis in children. *Pediatr Infect Dis J.* 1991;10(2):122–125 PMID: 2062603

8. Bradley JS, Jackson MA; American Academy of Pediatrics Committee on Infectious Diseases. The use of systemic and topical fluoroquinolones. *Pediatrics.* 2011;128(4):e1034–e1045 PMID: 21949152

9. Jacobs RF, Maples HD, Aranda JV, et al. Pharmacokinetics of intravenously administered azithromycin in pediatric patients. *Pediatr Infect Dis J.* 2005;24(1):34–39 PMID: 15665708

10. American Academy of Pediatrics. Pertussis. In: Pickering LK, Baker CJ, Kimberlin DW, Long SS, eds. *Red Book: 2012 Report of the Committee on Infectious Diseases.* 29th ed. Elk Grove Village, IL: American Academy of Pediatrics; 2012:553–566

11. Nambiar S, Rellosa N, Wassel RT, Borders-Hemphill V, Bradley JS. Linezolid-associated peripheral and optic neuropathy in children. *Pediatrics.* 2011;127(6):e1528–e1532 PMID: 21555496

Index